Medicine That Walks

Disease, Medicine, and Canadian Plains
Native People, 1880–1940

MAUREEN K. LUX

UNIVERSITY OF TORONTO PRESS
Toronto Buffalo London

© University of Toronto Press 2001
Toronto Buffalo London
Printed in the U.S.A.

Reprinted 2007, 2011, 2012

ISBN 0-8020-4728-9 (cloth)
ISBN 0-8020-8295-5 (paper)

Printed on acid-free paper

National Library of Canada Cataloguing in Publication Data

Lux, Maureen K. (Maureen Katherine), 1956–
Medicine that walks : disease, medicine and Canadian Plains Native
people, 1880–1940

Includes bibliographical references and index.
ISBN 0-8020-4728-9 (bound)   ISBN 0-8020-8295-5 (pbk.)

1. Indians of North America – Health and hygiene – Prairie Provinces –
History.   2. Indians of North America – Medicine – Prairie Provinces –
History.   3. Indians of North America – Prairie Provinces – Government
relations.   4. Indians of North America – Prairie Provinces – Social
conditions.   I. Title.

E78.P7L89 2001   362.1'089'970712   C00-933159-X

University of Toronto Press acknowledges the financial assistance to its
publishing program of the Canada Council for the Arts and the Ontario Arts
Council.

This book has been published with the help of a grant from the Humanities
and Social Sciences Federation of Canada, using funds provided by the
Social Sciences and Humanities Research Council of Canada.

University of Toronto Press acknowledges the financial support for its
publishing activities of the Government of Canada through the Book
Publishing Industry Development Program (BPIDP).

For Glen, Molly, and Sarah

Contents

List of Tables

x List of Tables

Acknowledgments

This study began as a doctoral dissertation, and I would like to acknowledge the help and patient advice of my supervisors Robin Fisher, John Hutchinson, and the late Douglas Cole, and the financial support of the Social Sciences and Humanities Research Council in the form of a doctoral fellowship. The transformation from dissertation to book was eased by the generosity and kind support of the good folks at the Hannah Institute for the History of Medicine. The post-doctoral fellowship and a teaching fellowship (which allowed me to try out some of these ideas on unsuspecting students) have made this work not only possible, but much better. Supervisors J.R. Miller and Stuart Houston kindly corrected some (but certainly not all) of my many errors. The staff and faculty at the University of Saskatchewan's history department, especially Bill Waiser, Michael Hayden, Larry Stewart, and the late Geoff Bilson, have always been supportive and encouraging. Archivists at the Glenbow Archives, the United Church Archives, the Alberta Archives, and the National Archives, and especially Nadine Small and D'Arcy Hande at the Saskatchewan Archives Board, have been unfailingly helpful and wise. I would also like to thank the Saskatchewan Lung Association for making their invaluable records available. Portions of Chapter Five appeared earlier as 'Perfect Subjects: Race, Tuberculosis and the Qu'Appelle BCG Vaccine Trial' in the *Canadian Bulletin of Medical History* 15, no. 2 (1998): 277–96. I am grateful for permission to reprint this material. And finally, thanks to Bev Towstiak for her insight and wit, which helped to keep the process in perspective.

The most fascinating and enlightening aspect of a study like this is the opportunity to meet with Aboriginal elders. Not all elders whose words appear in this book are named. That was their choice. They were good enough to share their stories and knowledge, and if they chose anonymity that must be respected. Visits and interviews with elders are a truly humbling experience. They carry knowledge of some of the worst indignities endured by their people, yet remain gracious when asked to recall them. I respectfully thank elders from the Carry the Kettle, Pasqua, Blood, and Peigan First Nations.

I would also like to thank my family, especially my parents, Joseph and Mary Grace, whose enthusiasm and love for learning inspires us all. And thanks to my husband Glen and our daughters Sarah and Molly, who patiently endure, and loudly encourage, all that I do. This book is dedicated to them.

MEDICINE THAT WALKS
Disease, Medicine, and Canadian Plains Native People, 1880–1940

Introduction: Beyond Biology

Mi'k ai'stoowa, Red Crow, cast in stone, graces the entrance to the Blood First Nation's new Kainai Continuing Care Centre with its massive ceremonial lodgepoles pointing to the sky. I leaned into the strong December wind and passed under his shadow and entered the newly opened sub-acute hospital. The great lodge room was flooded with natural light and the crystal voices of children singing to their elders. There I met with a Blood elder, who, with his infant grandson, welcomed me to the reserve and the hospital. The medicine practised there is both ancient and modern; smudges, face paint, and herbal 'brews' exist easily alongside intravenous poles and heart monitors. The elder began by explaining the continuing importance of the Sun Dance in healing. As he spoke, the baby was lulled to sleep in his grandfather's arms, with stories of the Blood people beating in his ear. It has been more than a century since Red Crow signed Treaty Seven, and it has been a hard century. The 'queen's generosity' promised in the treaties was mostly small and cruel. The notion of keeping balance between opposite spiritual and physical forces in order to be healthy – or, as the Blood people say, in order to be a 'real person' – has endured. But many 'real people' have been lost.

An Assiniboine elder puts it bluntly:

From the Treaty they took everything away, the diet, the way of life; all that was put on earth by the Great Spirit. The new diet made the people weaker. It was too much change, too quickly ... [The old people] say that they brought sickness over from across the water; sickness like typhoid fever. And after they got rid of Indian medicine and the people had to take white medicine, and some of it made us real sick. They kind of damaged our bodies through pills and their side-effects. They were experimenting on us. It was the tame food, too. We were used to eating wild game. That's why they figure our bodies lacked the strength they had before.[1]

The warmth of the spring of 1884 should have been welcomed. The winter had been especially severe; everyone was hungry and many were sick. Forced from Fort Walsh in southern Alberta to Indian Head in eastern Saskatchewan, the people counted their dead – 130 children and adults lost to sickness and starvation. The Indian Department offered cod liver oil but no food. Long Lodge was incredulous: 'I want no government medicine. What I want is medicine that walks. Send three oxen to be killed and give fresh meat to my people and they will get better.'[2]

Similar words were heard across the prairies in those days. Without the basic neccessities for life – food, clothing, and shelter – the Native peoples of the plains could not escape the descent into illness and death. They experienced a profound population decline in the four decades following the signing of Treaties Four, Six, and Seven in the 1870s. The Cree, Assiniboine, and Saulteaux of the central plains, and to the west the Siksika (Blackfoot), Kainai (Blood), Tsuu T'ina (Sarcee), Stoney, and Piikani (Peigan), suffered hunger, poverty, disease, and death in their homeland. The Canadian government's attempts to open the west for settlement and assimilate the people, at the least possible expense, created a perilous situation. Overcrowded and poorly venti-lated houses and schools bred a startling variety of diseases including measles, whooping cough, influenza, and tuberculosis; inadequate clothing and a deficient diet undermined recovery. Bureaucrats, mis-sionaries, and especially physicians explained the high death rates and continued ill health in the quasi-scientific language of racial evolution which inferred that only the fittest should expect to survive. The peo-ple's poverty and ill health were seen as an inevitable stage in the strug-gle for 'Christianity and civilization,' and as further evidence that assimilation was the only path to good health. This conclusion was not shared by Native people, who consistently demanded the economic and political freedom to redress their plight. Yet any resistance to govern-ment policy or to the casual humiliations of the reserve system was inter-preted as proof that only rapid assimilation could save the people.

The social history of medicine studies how disease and its treatment are framed by societies and cultures. In scientific terms, diseases such as tuberculosis and measles are discrete biological entities; in social terms, disease cannot exist without someone getting ill. The experience of illness sets in motion a train of events that usually begins with diagnosis, wends through treatment, and ends somewhere between recovery and death. The meeting between the ill and the well is a social exchange during which reference is made to categories such as gender, class, and race. Examples: the limited role of women as wives and mothers in Victorian Canada was reflected in, and reinforced by, the medical care and advice they received. In the name of good health, doctors warned women away from higher education and urged them to stay in their homes. Likewise, physicians, volunteers, and scientists in the twentieth century attempted to control and treat tuberculosis through social reform – an effort that was central to the formation and consolidation of the middle class.[3] In the same way, race and ethnicity have served as constants in framing disease, and never so much as in the relationship between Europeans and Aboriginal people. This study will trace that relationship, and the government policies that flowed from it, from the 1880s when Aboriginal people were perceived as a vanishing race doomed to extinction, to the 1940s when they came to be seen as a disease menace to the Canadian public. I will show, first, that the early hunger crisis in the 1880s and 1890s had long-term effects, both on health and on policymakers' perceptions that Aboriginal people were 'racially' flawed. Second, that despite the efforts of Aboriginal leaders, those perceptions were never questioned, because they served the larger goal of assimilation. Third, that the goal of assimilation justified the repressive economic, political, and cultural policies that resulted in terrible living conditions and subsequent poor health, which in turn justified the position that Aboriginal people were biologically inferior. Fourth, that the medical care the Euro-Canadians practised among Aboriginal people was self-serving, and was perceived as such by the people. And finally, that plains Aboriginal people created a place for themselves that allowed them to retain their humanity and faith while adapting to changing circumstances.

Aboriginal people were different: their languages, cultures, and religions, and especially their appearance, did not conform to Canadians' dreams of a west that would mirror the societies of the east.[4] The Canadian government donned the cloak of imperial power when it acquired the North-West Territories, and in doing so embraced the imperialist rhetoric that stressed the white man's burden to protect and elevate inferior races. Alexander Morris, treaty negotiator and lieutenant-governor of Manitoba and the North-West, typified the optimism of the righteous. As he said in 1880, 'Let us have Christianity and civilization to leaven the mass of heathenism and paganism among the Indian tribes ... and Canada will be enabled to feel, that in a truly patriotic spirit, our country had done its duty by the red man of the North-West, and thereby to herself.'[5]

From the 1880s until after the Second World War, Canadians – along with much of the western world – were preoccupied with race. In the nineteenth and twentieth centuries a great variety of meanings were given to the term 'race' – meanings that were applied to cultural, religious, ethnic, and social groups. Millions of people had their heads measured by scientists, who hoped to correlate brain size, and therefore intelligence, with degree of civilization. By the middle of the nineteenth century, race was considered a biological fact, a law of nature, and the ranking of races from inferior to superior was seen as scientifically valid. At the root of the preoccupation with race were the efforts of various branches of the natural sciences – including physical anthropology, comparative anatomy, and genetics – to explain diversity among humans. Race science grew out of advances in the biological and social sciences in the nineteenth century, and as knowledge increased about the different peoples of the globe, its findings were increasingly accepted as fact. Physical differences were associated with cultural differences; soon enough, rankings were being justified by biology. Undoubtedly, colonial domination was aided by biological 'proofs' that subject peoples were inferior.[6]

Christian faith and doctrine held the monogenist view that all the world's people emerged from a single family; thus, the Aboriginal of the New World was both rational and the possessor of a soul, and in theory at least was not to be enslaved or abused. The polygenist view that gained acceptance as the nineteenth century progressed held that races were distinct types. Race science attempted to explain observable and measurable differences such as skin colour and skull shape and size, as well as perceived differences in levels of culture and civilization. The ideas of American and British race scientists were well received in Canada, and popular and scientific interpretations of their ideas were used to explain the role and nature of this country's Native people. Race science was never isolated from the ideological questions of the day; indeed, it hoped to resolve those questions through science and scientific methods. Thus, quesitons about the government's role in the affairs of Aboriginal people occupied the anthropologist and the physician as much as the politician. Also, scientists as intellectuals commanded a public role whether or not they were commenting on science. Evidence of the intellectual or physical worth of human groups was often manipulated to fit stereotypical and preconceived notions. Race science was considered good science, at least until the 1930s, when scientists (especially biologists) found that their attempts to quantify race were rendering their work more and more irrelevant. The public rejected race science after Nazism was defeated, by which time it was clear what horrors could be perpetrated in the name of science and eugenics. Racism, or hatred based on race, unfortunately remains very much alive. Race science was not a discipline as such; rather, it was a tool used by many sciences to explain a social construct. The term 'racialism,' used at the turn of the century to denote prejudice based on race, was rarely resorted to because it was assumed that races existed and that the differences between them were natural. There were always bigots, but to use race to explain the physical and cultural differences in humans, and to assign rankings from inferior to superior, was not seen as evidence of bigotry (at least among those who were considered superior).[7]

One of the central figures in British race science was a Canadian. Reginald Ruggles Gates, botanist, geneticist, and anthropologist, was born in Nova Scotia to staunch Loyalist stock. But Gates found his 'spiritual home' in Britain in 1910 and took a teaching position at King's College, London, where he remained until the Second World War. Gates was the author of several influential books on race and genetics in the 1920s and 1930s.[8] His ideas on race in the 1920s linked skin colour to mentality and suggested that mental capacity increased with the addition of white ancestry. As with other race scientists of the day, his research questions were often influenced by racial stereotypes and his conclusions were preconceived; but as an academic and scientist, his opinions carried some weight. In a 1928 article, 'A Pedigree Study of Amerindian Crosses in Canada,' he was ostensibly studying the inheritance of individual differences such as eye, skin, and hair colour in 'hybrids'; however, the real issue was the burning eugenic question of the day: were the 'civilized' races always degenerated through mixture with the less evolved, and conversely, were 'primitives' elevated through the addition of 'white blood'? He noted at the outset that miscegenation in general 'is to be deprecated' when it occurs between advanced and backward races.[9] He touched on accepted measures such as the Cephalic Index, which supposedly proved race superiority by measuring face breadth to head breadth, expressed as a percentage, and concluded that in some times and places – especially the rough country of northern Canada – human crosses ('intermediate races') were better adapted to their conditions than either of the races from which they sprang. The distinct differences remained, but were recombined, and certain features predominated through sexual and natural selection. Gates's methods were probably typical of the discipline. In August 1924 he had spent 'a few days' at Bear Island after the conclusion of the British Medical Association meeting at Ontario's Lake Temagami. He hoped to document the 'pedigrees' of a number of Bear Island residents and their ancestors back six generations to the original marriage between an Ojibwa or Cree woman and a non-Native trader. His research became considerably muddled by the discovery that one of the 'pure white' ancestors was in fact a 'half-breed.' Furthermore, he used black-and-white photographs and a fair amount of guess work such as 'black eyes and doubtless a dark skin' to describe an Aboriginal ancestor, and 'probably blue-eyed' to describe a white ancestor. He distinguished between the Cree and Ojibwa on the basis of body type, head shape, and facial features and concluded that the Ojibwa 'look more stodgy and less intelligent' than the Cree. As well, they were 'inclined to be lazy, improvident and unreliable' while the Cree were 'thrifty and show greater ambition under white influence.' He also noted that the Ojibwa were Roman Catholic, whereas the superior Cree were Protestants. In 1928 his peers in the scientific community would not have questioned his methods, reasoning, or conclusions; indeed, he was one of the authorities in the field. Gates's importance is not in what he wrote, but in his position as an exemplar of the science. He only became 'rigid' Reginald Ruggles Gates when he clung to his views while his contemporaries discarded many such notions in the years surrounding the Second World War.[10]

Sir William Dawson, geologist and president of McGill University, was Canada's leading anti-Darwinist; he believed that the study of nature and science was the revealed hand of God, and that the survival of the fittest as applied to humans was 'nothing less than the basest and most horrible superstition.' However, Dawson was not representative of science in Canada, which quickly accepted the theory of evolution.[11] Darwin's own opinion, that racial differences are not very important in evolution, was ignored by his contemporaries. Social Darwinism, or the extension of evolutionary ideas to human societies – especially the idea that through natural selection the white (probably British) race had risen to a position of superiority – was a popular and ultimately dangerous notion. It was used to explain the class structure (viz., that the lowest classes were less evolved), and to justify the sterilization of 'undesirables' and the mentally 'unfit,' who threatened the purity of the race. Still later, the Nazis would use it to justify their horrific medical experiments. Even the differences between men and women – especially women's supposed inferiority – were explained through evolutionary theory and notions of the survival of the fittest.[12] By the early twentieth century, Anglo-Saxon Canada was supremely racist. Canada's open-door policy led to massive immigration, and it was left to self-appointed social reformers – social Darwinists – in medicine, the churches, and government to mitigate the impact of 'foreigners' on Canadian society. Church missionary societies established 'foreign missions' to Aboriginal people; their evangelical work among immigrants and Native people implied that there was hope that the most objectionable aspects of their behaviour, culture, language, and 'race' might disappear under careful guidance. The government, and the Canadian public generally, assumed that Aboriginal people needed a strong hand if they were to embrace a new economic, cultural, and physical reality. That these people's health seemed to deteriorate under the new regime was invariably put down to their race. The 'white man's burden' to assimilate the people was of course both circular in logic and self-serving in nature, and was based on the presumption that Aboriginal cultures were inferior and without structure or purpose.

At this time, the Cree and Assiniboine were relative newcomers to the western plains. In the seventeenth century they had been living in contiguous territories in present-day Manitoba and Ontario. When the Hudson's Bay Company (HBC) opened its bayside fur trade forts such as York Factory on the edge of their territories, the Assiniboine and Cree became both its customers and its wholesalers, and determined the form and terms of the trade. In their role as middlemen between the HBC and western groups, they moved farther west and south to the parklands of the central prairies. As they did so, the Ojibwa (Saulteaux) moved into the southern Manitoba regions they had vacated. The fur trade also brought the Cree into contact with the Blackfoot Confederacy, the Siksika (Blackfoot proper), Kainai (Blood), Piikani (Peigan), and Tsuu T'ina (Sarcee), who in the mid-eighteenth century occupied central Alberta and purchased guns from the Cree in return for horses, bison robes, and wolf and other furs.[13]

The Cree and Assiniboine incorporated the fur trade into their annual migrations. Those closely involved in the fur trade at York Factory spent their summers in the forest gathering food and trapping and hunting fowl, and their winters in the parklands hunting bison (or rather capturing them in pounds), and their springs fishing and trapping and trading with the HBC. Those Assiniboine not directly involved in the HBC trade maintained a grasslands home, in summer hunting bison, in autumn trading to the south, in winter pounding bison in the parklands, and in spring fishing and trapping. Likewise, the Blackfoot, who were more dependent on the bison for food, clothing, and housing, ranged south through the grasslands in American territory in summer and north to the parklands in winter. In this way the plains groups utilized the resource zones of the prairies.[14] The grasslands provided more large game than the woodland zone for besides bison, there were elk and deer; in the forest zone, small game – beaver, lynx, and muskrat – were used as food as well as for trade. Both groups rounded out their diet with wild fruits and vegetables. As Montreal fur traders penetrated the interior, the HBC was forced to do the same; as a result, in the 1770s the Cree and Assiniboine were forced out of their middleman role and compelled to compete with other Aboriginal groups for trade furs. The burgeoning fur trade required a large supply of provisions, and the Cree and Assiniboine groups that had previously accessed the bison herds on a seasonal basis moved into the grasslands to create a new role for themselves as provisioners to the fur trade. Warfare ensued as the Blackfoot, who also traded to the south with the American fur trade posts on the Missouri River, tried to protect their bison territories. In this way a large Native trading network between the plains and the upper Missouri was established that led to increased interethnic contact. When the Red River Colony was founded in 1812, it became a reservoir for infectious diseases. By the nineteenth century, the population shifts had created a pattern: the Plains Cree occupied the parklands in winter to access the bison; in summer they occupied the grasslands, and abandoned their woodland home almost completely. The Blackfoot had fewer connections to the woodlands and moved seasonally from parkland to grassland. The bison was important to them as a source of food, and also had a cultural importance that resonated in their religious symbols.

As fur trader Daniel Harmon remarked in 1804, 'These Indians who reside in the large Plains are the most independent and appear to be the happiest and most contented of any People upon the face of the Earth. They subsist on the Flesh of the Buffalo and of the skin they make the greatest part of their cloathing which is both warm and convenient.'[15] The successful hunter was rewarded with plenty. The flesh was eaten fresh, or dried and stored. Hides were made into great sheets for lodges, or cured and then sown into shirts, leggings, skirts, and moccasins. The tongue and skull were used in religious ceremonies. In short, the bison provided much that was necessary to life on the plains. But Aboriginal groups on the plains also utilized a wide variety of plants to maintain a balanced diet. Onion bulbs (*Allium cernuum; A. stellatum*) were widely used by the Cree, Assiniboine, and Blackfoot either raw or boiled in stews. Blue camas (*Camassia quamash*) was one of the most important and widely traded foods for the Blackfoot, who obtained it from the Kootenay people to the west. Cow parsnip or 'Indian celery' (*Heracleum ignatum*), a perennial taproot that was called the 'boss of all the green vegetables,' was harvested by all plains groups in the spring and was usually eaten raw; but the Blackfoot also cut the stems into pieces and stored them in blood to be used later in soups and broths. The prairie turnip or 'Indian breadroot' (*Psoralea esculenta*), a taproot gathered in late spring and summer, was probably the most important wild food gathered by prairie Aboriginal groups. The Blackfoot used it raw or roasted; the Cree peeled, shredded, and sun-dried it for use in a pudding mixed with saskatoon berries. Other greens, such as mint, were eaten for flavouring, raw or dried. The plains and parklands also were a rich source of berries and wild fruits. The most important was the saskatoon berry, which was mixed with fat and dried meat to make the pemmican that literally fuelled the fur trade. The Assiniboine also mixed saskatoon berries with dried prairie turnip and stored the mixture to provide food for winter. The Blackfoot used them as food, or mixed them with blood and meat for a ceremonial soup. Wide experience was necessary to know which plants and roots were edible and which were toxic.

Education in this crucial area, as in all the skills necessary to prepare children for adulthood, was given informally, with the children accompanying and mimicking their parents and elders. For example, while Indian celery was a good source of calcium and vitamins C and A, it looks very similar to water hemlock and poison hemlock. Moreover, special methods were developed to utilize the food sources available. For instance, the pit method of roasting was developed to prepare the many roots and bulbs in their diet that contained inulin, a long-chain sugar that is neither palatable nor easily digestible. Inulin breaks down under prolonged cooking (up to a day or more); the carbohydrates can then be digested. As well, drying was a practical method of preserving fruits and meats; it used only the sun's energy and made provisions light and easy to carry. Many leaves, tree barks, and seed kernels contain cyanide-producing glycosides that can cause nausea and even death, but these compounds can be dispelled through proper cooking and sun drying.[16] The resource zones were also important sources of the plants, leaves, and roots the people needed to meet their spiritual and medical needs. Isolated ecosystems such as the Touchwood Hills and Turtle Mountain in southeastern Saskatchewan, and Cypress Hills and Wood Mountain in southwestern Saskatchewan, supported a number of plants not commonly found in the surrounding shortgrass prairie. The plains people also used these 'outlier' ecosystems for warfare and scouting and as sites for winter camps, for Sun Dance camps, and for vision quests. In the Cypress Hills alone there were at least eighteen species of plants for horse medicine, and fifty-one species for human medicine.[17] The plains groups exploited these zones on a seasonal basis for food and medicine and also used them to access Native and non-Native trading networks. But with increasing contact with large population centres along the Red River and the upper Missouri came greater opportunities for disease transmission.

A lively debate concerning the impact of disease on Aboriginal peoples in the Americas has long been carried on and shows no signs of abating. There is no doubt that epidemic diseases – smallpox, influenza, whooping cough, tuberculosis, and others – swept through Aboriginal groups. The debate centres on the extent and impact of these Contact (post-1492) epidemics. One view, that Aboriginal people were uniformly devastated by imported diseases that were carried to them through trade contacts – often prior to actual contact – contends that the population levels recorded by Europeans represented the vestiges of what was once a much larger population.[18] Another view, the gradualist one, contends that the demographic decline began later, was more prolonged, and occurred only after sustained European contact that caused severe social and economic disruption.[19] The debate also hinges on the size of pre-Contact populations in North America. The collapse theorists estimate 7 to 18 million; the gradualists suggest a pre-Contact population in the 1 to 2 million range. Evidence for either view is sketchy, speculative, and generally extrapolated from very small samples. The statistical controversy tends to reflect the growing interest among academics in the social and political consequences of Native immigrant relations. The comparatively low pre-Contact estimates imply that European expansion was less destructive to Native people; the higher estimates suggest that the initial contact and subsequent interaction were much more devastating. Political and theoretical factors have influenced the debate, especially in recent years. At root is an assumption that pre-Contact Aboriginal people lived in a disease-free environment and thus had little immunological experience with introduced diseases. That position has been challenged recently by new archaeological and epidemiological research and methods, but the scope and nature of the archaeological evidence is admittedly very limited.[20] Nevertheless, it does promise to extend our understanding of pre-Contact Aboriginal communities as changing and dynamic, rather than (as so often presented) idyllic but static.

Associated with the sudden collapse theory is the argument that epidemic diseases not only caused demographic devastation, but also the death of indigenous cultures and forms of spirituality as their gods were abandoned in favour of the Christian God, who could protect His followers. Europeans with immunity to disease were able to overpower indigenous societies and then settle the depopulated lands: 'It was their germs, not these imperialists themselves, for all their brutality and callousness, that were chiefly responsible for sweeping aside the indigenes.'[21] Evidence for this conclusion rests not so much on the historical record as on the assumption that, if Aboriginal people converted to Christianity, they no longer practised their own spirituality; and that they no longer practised Native spirituality and medicine because these were insufficient to conceptualize and treat unknown diseases.[22] Very often, however, the veneer of Christian conversion was adopted in order to wrest advantages from colonial authorities. The rationale for the 'disease as spiritual disaster' theme derives from the principles of immunology, not from careful research on specific Native groups. For example, ethnohistorical research on the Huron has led to a significant revision of this view. Bruce Trigger argues that there is in fact little evidence that 'epidemics seriously undermined native religious beliefs or that Indians turned to Christianity during these epidemics because it promised them a more attractive form of immortality.' Epidemics in non-Native communities did not lead to a questioning of traditional faith; in fact, widely held beliefs were usually reinforced, not destroyed. Faced with epidemic disease, trusted healers and their cures were just as likely to be celebrated as debased. The failure of a particular treatment spurred the healers to look harder for a cure. When the epidemic waned, as each epidemic did, the rite performed at the time was credited with success.[23] The underlying assumption behind the collapse theory is that physically, culturally, and spiritually, Aboriginal societies were particularly fragile. To understand the impact of disease, we must examine specific Aboriginal groups within their historical, economic, geographic, and political contexts.[24]

The first well documented smallpox epidemic broke out along the upper Missouri in 1781. Smallpox is unlike other viruses in that it can remain infectious outside the body, on clothing and corpses, for several weeks. It also has a long incubation period – one to two weeks from the time of exposure to the acute stage where symptoms (headache, rash, and fever) appear. If death is to intervene, it is during this stage. Therefore, even considering the rather slow pace of travel by canoe or horse, smallpox can range far and wide carried on infected clothing or by infected but symptomless travellers.[25] The Cree and Assiniboine likely contracted the disease from the south at the Mandan trade mart. From there it quickly spread across the grasslands to the Blackfoot and north and east into Manitoba. The epidemic affected some more severely than others. Although the Assiniboine lost perhaps one-third of their population, they rebounded quickly. It is necessary to distinguish between ordinary epidemics, which are outbreaks that cause higher than normal mortality, and *depopulating* epidemics, which are defined by continued susceptibility to infectious disease with high mortality, and are age-specific in that they strike at those in their childbearing years. The 1781–2 smallpox epidemic certainly caused increased mortality, but in the thirty-three-year period from 1776 to 1809 the estimated Assiniboine population quadrupled. Their grassland Cree neighbours were more severely affected, and by 1822 they still had not recovered to their pre-1780 population. The Assiniboine population structure, with children comprising nearly half the population, was able to recover quickly. Perhaps the Assiniboine were more familiar with life on the plains than the Cree and had more reliable and abundant food supplies.[26]

People's reactions to disease are also significant. Non-Native observers and commmentators rarely cited effective responses. Instead they reported that Aboriginal people often attempted to relieve the high fever associated with smallpox by throwing themselves into lakes and rivers – usually to fatal effect. Or that at other times they hastened their own demise by practising blood letting or frequenting the sweat lodge.[27] Certainly, healers were hard pressed to cure smallpox, but relief from the symptoms was at hand: a febrifuge was prepared by mixing equal quantities of catnip (*Nepeta cataria*) and tansy; this caused profuse perspiration, which in turn broke the fever.[28] A tea made from willow bark, which contains salicin (the active ingredient in aspirin) was also used to treat fever; and the willow branches used to build sweat lodges would release salicin when subjected to the steam of the lodge. Mountain mint and goldenrod were also used to treat fevers, and sagebrush leaves, roots of the angelica or prickly ash, and potentilla were used on the blisters and sores. The Blackfoot alone had at least thirty-eight treatments for respiratory disorders and thirty-three for skin disorders and swelling.[29] A smallpox epidemic would burn itself out eventually, and the healer might then claim success. In Peigan oral tradition there is an interesting variation on the idea behind inoculation: when smallpox first arrived among the Blackfoot (Confederacy), 'an old one dreamed that to eat small bits of the [smallpox-infested] blanket the people could save themselves.'[30] Epidemics must surely have raised questions about whether the people should continue to interact with fur traders; but there is little reason to suggest that they caused peoples to question their core beliefs. According to one witness, the survivors of the epidemic believed that 'the Great Master of Life had delivered them over to the Evil Spirit for their wicked courses; and for many years afterward those who escaped the deadly contagion strictly conformed themselves to their own code of moral laws.'[31]

Smallpox was followed by recurring epidemics of measles, whooping cough, influenza, and smallpox again in 1837–8. The fifty- to sixty-year cycle between smallpox epidemics reflects the nature of the disease. Exposure confers life-long immunity, so smallpox could not again establish a secure foothold until those with a natural immunity had died; also, without a large concentration of people in one area, smallpox cannot become endemic. In April 1837, smallpox was carried upriver by steamer from St Louis, Missouri, and eventually infected the Sioux, Arikara, and Hidasta. But it was the Mandan, who lived in densely populated villages, who suffered the most devastation, losing up to seven-eighths of their population. Smallpox moved up the Missouri Valley, where it attacked Blackfoot and Peigan trading parties, and then onto the Canadian plains. In September 1838, when news of the epidemic reached Fort Pelly near the forks of the Qu'Appelle and Assiniboine rivers, the HBC trader William Todd began vaccinating the Cree who visited his post.[32] The cowpox vaccine material, which produces a mild infection but does not render the individual infectious, was supplied by the company for economic and humanitarian reasons. Todd sent several Native leaders among their followers with instructions and supplies to carry out the vaccination program. Consequently, the Cree suffered few losses during the epidemic. But the Blackfoot and the Assiniboine sustained considerable losses from smallpox. According to the Bad Head Winter Count (a method for reckoning the passage of time by recording significant tribal events), two-thirds of the Blackfoot nation – six thousand people – died from smallpox in 1837–8; although other estimates suggest that the loss was a little lower, more in the range of 50 per cent. So many Blood people died from smallpox near the confluence of the Oldman and St Mary rivers that the Blood named the place *Akaisakoyi* or 'Many Dead.'[33] The sorrow and anguish of the survivors must not be minimized. Families were torn apart as parents mourned for their lost children; orphans were taken in by relatives. The personal tragedy was devastating, yet the collective survived. Provided the epidemic caused uniform mortality across all age groups in the population, the age structure would remain the same, and within a few years births and deaths would return to their pre-epidemic levels. The Blackfoot population had been increasing prior to the epidemic and would begin to increase again within a few years.[34] By the spring of 1839, the warriors, at least, were sufficiently recovered to strike a blow at the Cree and Assiniboine. In the sixty years between 1780 and 1840, no Canadian plains group experienced a continual population decline, despite at least nine major epidemics. Indeed, in the forty years between 1823 and 1863, the Cree population in southern Saskatchewan, Manitoba, and Alberta grew by over ten thousand as a result of natural increase and immigration. The disease type, the season of the outbreak, the route of transmission, population densities, previous immunity, and the state of nutrition and general health all mitigate the severity and demographic impact of epidemics.[35]

In the summer of 1869, smallpox once again appeared on the upper Missouri. There was no vaccine at the posts in Saskatchewan and Alberta, so trader Isaac Cowie at Qu'Appelle attempted to use inoculation to prevent an epidemic. Inoculation differs from vaccination in that it introduces pus or powdered scab material to induce a mild infection, but renders the individual infectious:

> I at once asked Mr Breland [a Metis] to allow me to take the lymph from his grandchild's arm, and he gladly gave the permission. I rode out to their camp with them ... and from a fine healthy child I secured, on bits of window glass, enough vaccine to protect everyone requiring it in the Fort, from whom the supply was increased sufficiently to vaccinate all the people about the lakes and the Indians visiting them that fall. With the fear of the

former visitation before them, those who had been vaccinated at the fort took it out to the plains and spread it so thoroughly there among the Qu'Appelle and Touchwood Hills Indians that not one single case of small-pox was ever heard among them.[36]

Mortality from smallpox among the Blackfoot in 1870 has been esti-mated at between 600 and 800 out of a total population of less than 5,000, for a mortality rate of between 12 and 16 per cent; however, the Indian Department estimated the population of the Blackfoot nation at 9,200 in 1871.[37] But Father Lacombe at St Albert estimated that 'neither the Blood nor the Blackfeet Indians had, in proportion to their num-bers, as many casualties as the [North Saskatchewan River] Crees, whose losses may be safely stated at from 600 to 800 persons.' Captain William Butler of the British army was sent by Manitoba Governor Archibald to estimate (among other things) the extent of smallpox in the North-West. He stated that along the North Saskatchewan about 1,200 people died from smallpox in the summer of 1870. It is not clear whether this larger estimate includes the Lacombe estimate. In any case, there are no total population estimates that would put the losses from the epidemic in perspective. If we use Palliser's 1860 estimate that the pre-epidemic Cree population was about 11,500, the Cree losses were in the order of 10 per cent. On the other hand, if we accept Butler's population esti-mate, which puts the 1870–1 Cree population at 7,000, then the Cree losses were about 17 per cent. But presumably, Butler's estimate is a post-epidemic total. The difference between Butler's population esti-mate for the Cree of 7,000, and Palliser's 1860 estimate of 11,500 (a 40 per cent decrease), may be the actual extent of the Cree losses from the smallpox epidemic.[38] Although a 40 per cent mortality rate is in keeping with other estimates of smallpox mortality in initial epidemic cycles, smallpox was not unknown to the Cree and Blackfoot, and inoculation was used in the 1870 epidemic. It is highly questionable, therefore, whether we can accurately assess the extent of population losses.

There is no doubt that smallpox caused significant mortality, espe-cially coming as it did while plains people were pushing farther and far-ther west in pursuit of the dwindling bison herds. The American bison robe trade, with its particularly destructive medium of exchange – rot-gut whisky – further reduced Blackfoot living standards. Violence between the Cree and Assiniboine and the Blackfoot had increased in the previous decades; non-Native hunters and robe traders, along with Metis hunters from the Red River, were all pushing hard against Blackfoot territory. In the belief that the Blackfoot had suffered massive losses during the epidemic, a combined Cree and Assiniboine force of more than six hundred warriors led by Little Pine, Big Bear, Piapot, and Little Mountain invaded their territory. But the invaders were met at the Oldman River by a well armed, well deployed Blackfoot force, which easily repelled them and pursued them back across the river.[39] The Cree lost between two and three hundred warriors; the Blackfoot lost only forty, with fifty more wounded. Emissaries from each group met on the Red Deer River in 1871 and reached a peace that would not be broken. Epidemics in the nineteenth century increased in frequency and resulted in greater mortality as non-Natives increasingly penetrated the plains and competed for dwindling resources.

Despite significant population losses in the epidemics, the Aboriginal societies of the plains did not collapse. Their effective social and political organization may have been a factor in this. The band – a group of families that lived, travelled, and hunted together – was the central organizational feature of plains Aboriginal societies. Band leadership was decided by consensus, and usually went to an individual who had proven himself as a warrior or hunter and as a generous provider. There were also leadership positions for specialized tasks, such as a war leader and a hunt leader. If a leader failed to fulfil his promise, people simply moved off under new leadership that more closely met their needs. Larger gatherings of a number of bands took place in summer, when the saskatoon berries were ripe, for the Blackfoot Sun Dance or Cree Thirst Dance. The flexibility of the band form of organization made it particularly efficient. In winters when hunting was poor, family groups split off in order to pursue resources, to reconvene when one group had success. In the wake of epidemics, small groups likely joined larger, less affected groups; and cultural traits and symbols from one group were incorporated by others through marriage following population losses.[40] There is little evidence that infectious disease altered the core beliefs in the healer, who held the keys to the natural and supernatural worlds and who interpreted signs, diagnosed disease, and provided medicines from the grassland, parkland, and woodland pharmacopoeia.[41]

All of the plains groups recognized that good health was secured by acknowledging and respecting both the spiritual world and the physical world: in practice, little distinction was made between the two. Illness was a manifestation of the body and soul in search of harmony or balance. Disease and medicine was framed by plains Aboriginal cultures in a world view that placed people and their ills in a much larger circle of life that was populated by the animate and inanimate, the natural and supernatural. The ability to heal was recognized as a spiritual gift that allowed people access to the other world and some control over it. The prairies were a harsh environment that offered little room for error for those attempting to live off it. The plains peoples had adapted and indeed thrived by utilizing a complex set of economic, cultural, and spiritual structures. The process of adaptation did not halt with the fur trade, the gun, or the horse. Indeed, flexibility and adaptability were the basis of survival. But on the plains after 1880 the Blackfoot, Cree, and Assiniboine were without what had always been their main source of food, clothing, and shelter – the bison. Their economic base had eroded, and their treaties with the new Canadian government would soon be understood as failing to provide for their basic human needs. As the diseases of poverty rushed in, those who administered their lives would frame disease as a function of their race and their supposed 'stage of civilization.' From that point on, Christianity and assimilation were the paths to good health. That the people were nearly destroyed in the process was rarely seen as a fault of the policy; rather it was the fault of the people's character and customs – of their 'race.'

Chapter One

'The First Time We Were Poisoned by the Government': Starvation and the Erosion of Health

Few could imagine that the vast herds of bison would never return. Deep ruts still scarred the prairies where the huge beasts had passed. But in 1876, Cree Chief Mistawasis lamented to his people the loss of the 'ancient glory of our forefathers,' when the herds were so large that 'our fathers could not pass for the great numbers of those animals that blocked their way; and even in our day, we have had to choose carefully our campgrounds for fear of being trampled in our teepees.' But the herds could no longer sustain them: 'Gone they will be before many snows have come to cover our heads or graves if such should be.'[1] To the people who lived and died by the bison, it was clear that the plains economy was in transition. At treaty negotiations across the prairies, Aboriginal people were accepting 'the Queen's hand' and entering into pacts of friendship for the sake of receiving government support for their transition from hunting to agriculture. But the government understood the treaties as primarily land surrenders, and so grossly underestimated the commitments and financial costs of treaty making. The people were left without even the basic necessities of life – food, shelter, and clothing – that were once provided by the bison. The government issued rations and relief only reluctantly, for reasons of economy and also to discourage what officials perceived as the people's natural indolence. Soon enough, power in west shifted to those with access to food and resources, and the government pressed its advantage to enforce its vision of the prairies as a frontier for investment and settlement. As a result of all this, the Aboriginal people of the plains were plunged into a hunger/disease nexus, the impact of which would be felt for many years after the initial food crisis had passed.

The bison herds, the foundation of the prairie Aboriginal economy, were a storehouse and pantry on the hoof, but first they had to be found. Although the herds were at times huge, their ranges in the grassland and parkland were even larger. Migrating herds could be redirected by swollen rivers, prairie fires, or storms. No one understood that better than the Aboriginal people who depended on the herds not only for food, clothing, and housing but also for many of their cultural and spiritual symbols. Kapitikow, who would become Chief Thunderchild, told the story of a starvation winter in the 1850s when he was a young boy. There was nothing to hunt, and travelling became more difficult as the people weakened, and wolves killed their dogs at night. Kapitikow dreamed that their salvation lay to the south, and when he told his father of the dream, his father said, 'Dreams count, my son. Try to go south, all of you.' First they found an old bison bull whose meat was so tough the women could only boil it to make a soup, but their fortunes improved, and as spring arrived on the plains all were well fed. Kapitikow's father repeated, 'Dreams count, my son. The spirits have pitied us and guided us.'[2] It took skill, insight, and a close spiritual connection to the land to judge when to move camp in order to intercept the herds. When the animals were found, they were usually massed together, and the planned kill could begin, with care taken not to alarm the herd. In the days before horse and gun, herds were funnelled into log pounds or corrals, or driven over the edge of one of the many cutbanks that defined the prairie river valleys. After the horse was introduced, hunters were more mobile, but bison running still tested the skill of even the most experienced. Charging at full gallop through the snorting, stampeding herd, dust flying, the hunter had to reload his gun, first ramming the powder into place, then loading the shot, which he carried in his mouth, all the while choosing an animal and watching that the herd didn't turn and hunt the hunter. The most accomplished hunters still preferred using a bow and specially marked arrows so that the women who followed the hunt would know which animals to dress. In Aboriginal societies the successful hunter enjoyed honour, esteem, and political power.

By the 1860s, Cree and Assiniboine hunters were being forced farther and farther west into Blackfoot territory in pursuit of the herds, while the Metis ranged far from Red River to provision the fur trade. Not until the early 1870s were the Canadian herds being threatened, because the animals were still used much as they always had been, for the needs of the Native people and to provision the fur trade. It was in the United States that the carnage began in earnest; after the Civil War ended, the killing moved westward, targeting the bison herds and the Aboriginal people who lived by them. The hunt turned to slaughter, with hide and robe traders concealing themselves in bushes and indiscriminately emptying their repeating rifles into the herds. Ox teams and chains ripped hides from the still-warm flesh. Settlers and railway construction crews lived off the herds even while they sliced into bison habitat. Hunters, traders, and sportsmen ravaged the southern herds for the increasingly lucrative robe, hide and (later) bone trade. It has been estimated that a single American firm traded in the slaughter of more than *two-and-a-half million animals annually* from 1870 to 1875. The real pressure on the Canadian herds came when the robe and hide trade opened an overland route south from Blackfoot territory and into the Missouri River trade network.[3]

By the 1870s the Cree chiefs were edgy. The growing scarcity of game, the recent smallpox epidemic, the arrival of Canadian troops on the Red River to meet Louis Riel's challenge, and rumours that all of the people's land had been sold to the new Canadian government made for a tense meeting at Edmonton House in 1871 with Hudson's Bay Company factor William Christie. The respected Cree leader Sweet Grass outlined the chief's position: 'We heard our lands were sold and we did not like it; we don't want to sell our lands; it is our property, and no one has a right to sell them. Our country is getting ruined of fur-bearing animals, hitherto our sole support, and now we are poor and want help – we want you to pity us. We want cattle, tools, agricultural implements, and assistance in everything when we come to settle – our country is no longer able to support us.'[4] Sweet Grass, the foremost chief of the Fort Pitt people, had been a skilled hunter and a courageous warrior in the Blackfoot wars. He was admired by the younger Big Bear, but Sweet Grass was falling increasingly under the influence of Catholic missionaries in the area. Nevertheless, Sweet Grass was speaking for all of the Fort Pitt and Carlton people in 1871. Agriculture was beginning to be seen as a viable economic option for the Plains peoples. Two years later, in 1873, Cree and Assiniboine at Qu'Appelle interfered with survey and construction crews to press their demands for a treaty.

The precedent for treaty making stretched back to the British Royal Proclamation of 1763, which acknowledged Aboriginal people's right to the land. To clear the path for expansion, the Crown – and only the Crown – would negotiate treaties. The seven treaties that were signed in the 1870s opened the newly acquired Rupert's Land for settlement from the western shore of Lake Superior to the Rockies. But the treaty-making process was rooted as much in the Native people's need to protect their lands and future, as in the government's desire to honour precedent. Treaties One and Two in southern Manitoba were signed in 1871; at the insistence of the Saulteaux (Ojibwa) negotiators, they included provisions for schools, hunting and fishing rights, and agricultural aid, even though the government had come to the table only with offers of reserves and annuities. Treaty Three, relating to the lands between Lake Superior and the Red River (intended by government to be the first treaty), was not concluded until 1873 because the Saulteaux negotiators repeatedly refused the government's terms. The terms of Treaty Three built on the promises of the previous treaties and included increased annuities, larger reserves, and more financial aid.[5] These first three treaties created a corridor for travel from old Canada to the west.

On 15 September 1874, the Qu'Appelle Treaty, or Treaty Four, was negotiated between representatives of the Cree, Saulteaux, and Assiniboine of the area and three commissioners: Lieutenant-Governor Alexander Morris, Minister of the Interior David Laird, and William Christie, the former chief factor of the Hudson's Bay Company. These three were accompanied by a militia escort. Negotiations were strained by disagreements between the Cree and Saulteaux, and then halted altogether when the Saulteaux spokesman, Gambler, announced he would not proceed until the role of the Hudson's Bay Company had been clarified. He demanded that treaty negotiations be moved from the company fort to a neutral site, and that the government restrict the company's holdings and trading rights within the people's acknowledged territory. Pasquah contended that the £3,000,000 paid by the government to the company for their trading rights in the territory rightfully belonged to the Aboriginal people. Kakeesheway, or Loud Voice, the principal spokesman for the Cree, attempted to find a consensus between the Cree and the Saulteaux. Not until the sixth day of meetings were terms of the treaty discussed; however, Cree spokesmen Kanocees and Cheekuk were still reluctant to speak on behalf of important Qu'Appelle chiefs Piapot and Okanese, who were hunting on the plains.[6] Piapot, Okanese, and Cheekuk entered the treaty the following year, 1875. Only after further attempts to negotiate were rejected by the commissioners did the assembled chiefs finally agree to the same terms as in Treaty Three. But Treaty Four actually provided less financial assistance than Treaty Three.

It is difficult to know exactly what the Aboriginal people understood by the treaties. However, Gambler's approach to the negotiations suggests what must have been motivating the Saulteaux. His people lived in the parklands and forests in dispersed groups and had been skilled trappers and traders for generations. In the 1870s they were not faced with the same threat that the destruction of the bison economy posed for their Plains Cree and Assiniboine counterparts. Thus the Saulteaux negotiators argued for greater material benefits from any treaty, while the plains Cree and Assiniboine stressed their fears for the future and their need for an ongoing relationship with the government. As the Cree spokesman Kanocees asked, 'Is it true that you are bringing the Queen's kindness? ... Is it true that you are going to give my child what he may use? Is it true that you are going to give the different bands the Queen's kindness?' Clearly, the Cree and Assiniboine wanted the treaty to inaugurate a relationship with the government that would ease their transition to a new way of life.[7]

As far as the government was concerned, all of the numbered treaties were primarily surrenders of land. Yet the treaty talks rarely dealt with this aspect; instead, discussion always emphasized what the Aboriginal people would receive. They were promised they could continue to live as they always had, and to hunt and fish throughout their territory; but the written treaties all stipulated that those rights were subject to government regulation. It is clear, however, from the testimony of many elders that the Aboriginal people did not view the treaties as land surrenders at all, but only as promises that they would share the land with settlers.[8] Nevertheless, the text of every treaty stated that the people had agreed to 'cede, release, surrender and yield up to the Government ... all their rights, titles and privileges whatsoever to the lands.' In Treaty Four, that meant all of present-day southern Saskatchewan and parts of western Manitoba – more than 192,000 square kilometres. The land surrender clauses have created disagreement and distrust ever since. Subsequent events would turn on these fundamentally different interpretations of the treaties.

The people of Treaty Four were promised cash and clothing, as well as tools and equipment to be supplied 'once for all.' Each family was to receive two hoes, one spade, one scythe, and one axe, as well as enough seed – wheat, barley, oats, and potatoes – to plant the cultivated lands. One plough and two harrows were promised for every ten families, and to each chief for the benefit of all, one yoke of oxen, one bull, four cows, saws, a grindstone, and a chest of carpenter's tools. Also, a school was promised on the reserve for each band. Reserve land was to be apportioned on the basis of one square mile for every family of five. The reserve lands might be 'sold, leased, or otherwise disposed of by said government' for the people's use, with their consent; however, the people themselves were not 'entitled to sell or otherwise alienate' any of the reserve lands. Annuities of $25 for chiefs, $15 each for no more than four councillors, and $5 for band members were to be paid.[9] The government also promised to distribute $750 annually for shot and twine; Treaty Three adherents were to receive $1,500 annually. The distribution of implements and seed was contingent on the people actually cultivating the soil, though this would be difficult until the people received the implements. Unfortunately, the government was slow to send out surveyors to establish reserves so that cultivation might begin; and there was rarely enough food on hand to feed those who were ready to cultivate in the spring, which forced families to leave the reserve to hunt and fish. Seed and implements were distributed too late in the year to be of any use. Cattle were eaten rather than kept over the winter, because scythes were not available to put up hay. In all, very little progress was made toward farming in the first years after Treaty Four was signed.

The distinct lack of agricultural progress may account for the marginally better terms demanded, and won two years later, by the Woodland and Plains Cree at Carlton in Treaty Six.[10] It had been five years since Sweet Grass and other chiefs had requested a meeting with Canadian representatives, and Cree concerns about the failing bison hunt and their desire to restructure their economy had only increased in the meantime. When their concerns were ignored, they stopped the work of survey and telegraph construction crews to make their point. The Woodland and Plains Cree were not desperate for a treaty at any cost. They were a strong people, and with their Assiniboine and Saulteaux allies, had controlled much of the trade on the prairies for two hundred years. At Carlton in the valley of the North Saskatchewan, the commissioners were met by senior chiefs Mistawasis and Ahtahkakoop representing the 'House People,' so called because they traded at Hudson's Bay Company forts. Mistawasis and his people lived exclusively on the plains as bison hunters and also provisioned Carlton House with meat and robes; Ahtahkakoop's band were transitional Cree who trapped the forests to the north in winter and hunted bison in summer.

The meeting with the treaty commissioners on 18 August 1876 began with the sacred Pipe-Stem Ceremony. Chiefs and at least two thousand followers advanced in general celebration toward the commissioners, led by an elaborate display of horsemanship. The Pipe-Stem bundle, said to have been presented to the first human by the Great Manitou, was now brought forward by Strike-Him-On-The-Back – an honour that recognized his truthfulness and bravery. The Pipe-Stem was then raised to the sky and presented to all of creation by pointing it in each of the four cardinal directions. Prayers, chants, and drums accompanied the ceremony as the group again moved forward. The Pipe-Stem, beautifully carved and adorned, was then presented to commissioners Morris, Christie, and James McKay (a former HBC employee), and to Dr Jakes, the commission secretary, all of whom were invited to stroke the sacred object. The rite was a clear indication of Cree intentions and expectations: nothing but the truth could be spoken in the presence of the Pipe-Stem, and any treaty commitments made would be final and absolute. The significance of the ceremony was mostly lost on the commissioners, who considered it 'picturesque' and 'peculiar,' although they did recognize that the rite was intended to show friendship.[11] The commissioners put much more store in the signatures that finalized the process.

The terms of the treaty were similar to those of Treaty Four, with some important additions which indicated, first, that the Cree recognized that the prairie economy was deteriorating quickly, and second, that the treaty commissioners well realized that agricultural progress would be difficult given the promised supplies and tools. During negotiations, Poundmaker – not yet the influential chief he would become – made that very point, asking how they would be able to feed and clothe their children with the aid promised. As in the Treaty Four discussions, a Saulteaux negotiator, Joseph Toma, intervened and suggested that the lands being discussed were more valuable for farming and thus worth more: 'I do not want to keep the lands nor do I give away, but I have set the value. I want to ask as much as will cover the skin of the people, no more or less. I think what he has offered is too little.'[12] Although Toma was repudiated, the point was made. Besides promising twice as many tools (for instance, four hoes per family instead of two; two spades instead of one), Treaty Six allowed for $1,000 to be distributed annually for three years to purchase provisions for those who were cultivating the soil. The treaty also promised that in the event of famine or pestilence, the government would 'grant to the Indians assistance of such character and to such extent ... to relieve the Indians from the calamity that shall have befallen them.' The negotiations on this item lasted one whole day. Morris insisted that although the government might promise famine relief, 'I cannot undertake the responsibility of promising provision for the poor, blind, and lame. In all parts of the Queen's dominions we have them; the poor whites have as much reason to be helped as the poor Indian; they must be left to the charity and kind hearts of the people. If you are prosperous yourselves you can help your unfortunate brothers.'[13] Morris's comments betrayed an underlying attitude toward Native people that would inform much subsequent department policy. As time went on, the fulfilment of treaty promises was increasingly seen as a charitable enterprise, instead of the legal responsibility that it was, and the provision of charity was seen as an individual undertaking, not the purview of government. There were concerns that poverty, while always present, might easily turn to 'pauperism' (or a lack of industry and initiative) if indiscriminate charity went unchecked.[14] As Morris pointed out, there were limits to what the government could or would do.

The senior chiefs of the Carlton people, Mistawasis and Ahtahka-koop, and their councillors had prepared a list of specific items to present to the treaty commissioners. Included in that list was a demand for exemption from compulsory military service, and another for a medicine chest to be 'placed in the house of every agent for the free use of the band.' Despite the care Mistawasis took to confirm that the text of the treaty exactly represented the promises, the treaty made no mention of military service, and the medicine chest clause read 'that a medicine chest shall be kept at the house of each Indian Agent for the use and benefit of the Indians, at the discretion of such Agent.'[15] The medicine chest clause was a departure from the standard clauses in the preceding five western treaties. Possibly the treaty negotiators on both sides had in mind the HBC's custom of providing medical assistance to its hunters and trappers, as in the vaccination program during the 1837–8 smallpox epidemic. The treaties had shifted the other social costs of fur production (such as the provision of relief and medical assistance) from the HBC to the government.[16] The presence at the negotiations of significant numbers of Woodland Cree hunters and trappers, as well as former HBC chief factor William Christie, lends credence to this view. Nevertheless, the demand was made and accepted with little comment, while requests for rather more minor items, such as cooking stoves for chiefs, were rejected by the government negotiators as too lavish.[17] The medicine chest clause has been the subject of contention ever since: Aboriginal people insist that it was a promise to provide health care; the government has favoured a narrower interpretation that a medicine chest is to be provided, although it created a huge medical bureaucracy in the next decades.

The treaty commissioners could ill afford to be lavish. Their superiors in Ottawa were ever mindful of the costs of the treaties; they were unfamiliar with local conditions and saw the distribution of necessary implements and seed as too generous. In response to criticisms of his negotiations, Morris replied that the increases were 'right and proper' because the Native people were anxious to begin farming. Furthermore, Morris was convinced that the provisions promised in Treaties Three, Four, and Five were inadequate to enable the people to farm successfully – which was exactly Poundmaker's point in treaty discussions.[18] The prepared copy of Treaty Six that the commissioners had brought with them was amended to include the new promises and duly signed. The treaty commissioners then moved up the North Saskatchewan River to Fort Pitt (*Waskahikanis* in Cree) to meet with Sweet Grass.

The Fort Pitt meeting was the scene of an even more elaborate Pipe-Stem Ceremony, but it seems it was also the site of an attempt to orchestrate a quick adhesion to the treaty. Sweet Grass had to be sent for because he was out hunting on the plains, but no attempt was made to send a messenger to the other influential chief, Big Bear. Big Bear's following – the true measure of a chief's power and respect – had increased in the previous five years, partly at Sweet Grass's expense, because of Sweet Grass's reliance on the counsel of missionaries.[19] Big Bear had already been branded a 'troublesome fellow' by government emissaries for insisting in 1875 that a treaty be made before the Saskatchewan country was developed.[20] The treaty commissioners preferred to negotiate with Sweet Grass and the other Christian chiefs, and it is clear that Sweet Grass had decided to accept the treaty before he had even met with Morris. There were dissenting voices, however. Striped Gopher asked the commissioners if they truly understood the enormity of the task they were undertaking: 'Do you think you can truly shoulder the responsibility of looking after us?' An elderly woman also interrupted: 'Kitchikimaw, you have come to make a deal with your brother who is my child. I nursed him even as you derived your first nourishment from your mother's breast. She loves you as I love my son. Do not try to cheat him, for he deserves to live even as you do.' Both speakers were asked to withdraw.[21] By the time Big Bear reached Fort Pitt, the leaders had already signed the treaty. He was angry that they had not waited for him, but pressed Morris for assurances that the treaty would meet the people's needs and that the government would help preserve the remaining bison herds. He told Morris he could not sign the treaty because the people he represented were not there: 'I am alone; but if I had known the time, I would have been here with all my people ... I will tell them what I have heard and next year I will come.'[22] But Big Bear did not sign the treaty the following year; instead, he chose to wait and see if the promises were indeed enough to support his people. Later, the North-West Council made a weak attempt to preserve the bison with a hunting ordinance, but it was repealed a year later. Just months after he signed Treaty Six, Sweet Grass was dead, killed by a gun received from the treaty commissioners. Big Bear's granddaughter saw this as retribution for selling the land.[23]

There was still a large area – all of southern Alberta from the Cypress Hills to the Rocky Mountains and from the Red Deer River to the American border – that had not yet been ceded under treaty. This was the homeland of the Blackfoot Confederacy, comprising Blackfoot proper; the Blood; the Peigan; the Sarcee, a Dene people who had migrated south; and the Nakoda Stoney or Assiniboine, longtime enemies of the Blackfoot who had moved west to the foothills from the plains. These groups had different languages and cultures but had come to share a common set of problems, and they had been waiting a number of years for an opportunity to discuss urgent issues regarding their future. In 1874 the North-West Mounted Police (NWMP) arrived on their territory, sent by a nervous Canadian government that hoped to establish some form of sovereignty in the west to counter American incursions, such as the Cypress Hills massacre of Assiniboine people in the winter of 1872–3. With police in their midst, the robe traders, who peddled a particularly noxious whisky cut with water, tobacco, and painkiller, skittered away. The Aboriginal people welcomed the police presence because it enabled them to secure once again some hegemony over their lands and bison. But by 1875, Blackfoot, Blood, and Peigan leaders were petitioning Commissioner Morris for a resolution to a number of concerns: specifically, that hunters were decimating the bison herds and that settlers were claiming their lands. The government, for its part, was becoming increasingly worried that the American wars on the Nez Perce and on the Lakota led by Sitting Bull might spill over to Canadian soil. An Oblate priest, Constantine Scollen, who spoke Cree and had lived with the Blood for three years and who was present at the signing of Treaty Six, was asked to report on the Aboriginal people of southern Alberta. His 1876 report warned the government that although the Blackfoot peoples had been devastated by smallpox and whisky, they had lately recovered and were becoming increasingly intolerant of trespassers. In a postscript, he warned, 'I am also aware that the Sioux Indians, now at war with the Americans, have sent a message to the Blackfeet tribe, asking them to make an alliance offensive and defensive against all white people in the country.'[24] Although Blackfoot chief Crowfoot had met with Sitting Bull, Crowfoot had refused any alliance. Nevertheless, the government perceived the people as more 'warlike' than other plains people. They were also better armed and more likely to create trouble for the government.[25] The situation at Blackfoot Crossing in September 1877 was thus much different than at earlier treaty discussions. The peoples of the Blackfoot Confederacy had not cultivated the same close trading relationship with the HBC as the Cree and Assiniboine. Neither had they accepted the presence of HBC trading forts on their territory; instead, they had limited their contacts with the company to trading trips to Rocky Mountain House and Fort Edmonton, where they traded horses, robes, and meat for guns, ammunition, and cloth. The Blackfoot had for many years successfully protected their lands from incursions by other plains people, resorting to war in their defence. The treaty commissioners, David Laird and NWMP Lt-Col James Macleod, were made aware of the tense political circumstances.

David Laird, or Tall White Man, was hardly familiar with the plains or its people. Before being appointed Lieutenant-Governor of the North-West Territories in 1876 for a five-year term, he had been a journalist on Prince Edward Island, a Liberal MP, and for three years Minister of the Interior. He was present at the signing of Treaty Six and then replaced Alexander Morris as treaty commissioner to negotiate Treaty Seven. For this he was accompanied by James Farquharson Macleod, a Scot with a military background who established the first NWMP fort, Fort Macleod, in 1874, and who had recently been appointed police commissioner. The more than four thousand people who arrived at Blackfoot Crossing were a diverse group. Blackfoot leader Crowfoot was in his late forties, only a few years older than his friend Macleod, and it was because of this friendship that Crowfoot was pushed to take a leading role in the negotiations, even though he was neither the sole chief of the Blackfoot nor the chief of all the Blackfoot Confederacy, as the commissioners had assumed. Crowfoot was born to Blood parents but had been adopted by the Blackfoot and would remain with them his whole life. His leadership rested on his bravery in battle, his generosity, and his ability to deal with traders.[26] On 16 September the commissioners arrived at Blackfoot Crossing and found Crowfoot and the other Blackfoot chiefs and followers, and across the Bow River the Sarcee, the Stoney, Bobtail's

Cree band, and the various traders who made their money following the treaty parties. Neither the Peigan nor the Blood people had yet arrived.

Crowfoot listened to the terms of the treaty but refused to enter into any negotiations until the Blood chief Red Crow arrived. Red Crow, a lineal descendent of the great Blood chieftains, was the most powerful and respected chief to enter the Treaty Seven negotiations. In contrast to the more tempestuous Crowfoot, he was a quiet statesman. In the meantime, Medicine Calf (also known as Button Chief) spoke out against the terms of the treaty; he had experienced the treaty-making process in the United States and had seen promises routinely ignored. Laird was shocked and insulted when Medicine Calf told him that the people had already given much land and timber to the NWMP, for which they should be paid.[27] But most of the discussion of the treaty terms took place among the leaders in their own councils, out of hearing of the commissioners. With the arrival of the Blood and Peigan, the discussions grew heated as the chiefs discussed the government's offer. But what had they been told? According to the elders, the treaty that was negotiated at Blackfoot Crossing in 1877 was not reflected in its written text. Elders from all the Treaty Seven Nations insist that the treaty was mainly a treaty of peace, and that the issue of land surrender was never discussed. They were told they would share the land in peace with the newcomers but would be allowed to hunt and live as they always had. There were consistent problems with the interpreters: none of them spoke Sarcee or Stoney, and the commissioner's interpreters Gerry Potts and Jimmy Bird were likely unfamiliar with the commissioner's formal English. Red Crow and Crowfoot finally agreed to the terms as they were explained to them, over the opposition of war chiefs Medicine Calf, Many Spotted Horses, and White Calf. Given the international political situation and the people's growing uneasiness with incursions into their territory, in order to secure a treaty the commissioners may have allowed the Treaty Seven chiefs to believe that they were signing a treaty of peace and not a land surrender.[28]

According to Blood elder Louise Crop Eared Wolf, 'at the signing of the treaty at Blackfoot Crossing, Red Crow pulled out the grass and gave it to the white officials and informed them that they will share the grass of the earth with them. Then he took some dirt from the earth and informed them that they would not share this part of the earth and what was underneath it, because it was put there by the Creator for the Indians' benefit and use.'[29] According to oral history, annuities, provisions, rations, a medicine chest, and schools were promised, in return for a promise to keep the peace both with other Native people and with non-Natives. However, Treaty Seven made no mention of medicine or rations, and stated that the people had ceded 130,000 square kilometres of southern Alberta and a corner of southwestern Saskatchewan in return for annuities, seed or cattle, teachers, and reserves. At the time, in the autumn of 1877, neither side realized how differently the other understood the treaty; the people's greatest concern was to settle into their camps and wait for the winter hunt. But there was no snow that winter; instead, fires burned the prairies and kept the bison away. Crowfoot and his people remained near the Bow River that winter; most of the Blood and Peigan moved south in search of bison.

As far as the government was concerned, the treaties were land surrenders and had successfully transferred title of the prairies. The real work of settlement and railway building could now begin. Moreover, in 1876, even while treaties were being solemnly negotiated, the government had enacted a comprehensive piece of legislation, the Indian Act. It presumed to define who was and was not an 'Indian,' relegated Aboriginal people to the status of wards of the state, defined how reserves could be subdivided and surrendered, defined the political structure of bands, and established the Department of Indian Affairs. The Indian Act and the bureaucracy that it spawned presumed to direct and control the social, personal, political, religious, and economic lives of the people. The Indian Act defined the relationship between Aboriginal people and government and codified the assimilationist agenda. It would be years before Aboriginal people learned of its existence, and they certainly never agreed to its terms. What they had promised was to share the land; in return they were to receive aid, protection, and the 'generosity of the Queen.' Not long after the ink was dry, that generosity was needed. By April 1878 the government was receiving reports that bison were becoming critically scarce. Traders at Fort Benton, Montana, estimated that there was only one herd left, of about 100,000, which might supply the Treaty Seven people as well as the American Sioux and Crow. For the Cree and Assiniboine farther to the north and east the situation was deteriorating quickly. Farm instructors were needed to show the people how to grow crops, and provisions, seed, and implements were necessary to plant them.

Lieutenant-Governor Laird was aided by his assistant and agent for all of Treaty Six, M.G. Dickieson, and by Allan Macdonald, the agent for

Treaty Four. Macdonald, whose father was Archibald Macdonald, at one time the chief factor of the HBC, was raised in the west and lived in the Treaty Four area. He was aware of the enormous effort that would be involved in distributing the provisions, tools, and annuities promised in the treaties to more than 17,000 Aboriginal people spread across the prairies, and teaching them to farm. But officials in Ottawa were reluctant to consider the increased expenditure. David Mills, the Minister of the Interior, was convinced that stock and implements had been lavishly issued, that tools and implements were being sold, and that idle tools were rusting in the fields.[30] Laird, in residence at the territorial capital of Battleford, feared the consequences of the false economy being practised by Mills and the government. He warned that the government might choose one of three options: 'to help the Indians to farm and raise stock, to feed them, or to fight them.' Dickieson reported that the winter of 1877 was very hard on the people: 'The Indians were very poorly off, starving in fact,' and although not all the treaties included provisions for feeding the people,' we are on the eve of an Indian outbreak which will be caused principally by starvation, it does not do to scan the exact lines of the treaty too closely.' To put the situation in perspective for Mills, Dickieson noted that the cost to the American government to subdue the Sioux under Sitting Bull had been $2,300,000 and a large number of lives. In response, the minister struck from the department's estimates the provisions for people in Treaty Four, and cut in half the promised provisions for Treaty Six people, and allowed only $600 to hire farming instructors. The 1878 crop in Treaty Four could support only three bands, and in Treaty Six only four bands were able to rely on their garden produce and grain for at least a part of the winter.[31]

By the summer of 1879, widespread famine was imminent. Just two years earlier, in 1877, Dr D.W.J. Hagarty, the newly appointed medical superintendent for Manitoba and the North-West, noted the 'healthy appearance of the Indians, the freedom from disease, the general light-heartedness and the happiness and contentment.' By 1879 he found the same people emaciated. 'Hunger has shown its terrible effects upon them and scrofula and other kindred diseases are becoming deeply rooted.'[32] Hagarty was sent to vaccinate the Treaty Four people against smallpox, but first he had to feed them. The bands of Day Star and George Gordon ate their day's rations at one meal. A deputation told Hagarty that the people were still starving: 'You eat enough every day, and consequently do not eat much, but we have not eaten enough for the last two months and what you gave us yesterday only made us one meal.' Hagarty increased the rations for the next four days and then reduced them again. In June 1879, farther west at Qu'Appelle, government storehouses were raided for the flour and provisions left over from the treaty payments.[33] At Touchwood Hills on 11 August, Poor Man's band would not wait for Hagarty to dole out the rations stored there for their use, and took two oxen and some flour, 'although they were not to feed until the morning of the 14th.' As if hunger was not enough, the vaccine itself was making the people sick with serious side effects. The Sioux near Portage la Prairie suffered so much that they wondered whether Hagarty had been sent by the American government to kill them. On the Roseau River south of Winnipeg, Short Bear asked Hagarty to vaccinate only half the band in March and return later to vaccinate the other half: 'I want the well half to take care of the sick half.' Understandably, when Hagarty returned in July he had considerable difficulty persuading the people to submit. By the end of his vaccination trip, Hagarty was forced to admit there were serious problems with the vaccine and was recommending that vaccination should never again be attempted at the treaty payments in summer because it 'suffers or deteriorates on being exposed to atmospheric influences especially a heated atmosphere as we have on the prairies in summer.'[34] Hagarty had expected to vaccinate more people, but by early September most had gone south and west onto the prairie in a desperate search for food.

Hunger was also a threat to the more than one thousand people camped at Battleford. There were no bison north of the Red Deer and Saskatchewan rivers. The women were digging wild turnips and picking berries, but there was little meat and no flour in the territories. Laird expected that there would be trouble if the crops failed and recommended that the HBC posts on the North Saskatchewan be fortified and that the police force in the area be increased substantially.[35] Treaty Six agent M.G. Dickieson requisitioned 19,500 pounds of bacon for the people at Fort Carlton, Prince Albert, Battleford, Fort Pitt, Victoria, and Edmonton. By the end of the month he had increased the requisition to 20,000 pounds of bacon, plus 300,000 pounds of flour and an additional 100,000 pounds of beef. Agent Allan MacDonald at Treaty Four requested 7,500 pounds of bacon and 215 sacks of flour. By late August, the fear of famine seemed well grounded. Even if Laird could convince the government to send supplies, there was no guarantee that they would arrive before freeze-up and the close of shipping for the year. At the self-styled 'Starvation Committee' meeting in August, the urgency of the situation was clear to everyone. Besides Laird and Dickieson, the committee included the NWMP commissioner, James Macleod; a representative from the military, Lt-Col Hugh Richardson (who would later preside over the trials of Big Bear and Poundmaker in1885); and the new Indian commissioner, Edgar Dewdney. Dewdney, a civil engineer whose greatest qualification as Indian commissioner was his loyalty to the newly elected Prime Minister John A. Macdonald and the Conservative Party, was appointed in May 1879 to replace Laird, who had asked to be relieved of that part of his duties. The committee found that besides the supplies already requested, another 200,000 pounds of flour, and 100 to 200 ninety-five-pound bags of pemmican, and any fish that could be found, were now needed. Dewdney worried that all the supplies in the North-West would not be able to feed three-quarters of the Native people for more than one month.[36]

The food crisis was not limited to the people of Treaties Four and Six. By July 1879, the 1,000 people under Blackfoot chief Crowfoot were 'on the verge of starvation' and 'quite emaciated,' and out of desperation were eating the flesh of poisoned wolves and dogs. Some had nothing but old bones, which they gathered and broke up to make soup. Crowfoot's fellow Blackfoot chief Old Sun and the Sarcee chief Bull Head required immediate assistance for seventy lodges (about five hundred people) facing starvation. Their people had been forced to sell their horses and rifles and were eating dogs, gophers, and mice.[37] Crowfoot explained to Dewdney that his young men were difficult to control because they were hungry. They were threatening to kill settlers' cattle and telling him he should never have signed the treaty. In September, Dewdney sent enough relief supplies to Crowfoot for him to take his people east to the bison herd near Cypress Hills.[38] In October they followed the bison into Montana, where they remained for the winter.

In 1880, in reaction to the crisis, the Indian Department announced a new program that would have Native people settled on their reserves, with instructors at hand to help them learn farming and stock raising. Dewdney's appointment as Indian commissioner in 1879 was central to the administration of the farm program, which would establish seventeen farming agencies: six in Treaty Four, nine in Treaty Six, and two in Treaty Seven. Two 'government' or supply farms were also to be established in Treaty Seven, near Fort Macleod and Fort Calgary. Dewdney expected, unrealistically, that the cost to the government of the instructors and their families would easily be recouped in one year. It would fall to the farm instructors and agents to implement the new 'work for rations' policy – a policy informed by the perceived need to forestall pauperism. This new policy would significantly decrease the amount of rations provided, for only after instructors were satisfied that work had been done would they be issued. But as Dewdney admitted, 'my only fear is that so many will be anxious to work that we will not be in a position to keep them all going.'[39] In early 1880 his fears were realized.

Throughout the Treaty Four region, more than six years after the tools and seed were promised, the people were destitute. In present-day southeastern Saskatchewan, Okanese's band was starving. Those who had taken up farming found that the system of farm instructors was not working. The oxen they had been promised in the treaty had not been supplied, and as a result no crops were produced. Twenty people were slowly starving to death, too weak to keep up fires in their tents in temperatures of minus 45°F. Agents reported that fur-bearing animals that might have provided clothing were scarce, and besides, the people could not hunt for they 'were naked and the cold was intense.' They were eating their horses and dogs. At Qu'Appelle the men went out onto the prairie in an attempt to hunt while the women and children remained at the reserve. But without clothing, the women could not even fish.[40] At White Bear's reserve near Fort Ellice, the Cree and Assiniboine were dangerously short of clothing and food. They covered their lodgepole frames with mud because skins were unavailable. Three more people starved to death in January 1881. Farm instructor James Scott considered the department's pork rations as 'both musty and rusty and totally unfit for use – although we are giving it out to the Indians, in the absence of anything better, but we cannot use it ourselves.'[41]

In response to the deteriorating situation, over 4,000 people led by Big Bear, his fellow non-treaty chief Little Pine, and other Cree leaders migrated to the Cypress Hills near Fort Walsh in search of bison. And thousands from Treaties Six and Seven moved to Fort Macleod, where they were given small quantities of beef and flour every other day.[42] Rations were provided only to those who had taken treaty. Little Pine and his people could hold out no longer and took treaty in 1879. A number of Big Bear's followers left him in order to eat and joined Lucky Man and Thunderchild. In all, more than one thousand Plains Cree took treaty for the first time in 1879.[43] Shortly afterwards, they chose contiguous reserves at Cypress Hills. The mass migration then moved into the United States.

The people really had little choice. Starvation was a certainty on the reserves in Canada, their only hope was to take their chances hunting on the coteaux and in the valleys of the Milk and Missouri Rivers. Had there been food in Canada, they would have stayed in Canada, because south of the border they had to vie with hostile Crow and south Peigan, all in pursuit of the remaining bison herds. It did not take long for the inevitable to happen: disease ravaged the camps. As the people lost strength, measles and scarlet fever broke out among 350 lodges (at least 2,800 people) of Blackfoot, Peigan, and Cree at Meagher and Choteau in Montana. In one camp, 100 people died.[44] Then, in the spring of 1881, mumps swept through the camps. The stress of overcrowding, an inadequate diet, and the constant movement in search of game produced an out-of-control synergism between infection and hunger. Hunger can weaken human immune systems to such an extent that the severity, duration, and complications from minor infections are enhanced, with a resulting rise in mortality. Minor infections turn fatal in the presence of hunger and yet more infections.[45] When Crowfoot and 1,064 of his people returned to Fort Macleod on foot in July 1881, they were desperate.

As summer turned to fall, more and more people crossed back into Canada to Fort Walsh in the Cypress Hills. They were fleeing the hostile American bands, the American military, and ranchers who claimed to have lost cattle to Canadian Native people. Overcrowding became extreme, with more and more families forced to live in fewer and fewer lodges.[46] Treaty Seven agent and NWMP inspector Cecil Denny gave out ammunition, tobacco, tea, and hooks for fishing to the able-bodied. More than four hundred people were starving, yet Denny still had to justify the distribution of rations to his superiors: 'They are getting the very smallest quantity of food that can be given them ... I of course give no sugar to Indians. And other things I give as sparingly as possible.'

Piapot, chief of the Young Dogs, a mixed band of Cree and Assiniboine, was one of the most influential leaders of the Qu'Appelle Cree. He accepted Treaty Four in 1875 and in 1880 chose a reserve near the Cypress Hills next to Little Pine's. When he arrived back at Fort Walsh in the fall of 1881 with twenty-three lodges – at least 184 people – he was 'very badly off.' Thirty of his people, mostly children, had died in August from scarlet fever. By this time it was clear to Dewdney that Cree leaders, including Big Bear, Piapot, and Little Pine, were attempting to maintain Cree autonomy by establishing a huge concentration of reserves near the Cypress Hills. This would effectively preclude Canadian control over the area – an area that the new transcontinental railway would have to cross.[47] Dewdney commented on the fatal results of government policy: 'I have no doubt the sudden change from unlimited meat to the scanty fare they received from the government has to some extent brought it [mortality] about.' Indeed, he was under orders from the deputy superintendent, Lawrence Vankoughnet, to keep Fort Walsh to starvation rations.[48] Vankoughnet had been appointed in 1874 through family and political connections. It was he who managed the everyday work of the department; the superintendent general (or minister), Prime Minister John A. Macdonald, oversaw his work. Vankoughnet's administration of the department was described as completely inflexible and short on 'common humanity.'[49] The starvation at Fort Walsh was a cynical and deliberate plan to press the government's advantage and force the Cree from the area to allow the government a free hand in developing the prairies.

The department was well aware of the horrific effects of its policy. The year before, Dr John Kittson of the NWMP had warned the Indian Department that the rations were inadequate for subsistence. Working from figures he received from prisons and asylums in Europe, Kittson reckoned that a minimum daily ration for a man in moderate health with an active life should be one pound of meat, 0.2 pounds of bread, and 0.25 pounds of fat or butter. State prisoners in Siberia were given more than twice the ration. In severe weather or hard labour, the NWMP minimum daily ration was 1.5 pounds of meat, and 1.25 pounds of bread, plus tea, coffee, sugar, and abundant beans and dried apples. The daily ration for Native people of a half-pound of meat and a half-pound of flour was, according to Kittson, 'totally insufficient.' And the consequences were appalling: 'Gaunt men and women with hungry eyes were seen everywhere seeking or begging for a mouthful of food – little children ... fight over the tid-bits. Morning and evening many of them would come to me and beg for the very bones left by the dogs in my yard. When I tell you that the mortality exceeds the birth rate it may help you to realize the amount of suffering and privation existing among them. The only surprise is that they remain so patient and well disposed ... but human suffering must have its limits.'[50]

By the summer of 1882, Dewdney, in violation of the 1874 and 1876 treaties, which allowed leaders to choose reserves where they wanted, was determined to force the Cree and Assiniboine off the reserves they had chosen in the Fort Walsh district and onto reserves farther north at Qu'Appelle, Battleford, and Fort Pitt. The people were ordered to leave Fort Walsh or starve. Piapot left Fort Walsh for Qu'Appelle with 470 people, most on foot, with rations for 17 days. For the 360-mile trip they were allowed one half-pound of flour and a small amount of pemmican per person. When they arrived at Qu'Appelle, they found the people there starving. Piapot was incensed. He claimed that the food they received was killing them. The people were sick with dysentery. He wanted to choose his own reserve as the treaty had promised. By late summer he was back at Fort Walsh. The Assiniboine under Chief Long Lodge encountered similar conditions at the Indian Head reserve. Spoiled bacon caused severe diarrhoea and a number of deaths. Long Lodge and his band left the reserve in early August, refusing to return until fresh meat was issued. The assistant commissioner suggested that beef be supplied up to three times per week if necessary to keep the people on the reserve.[51] Piapot, Long Lodge, Lucky Man, Big Bear, and Little Pine, with more than two thousand followers moved back to Fort Walsh.

At Fort Walsh the winter of 1882–3 began in early October with blizzards and severe cold. Yet Dewdney was determined to force the people to leave the fort and travel to their reserves to receive their annuities – this, even though he could see they were in no shape to travel. Their clothes were little more than rags, their warm hide lodges had been replaced with torn cotton, and they were trying to survive on meagre rations. The children's clothes were in tatters and there were no robes or blankets for them to protect themselves from the biting prairie cold. Police surgeon Augustus Jukes was alarmed by the destitution at the fort: 'It would indeed be difficult to exaggerate their extreme wretchedness and need, or the urgent necessity which exists for some prompt and sufficient provision being made for them by the government.' Jukes warned that it was urgent that the government recognize the situation and make the annuity payments at Fort Walsh 'so that they may obtain requisite clothing and that immediate steps be taken that all alike may be furnished during the impending winter with sufficient food to rescue at least their women and children from death by cold and hunger.' Dewdney dismissed Jukes's alarmist tone; the doctor, he said, was unfamiliar with Native people and their 'indolence.' Rather than see the people starve, the NWMP took it upon themselves to issue rations at a rate of one-quarter pound of flour and a few ounces of meat. But as Inspector Frank Norman readily admitted, the people had to make two days' rations last seven days. Frederick White, the NWMP comptroller, urged Dewdney to take action on behalf of the more than two thousand people 'almost naked and [on the] verge of starvation.'[52] But the hunger crisis was not limited to those at Fort Walsh.

Across the prairies people were suffering, including those who were not ostensibly the targets of Dewdney's attempts to crush the Cree leaders. At the Moose Woods Sioux reserve near present-day Saskatoon, the people were without clothing and food, and four people who died there were 'actually skeletons.'[53] At Qu'Appelle, smallpox threatened to worsen an already bad situation. After one death in March, agent Allan MacDonald established a health district for seventy miles around the post because he feared an epidemic among the weak and hungry people. He advised that food was needed to avert an epidemic: beef and tea 'of course there will be the greatest economy used in these, and may be given by the advice of the medical officer.'[54]

In early November, MacDonald travelled to Fort Walsh to make treaty payments. He shared Dewdney's conviction that the people must relocate to other reserves, even though he knew full well what the conditions were across the prairies: 'I know they are not getting enough flour but I like to punish them a little. I will have to increase their rations, but not much.'[55] Such was the 'Queen's generosity.' Big Bear, who had refused to sign the treaty until he had an opportunity to judge its benefits and the intentions of the government, could hold out no longer – his people were hungry and weak. On 8 December 1882, he signed his mark on an adhesion to Treaty Six so that his people would receive rations. When Fort Walsh was finally closed in 1883, Big Bear moved north, though he still refused to choose a reserve; Little Pine and Lucky Man moved near Poundmaker at Battleford; and Piapot moved to Qu'Appelle. In this way they effected a modified form of their original plan to remain united on adjacent reserves. Cree efforts to hold the government to its treaty promises did not end with their move onto reserves, despite the ignominy of having to accept government rations.

When Piapot's people arrived at their reserve at Indian Head they were very weak. MacDonald reported that the exceedingly high mortality rate was largely due to 'consumption' (pulmonary tuberculosis). Farm instructor Richard McKinnon noted that in just five months, between November 1883, when the people settled on the reserve, and April 1884, 42 of Piapot's 550 people died, as well as 31 of 257 Assiniboines of Take the Coat band, making the death rates 76.3 and 120.6 per thousand respectively.[56] However, oral history holds that 130 adults and children died that winter from malnutrition and starvation. According to Goodwill and Sluman, the discrepancy can be accounted for by the department's desire to 'give the most conservative picture possible of the plight.'[57] According to elders, starvation was indeed the primary cause of death: 'They did a lot to starve the Indians. The first thing they did was to fence the reserve in ... The fence was to keep the people in ... When the people came here they were starving already. So many were sick that a doctor from Indian Head was called. The doctor got mad at the agent and told him the people are starving.'[58] Piapot moved his people off their reserve in May 1884 because, he claimed, so many of his people died there.[59] He wanted a site with fresh running water and plenty of fish, and headed for Pasquah's reserve. Fearing his motives, the government dispatched fifty-four policemen armed with a cannon to intercept him. He agreed to meet with officials at Qu'Appelle to defuse the situation, and in August 1884 settled his people on a reserve adjoining Muscowpetung's on the Qu'Appelle River.

Life at the Treaty Four reserves was difficult. The people were expected to work for rations when there were not enough tools, implements, or seed, although much of the necessary equipment was sitting in the government storehouse. The department was reluctant to issue tools and implements until the people, in the department's opinion, were ready for them. Rations suffered considerably in transit, and supplies that were issued were often so poor in quality as to be useless. By the end of 1883, Dewdney had been informed that the people in Treaty Four were poorly clad (most were without shoes) and 'afraid they are going to starve.' Agent MacDonald had warned Dewdney that January and February were likely to be very hard for the people because the fish would not take bait in the cold weather and rabbits would be scarce. Also, the potatoes stored for winter use and for seed were rotten, and the grain had not yet been ground into flour.[60]

Throughout the 1880s the two chief causes of death on the Treaty Four reserves were whooping cough among the children and pulmonary tuberculosis among the adults.[61] Morbidity and mortality from both diseases can be directly linked to economic conditions. Whooping cough, or pertussis, is an acute infection of the respiratory tract and is characterized by spasms of coughing and by a prolonged inspiration that gives the disease its name. During this stage the disease is highly communicable. The whoop is often followed by vomiting, and in infants cyanosis (bluish colour of the skin) may follow. Convalescence requires bed rest, a good diet, and adequate fluids; death follows complications such as bronchopneumonia, atelectasis (collapsed lung), convulsions, and haemorrhage. Like whooping cough, tuberculosis is a bacterial infection; while often associated with the lungs, it can affect almost any organ or tissue. Until the disease reaches its most advanced stages, many people are free of symptoms, or they experience only mild respiratory symptoms not unlike the common cold. It is likely that the general symptoms of tuberculosis – fatigue, lethargy, weight loss, and fever – are not even seen as unusual in undernourished communities. Tuberculosis is an environment-specific disease. Whether it develops once a person becomes infected depends on a number of factors, the most important of which are living conditions (including overcrowding) and quality of nutrition.[62] Sufficient food, warm clothing, and adequate housing are the three best guards against tuberculosis. Those with the least suffer most from the disease, and rising living standards greatly reduce mortality from it. Both whooping cough and tuberculosis are spread through droplet infection by talking, sneezing, and spitting. Once released into an enclosed space, the droplets can remain suspended in the air, much like smoke. For both diseases, closed, cramped living quarters help maintain high infection rates.

The desperate conditions on the prairies grew worse after Ottawa cut expenditures in 1883 in response to a general economic recession. Deputy Superintendent Vankoughnet directed the cost-cutting measures after a tour of the west, in the belief that agents were being irresponsible with the department's funds; he also ordered the dismissal of clerks, assistants, and instructors. Rations were to be distributed only in return for work and under no other circumstances. Also, he ordered the closing of the 'home' or government farms, despite the need for them, in the hope that increased settlement would provide seed, tools, and other services.[63] Dewdney did not endorse what he called Vankoughnet's 'Let them Suffer' policy toward the Native people. He warned his superiors that the people were already suffering and could ill afford any more deprivation. Harsh treatment, he cautioned, was ill-advised: 'the feeling among the Indians is such that they will not suffer without an effort to obtain what they consider is their right.'[64]

The 'work for rations policy' was to be implemented by Dewdney's new assistant commissioner, Hayter Reed. Reed, known as Iron Heart by the people, once referred to the Battleford Cree as the 'scum of the Plains.'[65] He was trained in the military, and in his work as agent for Treaty Six he expected complete obedience to his commands. Native people, according to Reed, were parasites and content to live off the government. As assistant commissioner he believed that the work-for-rations policy was fundamental to the larger moral purpose of shaking the people out of their supposed indolence and turning them into productive citizens. Although agriculture was far from thriving in Treaty Four, the young and able-bodied were to receive no government food

rations. In early 1884, Yellow Calf, leader of a band of Saulteaux fur trappers, with twenty-five men, approached the ration house on the Sakimay
reserve at Crooked Lakes east of Fort Qu'Appelle. He and his followers
were hungry and needed food for their families. When the farm instructor explained that Reed would not allow them any rations, they rushed
the warehouse and took flour and bacon. When NWMP inspector
Deane and his troops arrived, Yellow Calf demanded a meeting with
Dewdney to impress on him their need for food, clothes, and work. The
incident ended peacefully after seven hours of negotiations. Charges of
larceny were brought, but the sentences were suspended. Agent Hilton
Keith testified that the ration policy had caused the disturbance. Reed
argued back that the people had been dancing and had worked themselves into a frenzy, and when their food was gone they 'were in such a
state of excitement sufficient to subordinate all other considerations to
the craving for more.'[66] He would not admit that the ration policy was to
blame, although he later conceded that 'sickness was more or less rife'
among the people, that the hunting was poor and fishing impossible,
that they had no market for their grain crop, and that the winter was
very difficult. He wanted to dispel alarm among the settlers, however, so
he had the offenders taken to Regina. While the police were busy with
Yellow Calf, they received a telegram from File Hills reporting a similar
incident there.[67] Two years earlier, an equally ugly incident over food
between the ration issuer and Bull Elk, a minor chief in Crowfoot's
band, led to shots being fired and Bull Elk's arrest.[68] Such collective
actions to take food by force indicated high levels of distress. Families
forced into hunger and surrounded by disease had little patience for
Reed's social engineering, especially when food was available at the
ration house. Spokesman Louis O'Soup questioned Reed: 'If provisions
were not intended to be eaten by the Indians, why were they stored on
their reserve?'[69] The withholding of desperately needed food on
reserves led some to acts of violence. It was not the result of a people
who would not give up the chase and the fond memories of freedom.[70]
However, violent confrontations, were only the outward manifestation
of the ration policy.

   Chronic malnutrition, coupled with inadequate clothing and housing, had created a horrendous situation. Dr Oliver Cromwell Edwards at
the Treaty Four reserves noted many cases of 'bronchial troubles, ending in the spitting of blood and quick consumption and death.' He also
found what he termed 'land scurvy' caused by the exclusive use of salt
pork. The symptoms he described included swollen and enlarged

glands of the neck, and not the obvious scurvy symptoms of spongy, blackened gums and painful hardening of the leg muscles. Here, he may have been misdiagnosing 'scrofula,' a tubercular infection of the lymph glands. Nonetheless, it was apparent to Dr Edwards that the cause of the illness was the food, or lack of it: 'many of those who have died this winter have died from absolute starvation.'[71] It would do no good, he continued, to supply the people with ammunition because there was no game. Dr Edwards arrived in the west from Montreal in 1882 filled with romantic notions of the west and its primitive people. The romance died quickly at Fort Ellice, west of Brandon: 'The Indians are a disgustingly dirty crowd and I am fast becoming an American as to the best mode of dealing with them.'[72] In 1882, he was awarded the contract to vaccinate the Cree and Assiniboine people in Treaty Four. In 1884, he and his wife Henrietta joined the elitist settler society at Indian Head, which revolved around the Bell farm and the Indian Head Cricket Club. His work with the Assiniboine and Cree presented the Edwards family with the opportunity to indulge their Victorian passion for categorizing nature and collecting artifacts. They traded food and clothing to the starving Assiniboine in return for ceremonial clothing and spiritual bundles.[73]

Dr Edwards's report on the people's health was not well received by Reed, who was unwilling to admit the shortcomings of the ration policy and argued that the illness reported by Edwards was likely caused by the people's own 'immoral habits.' Apparently Reed believed that their plight was self-imposed, and a result of their overcrowded living conditions, where two or three families were forced to live in the same small log shack, which Reed perceived as immoral. Besides, he argued, 'when the doctor speaks of starvation [he] does not mean that the quantities issued were not sufficient but that the Indians were unable to eat the bacon.'[74] Yet, other doctors in the Treaty Four region were often using beef broth to treat those suffering from scarlatina and consumption. At Moose Mountain the main causes of death were consumption and scrofula, the contributing causes being cramped, poorly ventilated housing, and a poor diet consisting of bacon and flour.[75] MacDonald also noted that the extreme shortage of clothing was the cause of 'a great deal of suffering' during the winter. The hunting and fishing was poor in the winters of 1883 and 1884, and with increased immigration it was unlikely to improve substantially. At the Crooked Lakes reserves (Ochapowace, Kahkawistahaw, Cowessess, Sakimay, and Yellow Calf bands) between July 1882 and April 1883, only half the families had any crop, which left 670 people without farm produce. But only 534 received rations, and Yellow Calf's band received no rations at all. The daily ration was about 0.7 pounds of flour and 0.2 pounds of bacon per person, with children on half-rations. At File Hills the population was 476, but fewer than half (209) were engaged in farming. Only 232 people received rations. It was clear that farming did not produce enough to feed half the residents of the reserves, and that rations were woefully inadequate to stave off death from malnutrition and infection.[76]

Aboriginal people had been promised just eight years earlier that by 'taking the Queen's hand' in treaty, they would have a future. Instead they were caught in a vicious circle of malnutrition, which weakens the immune system, and infection. Nearly any endemic illness can become epidemic during famine – especially typhus, smallpox, dysentery, tuberculosis, influenza, and pneumonia. This synergism between common infections and malnutrition accounted for the increased mortality and morbidity.[77] The extent of the misery and suffering in Treaty Four is easily seen in the statistics. In the ten years from 1884 to 1894, the Crooked Lakes reserves lost 41.3 per cent of their population, while File Hills lost 46 per cent (Tables 1.2 and 1.4). The average child mortality rate surpassed the birth rate; for every child born, at least one and often two children died (Tables 1.1 and 1.3).

Population losses can be accounted for by three factors: decreased birth rates, increased death rates, and migration. At the Crooked Lakes and File Hills reserves, the death rate continued to rise during the first decade after settlement, while the birth rate remained constant or increased slightly. There is no real incompatibility between the two rates, however. As the population fell there may have been marginally more resources per person on the reserves, but considering the increasing death rate, that explanation seems unlikely. On the other hand, the rising birth rates may represent an especially odious cycle where increased birth rates and high infant mortality indicate deteriorating health status. Frequent child deaths promoted fertility for fear of not having any surviving children. But repeated cycles of pregnancy and lactation made major demands on maternal nutrition and promoted chronic malnutrition. Therefore, women tended to give birth to underweight babies, which increased the risk of infant and child mortality. Thus, high fertility resulted in undernourished women, and infants at high risk of contracting infectious disease and dying.[78] This cycle is clearly evident in the Treaty Four Reserves (Tables 1.2 and 1.4). The most significant population loss was suffered by children and the

TABLE 1.1
Crooked Lakes Reserves, 1884–1894: Birth and Death Rates

	Total pop.	Births	Rate per 1000	Total deaths	Rate per 1000	Child deaths	Child deaths % of births
1884	1001	29	28.9	60	59.9	52	179
1885	854	26	30.4	69	80.7	41	158
1886	803	22	27.3	47	58.5	39	177
1887	658	23	34.9	41	62.3	35	152
1888	632	27	42.7	28	44.3	19	70
1889	669	24	35.9	23	34.4	24	100
1890	612	20	32.7	53	86.6	32	160
1891	612	43	70.3	29	47.3	14	32
1892	574	20	34.8	36	62.7	27	135
1893	571	28	49.0	26	45.5	14	50
1894	587	27	45.9	23	39.1	14	52

Source: NA, RG 10, vols. 9417–27, Annuity Paylists, 1884–94.

TABLE 1.2
Crooked Lakes Reserves, 1884–1894: Population Distribution

	Total pop.	Men	Women	Boys	Girls	Other relatives*
1884	1001	140	219	259	293	90
1885	854	127	185	223	226	93
1886	803	134	181	198	212	78
1887	658	113	153	162	173	57
1888	632	115	153	147	169	48
1889	669	150	199	125	152	43
1890	612	140	195	120	119	38
1891	612	136	186	117	138	35
1892	574	139	172	103	128	32
1893	571	139	170	110	130	22
1894	587	136	184	114	131	22
change 1884–94**	−41.3%	−2.8%	−15.9%	−55.9%	−55.2%	−75.5%

Source: NA, RG 10, vols. 9417–27, Annuity Paylists, 1884–94.
*'Other relatives' were generally parents and grandparents of the family head receiving annuities.
**Percentage change between the 1884 figures and the 1894 figures.

TABLE 1.3
File Hills Reserves, 1884–1894: Birth and Death Rates

	Total pop.	Births	Rate per 1000	Total deaths	Rate per 1000	Child deaths	Child deaths as % of births
1884	476	10	21.0	11	23.1	7	70
1885	424	14	33.0	21	49.5	14	100
1886	337	10	29.6	27	80.1	22	220
1887	296	14	47.2	21	70.9	16	114
1888	300	12	40.0	24	80.0	14	117
1889	305	19	62.2	11	36.0	8	42
1890	283	15	53.0	45	159.0	34	227
1891	273	14	51.2	18	65.9	12	86
1892	276	13	47.1	16	57.9	10	77
1893	276	5	18.1	7	25.3	7	140
1894	257	11	42.8	9	35.0	2	18

Source: NA, RG 10, vols. 9417–27, Annuity Paylists, 1884–94.

TABLE 1.4
File Hills Reserves, 1884–1894: Population Distribution

	Total pop.	Men	Women	Boys	Girls	Other relatives*
1884	476	69	106	135	122	44
1885	424	65	105	114	98	42
1886	337	58	92	91	71	25
1887	296	52	82	76	62	24
1888	300	54	85	72	61	28
1889	305	65	95	66	60	19
1890	283	65	90	55	54	19
1891	273	66	92	45	55	15
1892	276	68	92	46	59	11
1893	276	70	93	45	56	12
1894	257	63	84	46	56	8
Change 1884–94**	−46.0%	−8.6%	−20.7%	−65.9%	−54.0%	−81.8%

Source: NA, RG 10, vols. 9417–27, Annuity Paylists, 1884–94.
*'Other relatives' were generally parents and grandparents of the family head receiving annuities.
**Percentage change between the 1884 figures and the 1894 figures.

elderly, which suggests that reserve life was particularly dangerous for those who were unable to command resources in their own right. It also indicates serious problems in the general state of health, since infant and child mortality rates are the most sensitive indicators of the overall health status of a community. The main determinant of infant and child mortality is the nature of the physical environment.[79] Infant and child mortality rates are also closely linked to family income. The less dramatic, albeit significant, decline among men and women indicates that the other major determinants of health – adequate nutrition, clothing, and shelter – were lacking.

Migration, the third determinant of population loss, was a significant factor between 1885 and 1888, in the aftermath of the Riel Rebellion. Although the Aboriginal people in Treaty Four played no part in Riel's violent attempts to force the Canadian government to respond to Metis concerns, the department used the rebellion to strengthen its control over most aspects of Aboriginal people's lives. During those years, the rate of loss across all population categories was constant. The Crooked Lakes reserves experienced their greatest net losses due to migration between 1885 and 1887, when 576 people left and only 195 entered. Over the same period at File Hills there was a net loss of 155 due to migration.[80] Most reserves in the west experienced significant population losses due to migration in these years.[81] It is therefore not possible that these people joined other Canadian bands; instead, they left their reserves (and perhaps the country) and rescinded their status in the eyes of the government because of social, political, and economic conditions on the reserves. In other words, they were chased out of the treaty.

The incidence of hunger and disease was slightly reduced by the availability of food sources other than government rations. On the short grass prairie of Treaty Four in southern Saskatchewan, other large game would have suffered the same loss of habitat as the bison, not to mention increased pressure from hunting. Women used a variety of resources to feed their families. They picked saskatoon berries, chokecherries, pin cherries, and wild strawberries, which they then crushed, dried, and stored in washed flour bags. They worked as domestics for settler families like the Edwards. And on the reserve some small game was available – rabbits, prairie chicken, and fish. As elders noted, 'the people would have died without that small game on the reserve. We weren't even allowed to shoot the jumpers [deer]. I don't know why.'[82]

Few plains people escaped the awful poverty that marked the first decades of government administration of their affairs. At the Peace Hills agency near Edmonton in the miserable winter of 1883, Cree chiefs Samson and Ermineskin, and others, tried to interest the government in their 'dire poverty' and utter destitution. They had not received the farming implements and cattle that were promised in the treaty because the employees at their reserves 'have robbed us of more than half of these things on which we were to depend for a living.' They had only received half the seed they were promised and none of the ploughs, harrows, axes, and hoes. They could not, they claimed, make their case to the agent because the interpreter would not translate their complaints. They had become 'mendicants at the door of every white man in the country.' They were slowly starving, and begged the minister: 'If we must die by violence, let us do it quickly.' In what had become a stock departmental response to criticisms of its policy, agent William Anderson dismissed the people's complaints and accused outsiders – in this case Father Constantine Scollen, the long-time Catholic missionary among the Blackfoot and Cree – of publicly fomenting trouble. Anderson suggested that the commissioner, Dewdney, might have the priest arrested. In his own defence, Scollen stated that the people were destitute and that when they applied to the agent for relief they were generally driven off with a growl. He added that the people were willing and anxious to work but had neither seed nor tools. To illustrate their dire situation, Scollen noted that the people could not even afford to bury their dead: 'I know of one corpse to have been eaten by dogs and wolves not a quarter of a mile from Edmonton.' He had recently brought in eight dead to be buried at the mission. The Hudson's Bay Company used to at least provide coffins, he said. Could the government not do the same?[83]

Further east, at the Treaty Six reserves near Battleford, the Cree were attempting to support themselves through farming. In the fall of 1882, Poundmaker's band had teased a wheat crop out of the dry prairie soil between drought in the spring and frosts in the fall, only to find that there was no way to grind it into flour: 'We do not know what to do with our wheat, and have to starve, beside our big sacks of grain.' The oxen, seed, and implements promised in the treaty were not forthcoming, so the people were forced to leave the reserve to hunt, which further slowed their progress on the farms. A serious shortage of clothing forced the Poundmaker and Thunderchild bands to abandon their farms and strike out onto the plains in search of game. As Poundmaker ably stated, 'It seems to me that we are as anxious to be independent as the

TABLE 1.5
Battleford Reserves, 1884–1894: Birth and Death Rates

	Total pop.	Births	Rate per 1000	Total deaths	Rate per 1000	Child deaths	Child deaths as % of births
1884	1956	46	23.5	85	43.4	61	132.6
1885	1952	38	19.4	87	44.5	81	215.5
1886	1614	49	30.3	194	120.2	108	220.4
1887	1559	33	21.1	89	57.0	56	169.6
1888	1395	36	25.8	76	54.4	39	108.3
1889	924	41	44.3	67	72.5	42	102.4
1890	874	36	41.4	59	67.5	19	52.7
1891	888	29	32.6	34	38.2	19	65.5
1892	875	33	37.7	40	45.7	17	51.5
1893	797	39	48.9	28	35.1	15	38.4
1894	856	30	35.0	52	60.7	27	90.0

Source: NA, RG 10, vols. 9417–27, Annuity Paylists, 1884–94.

TABLE 1.6
Battleford Reserves, 1884–1894: Population Distribution

	Total pop.	Men	Women	Boys	Girls	Other relatives*
1884	1956	293	419	561	599	84
1885	1952	281	488	539	566	78
1886	1614	261	415	411	438	89
1887	1559	252	422	385	403	97
1888	1395	206	372	365	362	90
1889	924	205	314	190	149	66
1890	874	186	292	189	144	63
1891	888	192	289	189	158	60
1892	875	199	274	182	167	53
1893	797	163	233	175	175	51
1894	856	188	268	179	171	50
Change 1884–94**	−56.2%	−35.8%	−36.0%	−68.1%	−71.4%	−40.5%

Source: NA, RG 10, vols. 9417–27, Annuity Paylists, 1884–94.
*'Other relatives' were generally parents and grandparents of the family head receiving annuities.
**Percentage change between the 1884 figures and the 1894 figures.

Government are to get rid of the burden of supporting us.'[84] Catholic missionary Father Louis Cochin at Poundmaker's reserve witnessed the starvation: 'I saw the gaunt children, dying of hunger, come to my place to be instructed. Although it was 30–40 degrees below zero their bodies were scarcely covered with torn rags ... The hope of having a little morsel of good dry cake was the incentive which drove them to this cruel exposure each day ... The privation made many die.'[85] Rations at Battleford allowed for only one meal a day, and many were too weak to work for them. Inspector Oulison of the NWMP noted that 'a good many of them are now ill and will likely die.'[86] Although crops were planted and harvested in some parts of the prairie that fall, many people were suffering the ill effects of the now five-year hunger. The nearby Stoney people of the Mosquito, Grizzly Bear Head, and Lean Man bands were the worst off, with seventy-seven deaths (including fifty children) in a population of only three hundred. One Arrow's band at Carlton suffered from exposure and starvation over the winter of 1883–4, when the weather across the prairies was more severe than usual. In a population of ninety-two there were two births and thirteen deaths, ten of whom were children.[87] The crude death rate was 141.3 per thousand. Population losses on the Battleford reserves were similar those suffered by the Treaty Four people (see tables 1.5 and 1.6). In each of the first ten years after settlement, the annual death rate was twice the birth rate. More than half of all deaths in the first ten years were of infants and children (Table 1.5), which suggests that living conditions were the cause of the high mortality rate. The strong and persistent inverse relationship between economic status and infant and child mortality was as clear among the Treaty Six people as it was among the people of Treaty Four.

The Cree led by Big Bear and Little Pine moved to reserves after the Fort Walsh debacle but did not abandon their efforts to have the treaty promises honoured and the clearly inadequate provisions in the treaties renegotiated. Indeed, conditions on the reserves only reinforced their determination. In June 1884, Big Bear arrived at Poundmaker's invitation to make a Thirst Dance at Little Pine and attend a general council of area chiefs, at which plans were made to press the government to keep its treaty promises. Big Bear had already been branded a troublemaker by the government for his consistent efforts to gain the most favourable reading of the treaty for the Cree people. But he was too much the savvy politician to believe that his people could ever benefit from violence against the government. As he once noted, his people should not fight the Queen with guns, but with her own laws.[88] The

Thirst Dance had just begun at Little Pine's reserve when two men, Kaweechatwaymat and The Clothes, approached instructor John Craig at the ration house. They had been ill and were hungry. Craig was attempting to push them out of the ration house when one of the men struck him on the arm with an axe handle. Craig called out the NWMP, who arrived the following day. The police and employees moved all the stored flour and bacon off Little Pine's reserve to Poundmaker's reserve, which was now deserted. One of those employees, Robert Jefferson, the instructor at Poundmaker's reserve, accompanied the police. The young Englishman had settled on the Red Pheasant reserve in 1878 as a teacher; then in 1884 he joined the Department of Indian Affairs as a farm instructor at Poundmaker's reserve. According to Jefferson, 'the trouble was all over a few pounds of flour.' In a fine bit of irony, the police and employees spent the night building bastions lined with full flour sacks for protection from the anticipated attack. Horses charged and reared, and men shouted, but no shots were fired as the Cree met with NWMP Inspector Leif Crozier's forces and the offenders were taken into custody. The following day, in an effort to ease tensions, there was a general distribution of rations. Crozier was publicly credited with the peaceful outcome. However, according to Poundmaker's deputy Fine Day, there was no trouble because Poundmaker did not wish it.[89] The chiefs knew that serious trouble would not advance their interests.

The chiefs' council met in early July 1884 at Carlton. Their demands were by now familiar. They pressed the government to deliver the farm implements and livestock promised in the treaty. They explained that their people could not work with the wild cattle they had been given, that the crops had been poor and the game scarce, and that all of their people had been 'reduced to absolute and complete dependence upon what relief was extended.' They lacked clothing and rations and so could not work; the promised medicine chests had not been delivered; their requests had been consistently ignored; and they were only barely able to restrain the young men who advocated violence. Reed admitted that many of the cattle were wild, but added that no record survived of what had been issued to whom. The tools issued were of good quality, he contended, but the people were very hard on them. He insisted that medicine chests had been promised for each agency, not each reserve, but admitted that no chests had been delivered. Later he suggested to his superiors that the unrest was the result of poor crops, and dismissed the remainder of the chiefs' statement as the work of the agitators Riel and Big Bear.[90] There were considerable grounds for complaint according to Jefferson, who suggested that Reed had calculated the absolute minimum ration and then deliberately kept the people hungry.[91] As well, the housing was deplorable. Log houses with mud walls and roofs let the rain in and washed everything inside with dirt. Jefferson added that the instructors' quarters were no better – some had a small cook stove. According to Fine Day, life on the reserves consisted of planting potatoes, cutting fence poles, putting up hay, and 'bothering the instructor for food ... The Indians saw that they were the slaves of the government – doing tasks and receiving bad food, and little of that.' Jefferson observed that the sickness that befell the people 'was the result of the radical change in their circumstance, especially the food.'[92]

If ever a people had cause to rebel in the spring of 1885, it was the Aboriginal people of the Canadian west. But there is no evidence that they conspired with Louis Riel against the Canadian government. It was not for Riel's lack of effort: for years his emissaries had been trying to involve Cree leaders in his plans. However, the Cree leaders had consistently rebuffed his overtures. On 3 March 1885, Riel, hoping to recreate his Manitoba resistance of 1869, proclaimed himself head of a provisional government that would administer the North-West. The Metis under him then began preparing for an attack from an NWMP column moving toward Carlton House. On 18 March they took over stores and ammunition and placed the local traders at Batoche in custody. The Riel or North-West Rebellion had begun. The events will not be discussed at length here as they have been treated by a number of excellent histories.[93] That being said, three separate incidents took place during the rebellion, unrelated to Riel's purposes, that would undo all the diplomatic efforts of the Cree leaders to bring about a favourable reading of the treaties. These incidents were a sad and perhaps inevitable consequence of government policy. People had been pushed to the limit of their endurance by hunger and disease, and too many children had died. The rebellion was the spark that ignited their desperation. Chief Poundmaker had no desire to join in Riel's increasingly violent cause, but he did sense that affairs were at a critical juncture, and so he decided to lead a deputation to Battleford to proclaim the people's loyalty, and to perhaps come away with much-needed rations and supplies. As the group made its way toward Battleford on 30 March, settlers and shopkeepers panicked and took refuge in the NWMP's Fort Battleford. After waiting for days to meet with the agent, who refused to leave the fort, the hungry people looted shops and quickly left town. While this so-called 'Siege of Battleford' was unfolding, just to the south, at the Stoney reserves of the Mosquito, Grizzly Bear Head, and Lean Man bands, a farm instructor and a farmer were shot and killed. As already noted, the Stoney had suffered terribly since settling on their reserves. One of the children who survived that awful winter was dangerously ill with tuberculosis in the spring of 1885, and when she died her father Itka struck out at the real source of power on the reserve, and killed the man who controlled the rations, James Payne. The next day, Barney Tremont, a local farmer who had also made himself hated by the people, was shot.[94] Farther north and west at Frog Lake, Big Bear's band had been suffering considerably since moving north from Fort Walsh. The chief's decision to wait before selecting a reserve site meant that the band was without even the meagre rations other bands had been receiving. Big Bear's leadership was melting away; his son Ayimassees and war chief Wandering Spirit were taking control of the increasingly desperate and discouraged band. That was the spark that began the tragedy at Frog Lake. The first to be killed by the raging and now drunken young men on 2 April 1885 was subagent Thomas Trueman Quinn, 'a very hard man. No one could ever make him change his mind once he shook his head and said "no."' The next killed was farm instructor John Delaney, who was roundly hated for his relationships with very young women on the reserve, and for his casual humiliations of the hungry people – 'we had to crawl or starve.' In all, nine men were killed, despite Big Bear's attempts to stop the carnage.

Most of the badly frightened Battleford area bands had taken refuge at Poundmaker's reserve at Cut Knife Hill and had stayed there throughout April. At dawn on 2 May, Colonel Otter attacked the camp with four hundred men, cannons, and a Gatling gun. Otter's men were forced to retreat by the fifty or so warriors sent out to meet them. Poundmaker allowed Otter's force to limp away: 'He said that to defend themselves and their wives and children was good, but he did not approve of taking the offensive. They had beaten the enemy off; let that content them. So there was no pursuit.'[95] By the middle of May, the Canadian militia and NWMP had defeated Riel's forces. The government was now intent on crushing any remaining traces of Aboriginal autonomy, even though it was clear that the Cree leaders had consistently counselled restraint and neutrality. Dewdney himself admitted that any Cree participation had been 'the acts of a desperate, starving people' and unrelated to Riel's purposes.[96] Nevertheless, the Native people of the prairies were to pay dearly for their supposed involve-

ment. In his annual report for 1886, Dewdney stated that the past policies of the government were not to blame for the Native people's
actions during the rebellion. They had rebelled, Dewdney explained,
because 'it is a peculiarity of their race to be extremely susceptible
to influence, to care little for the morrow if the day satisfies their
wants, and (perhaps from their nomadic tendencies) to welcome any
change.'[97] Yet it was hunger that had precipitated the violence. The
Indian Department had been warned over and over by its own officials
and by others that if food aid was not increased, there would be trouble.
The Natives' violence during the rebellion was not part of Riel's designs
to press Metis demands; rather, it was a reaction to, and evidence of, the
desperation of hungry young men.

The efforts by Big Bear and others to have the treaty promises kept
and perhaps even revised were crushed in the aftermath of the rebellion. Big Bear and Poundmaker were imprisoned for their supposed
involvement. Both died shortly after being released, which effectively
decapitated the movement. And if the Native people of the Battleford
reserves had any doubts about the government's intentions toward them
after 1885, those doubts were dispelled in November of that year, as they
watched eight men drop to their deaths from the gallows at Battleford.
The people could ill afford further hardship. The government now took
aim at what it considered disloyal bands, withholding annuities, confis-
cating horses and guns, suspending rations, and breaking up and dis-
persing bands. Even bands considered loyal were subject to new
regulations that severely limited their physical and economic freedom:
the pass system restricted their physical movement, while the permit system restricted their ability to market their agricultural produce. The
same living conditions that were killing Native children had also caused
the unrest among the Native people during the rebellion. The people
were frustrated by the prairie climate and inadequate tools, and they
seemed no nearer to making progress in agriculture. As a witness to the
events of 1885 noted, 'the chances were that the trouble would disappear under a shower of flour and bacon.'[98] But a 'shower' of food would
not be forthcoming.

There is little doubt that Canadian voters perceived the ration policy
as already far too generous. Battleford's Saskatchewan *Herald* claimed
that reports of starvation on reserves were unfounded. Native people,
editor P.G. Laurie claimed, were content to live off the government and
had to be compelled to settle and work on their reserves. 'Philanthro-
pists' were wrong-headed in their calls for greater aid to Native people,

he claimed, because relief only made the people 'more helpless.'[99] Laurie's estimation of the roots of the problem echoed a segment of public opinion that was more clearly expressed by the department itself: 'The provisions supplied them are so distributed as to encourage industry. Men who absolutely refuse to work are certainly not encouraged in their idleness ... for if they once acquire the notion that it is the duty of the government to maintain them they will never attempt to do anything for themselves.' The government described its difficult position as being caught between 'two hostile fires of criticism': the Opposition's charges that it was wasting money feeding 'idle vagabonds,' and criticisms that it was 'starving the poor Indians.'[100] An increase in rations, however unlikely, might well have forestalled the violence.

In the repression that followed the rebellion, the Edmonton reserves suffered along with the others even though they were not considered disloyal. The Edmonton chiefs appealed directly to the prime minister for some kind of aid. They admitted to killing and eating department cattle that were on their reserve to feed their families, adding in mitigation, 'We don't want to break the laws but we and our children are dying of hunger.' Reed asked Dr H.C. Wilson of Edmonton, who visited the people in January 1888, whether there was any starvation on the reserves. Wilson told him there was some evidence of it, but only in the very old people: 'No particular or special complaints were made to me, nothing but the usual grumbling about wanting more grub.' The register of deaths from October 1887 to March 1888 listed seven deaths. Two children had died from whooping cough and three from consumption; two adults had died of consumption. The agent supposed that the people were hungry because they had not exerted themselves sufficiently, and that they had been forced to kill department cattle to survive. The people were told, with no irony intended, that if they continued killing cattle to eat, the government would stop issuing food supplies to them. The story of starvation at Edmonton received widespread attention in the press.[101] Although Reed put the problem down to the pernicious influence of outsiders, he decided to increase rations temporarily. By December 1888 the agent was reporting that due to a fair crop and increased rations, the people's health had improved and they were 'very fortunate.' Reed immediately instructed the agent to decrease rations.[102]

At all of the Treaty Six reserves, the population losses were most acute between 1885 and 1889. At the Edmonton reserves, 30 per cent of the 1884 population had either left or died by 1889. At the

TABLE 1.7
Edmonton Reserves, 1884–1894: Birth and Death Rates

	Total pop.	Births	Rate per 1000	Total deaths	Rate per 1000	Child deaths	Child deaths as % of births
1884	976	35	35.8	15	15.3	7	20
1885	871	36	41.3	25	28.7	16	44.4
1886	697	26	37.3	58	83.2	40	153.8
1887	673	26	38.6	54	80.2	39	150
1888	670	35	52.2	41	61.2	30	85.7
1889	676	29	42.8	19	28.1	12	41.3
1890	695	28	40.2	13	18.7	5	17.8
1891	692	25	36.1	20	28.9	15	60
1892	688	20	29.0	55	79.9	32	160
1893	704	19	26.9	33	46.8	25	131.5
1894	726	38	52.3	22	30.3	11	28.9

Source: NA, RG 10, vols. 9417–27, Annuity Paylists, 1884–94.

TABLE 1.8
Edmonton Reserves, 1884–1894: Population Distribution

	Total pop.	Men	Women	Boys	Girls	Other relatives*
1884	976	177	200	281	284	34
1885	871	144	192	270	241	24
1886	697	125	161	206	187	18
1887	673	120	160	206	166	21
1888	670	115	154	202	179	20
1889	676	145	177	173	165	16
1890	695	155	187	177	160	16
1891	692	155	193	176	149	19
1892	688	154	193	173	148	20
1893	704	158	203	177	148	18
1894	726	160	201	185	165	15
Change 1884–94**	−25.6%	−9.6%	+0.5%	−34.2%	−41.9%	−55.8%

Source: NA, RG 10, vols. 9417–27, Annuity Paylists, 1884–94.
*'Other relatives' were generally parents and grandparents of the family head receiving annuities.
**Percentage change between the 1884 figures and the 1894 figures.

Battleford reserves, more than 50 per cent had left or died in the same years. Not surprisingly, there was a net loss due to migration out of the treaty – and for many people out of the country – in the wake of the 1885 troubles. For example, in September 1886 sixty-three men, women and children led by Jacob Red Deer 'deserted' Poundmaker's reserve for the Peace Hills reserves (the name was changed to Hobbema in 1893.) Agent Joseph A. Mackay and fifteen police officers forced them to return at least temporarily. In the meantime, twenty more left with Cut Lip. Mackay blamed the exodus on the peoples' destitution, on their knowledge that they would not receive annuities for another year, and on reports of better conditions in the United States, where the inducements were food and blankets.[103] Conditions south of the line were little better, however. But the government reserved its strongest wrath for those who remained in their own homeland. Living conditions deteriorated, if that was possible, and at the Battleford reserves in 1886 the death rate was nearly *four times the birth rate*; twice as many infants and children were dying as were being born. Between October 1885 and October 1886, out of a population of 1,952, 289 people left for personal and political reasons, 194 people died (108 of them children), and only 49 children were born. The birth rate was 30.3 per thousand, the death rate an astounding 120.2 per thousand (Table 1.5). At Edmonton in the same period, the starting population was 871; 142 people left the reserves, 58 people died (40 of them children), and 26 children were born (Tables 1.7 and 1.8). At both Battleford and Edmonton, the two years following the rebellion were the worst for population loss. The highest death rates occurred on the reserves most closely linked with the Riel Rebellion. The three Assiniboine bands suffered death rates of 178 per thousand (Mosquito), 306.4 per thousand (Grizzly Bear Head), and 117.6 per thousand (Lean Man). The rate on Red Pheasant reserve was 123.7 per thousand, while on Thunder Child and Sweet Grass reserves the rates were 233.5 and 185 respectively.[104] By way of comparison, the highest death rate in 1890 among Canadian cities was that of Quebec City (31.6 per thousand), and death rates in London and Paris at the time were 20 per thousand.[105] Although appropriations for relief were increased in 1886, those appropriations went specifically to those people who did not leave their reserves during the rebellion and were thus deemed by the department to have been loyal.[106]

Circumstances in the Treaty Seven areas were somewhat different. Certainly, the early years of the treaty were as desperate in southern Alberta as anywhere else on the prairies. At the Blood camps on the Belly River confusion reigned in the summer of 1881 when the hunters returned and the population jumped from 800 to over 3,000. The children were sick with measles and scarlet fever; corpses were suspended on scaffolds and hung in the trees. Necessities once provided by the bison were running short, especially clothing and housing. Lodges were torn and ragged. Log houses with mud roofs and dirt floors were a poor substitute, and very few were being built because of a lack of suitable lumber. As of 1881 there were more than 3,164 people on the Blood reserve, but only sixty-three houses had been built.[107] As more and more Native people arrived at their reserves, the food crisis grew urgent. However, Dewdney was most concerned about the impact of starvation on the settler's cattle. If the people were not fed, he noted, 'they will die of hunger, there being no game on the Plains ... and if they are to be encouraged to work their fields, they will have to be furnished with sufficient food to enable them to do so ... and if care is not taken to have a sufficiency of food on hand during the coming winter ... then white people's cattle will be killed and disorder spread throughout the country.'[108] Dewdney proposed a daily ration of three-quarters of a pound of flour and one-third of a pound of bacon for at least ten months; farms in the area would provide vegetables for two months. He complained that bacon was expensive because it had to be imported.

But the quantity of rations was not the only issue. Elders from Treaty Seven charged that the rations were contaminated. Tom Yellowhorn of the Peigan Nation tells how the agent directed the people to mix a yellow chemical into the flour for making bread: 'The people who lived around the agency camp were those who got sick. Those who were away at the time did not get sick ... So many died so fast they did not have time to bury them; they just left bodies on top of the ground. Today this place is known to the Indians as Ghost Coulee ... The Indians always used "The time the flour burned" for a counting date; that was around 1882.' Peigan elder Alan Pard explained that the yellow substance in the flour was believed to be sulphur: 'There was also lye in the meat, also bluestone in the meat.' Bluestone, also called blue vitriol, is a salt chiefly used as an insecticide or fungicide. 'My grandfather says it was sulphur in the flour. The people's bellies were distended.' Rations at the Blood reserve were also contaminated. A Blood elder explained: 'The food was treated with a kind of chemical. The Indians believed it was a poisonous substance. The meat discoloured with the use of this substance. This substance was mixed with flour, with this the people began to have stomach troubles, they called this "belly sickness." The people who died from this food poisoning were all buried at the Belly Butte site.' Blood elder George First Rider agreed: 'The meat was treated with some kind of chemical. Shortly after it would turn blue and would not be eatable. Those were the days when the people were dying off. Bodies were hauled out of the camps at a high rate and carried to the burial grounds. During the time of the issuing of rations, many people got sick and very many died ... That was the first time we were poisoned by the Queen and government. Those people were just about all wiped out by the first ration.'[109] It is impossible to know how the meat and flour nations became contaminated, although oral history tends to view it as a deliberate act. Chemicals added to the meat and flour may have been an attempt to preserve the rations, or this may have been an attempt to salvage already spoiled food. In any case, it is clear from elders' testimony that the people understood that they had been poisoned. Methodist missionary John Maclean was besieged with requests for food for the sick and dying. The nights resounded with beating drums and singing and with women wailing at the loss of their children and friends.[110] The women were in rags, forced to fight over old cotton flour sacks to make clothing for themselves and their children. Agent Cecil Denny reported dangerous levels of dissatisfaction.[111] That winter, among 2,270 at the Blood reserve, 50 children and 77 adults died while only 36 children were born – a death rate of 55.9 deaths per thousand.

The flour delivered to the Blackfoot and Sarcee reserves in 1883 was also substandard and was thought to have caused the deaths of thirty-five to forty people. Crowfoot's former favourable opinion of department officials began to erode as he watched his people weaken. When he complained to the department inspector, Thomas Page Wadsworth, about the flour rations, his concerns were dismissed as attempts to 'show off' his continued strong leadership. Death rates at the Blackfoot and Stoney reserves were 28 per thousand and 31 per thousand respectively.[112] Crowfoot must have been haunted by the warning he received the night before he agreed to sign Treaty Seven, when he sought out the council of a wise old man: 'Your life henceforth will be different from what it has been. Buffalo makes our body strong. What you eat from this money will put you buried all over these hills. You will be tied down, won't wander the plains, whites will take our land and fill it ... That's why I say don't sign. But my life is old, hence, sign if you want to.'[113] The old man's prophecy was painfully accurate. Once the people of Treaty Seven

TABLE 1.9
Blackfoot Reserve, 1884–1894: Birth and Death Rates

	Total pop.	Births	Rate per 1000	Total deaths	Rate per 1000	Child deaths	Child deaths as % of births
1884	2166	71	32.7	61	28.1	36	50.7
1885	2147	20	9.3	48	22.3	29	145
1886	2046	19	9.2	27	13.1	15	78.9
1887	1952	43	22.0	50	25.6	28	65.1
1888	1816	39	21.4	51	28.0	22	56.4
1889	1827	74	40.5	36	19.7	14	18.9
1890	1646	73	44.3	56	34.0	28	38.3
1891	1538	47	30.5	86	55.9	38	80.8
1892	1319	52	39.4	68	51.5	26	50
1893	1318	52	39.4	44	33.3	23	44.2
1894	1251	43	34.3	83	66.3	52	120

Source: NA, RG 10, vols. 9417–27, Annuity Paylists, 1884–94.

TABLE 1.10
Blackfoot Reserve, 1884–1894: Population Distribution

	Total pop.	Men	Women	Boys	Girls	Other relatives*
1884	2166	293	599	693	579	2
1885	2147	305	605	693	543	1
1886	2046	302	597	644	503	–
1887	1952	298	584	580	489	1
1888	1816	284	544	542	446	–
1889	1827	272	536	550	463	–
1890	1646	283	476	482	405	–
1891	1538	317	535	371	315	–
1892	1319	296	442	332	253	–
1893	1318	300	438	337	243	–
1894	1251	299	416	317	219	–
Change 1884–94**	−42.2%	+2.0%	−30.5%	−54.2%	−62.2%	–

Source: NA, RG 10, vols. 9417–27, Annuity Paylists, 1884–94.
*'Other relatives' were generally parents and grandparents of the family head receiving annuities.
**Percentage change between the 1884 figures and the 1894 figures.

had settled on their reserves they faced the same horrible living conditions as other plains peoples (see tables 1.9 and 1.10). Prolonged hunger, torn lodges, ragged clothes, and inadequate and contaminated rations provided an ideal environment for disease. Then a new infectious disease, erysipelas, caught hold and soon reached proportions that were described as epidemic by agent and former policeman William Pocklington. The presence of erysipelas indicates a dangerously infective environment. This disease is caused by the same type-A streptococci that cause scarlet fever and puerperal fever ('childbed fever.') Overcrowding and bacteria-laden dirt floors create ideal conditions for the disease to spread. The initial symptoms are a sore throat and coughing (which spray the germs into the air); these are followed by fever, chills, and reddish eruptions on the skin, which can spread infection to open wounds or to the reproductive tracts of women in labour. A description of erysipelas from the nineteenth century suggests its serious nature. Shortly after the appearance of a blemish on the skin, 'flesh [may] drop from [the] limb, or the whole member present the disgusting spectacle of a livid mass of putrefaction.'[114] At the same time, many other people were dying of a 'dangerous fever' that the government doctor seemed unable to diagnose or treat, but was likely associated with erysipelas. Death claimed many middle-aged and elderly people. Of 2,178 people on the reserve, 25 adults and 36 children died while 74 children were born.[115] The Winter Count, an Aboriginal method used to distinguish the most remarkable events of the year, noted for 1885, *ekorpipastsimasin*, or erysipelas.[116]

West of the Blackfoot, the Stoney people settled in the foothills of the Rockies. They were Assiniboine, survivors of the 1837 smallpox epidemic, who fled through forbidden Blackfoot territory making for Windigo Head, a promontory jutting out of the Rockies near what was to become Morley.[117] The Stoney who signed Treaty Seven – Bearspaw, Chiniki, and Jacob Goodstoney – assumed they would have separate reserves. But at the treaty negotiations, John McDougall, a Methodist missionary and interpreter (who spoke Cree, not Stoney), apparently indicated that all the bands would settle near Morley, where his mission was located. Elders state that Morley was only a wintering site and that they hunted and lived in the mountains, and that McDougall had his own interests in mind. John McDougall's father George had started the Methodist mission in 1873; after his death in 1876, John would continue his father's work for thirty more years. John saw himself as a great friend of the Aboriginal people, but the elders' evidence suggests that at Mor-

TABLE 1.11
Stoney Reserve, 1884–1894: Birth and Death Rates

	Total pop.	Births	Rate per 1000	Total deaths	Rate per 1000	Child deaths	Child deaths as % of births
1884	621	23	37.0	17	27.3	13	56.5
1885	642	28	43.6	9	14.0	4	14.2
1886	633	23	36.3	35	55.2	19	82.6
1887	614	26	42.3	64	104.2	40	153.8
1888	560	25	44.6	49	87.5	32	128
1889	585	13	22.2	32	54.7	18	138.4
1890	570	15	26.3	32	56.1	22	146.6
1891	424	22	51.8	18	42.4	13	59.1
1892	557	24	43.1	20	35.9	16	66.6
1893	573	23	40.1	19	33.2	14	60.8
1894	561	24	42.7	.32	57.0	24	100

Source: NA, RG 10, vols. 9417–27, Annuity Paylists, 1884–94.

TABLE 1.12
Stoney Reserve, 1884–1894: Population Distribution

	Total pop.	Men	Women	Boys	Girls	Other relatives*
1884	621	118	142	179	181	1
1885	642	127	150	189	176	–
1886	633	119	149	187	178	–
1887	614	114	137	178	185	–
1888	560	109	129	167	155	–
1889	585	109	138	176	162	2
1890	570	109	132	168	159	2
1891	424	92	105	120	102	5
1892	557	115	142	155	139	6
1893	573	120	147	153	148	5
1894	561	116	155	142	143	5
Change 1885–94**	−9.7%	−1.7%	+9.2%	−20.7%	−20.9%	–

Source: NA, RG 10, vols. 9417–27, Annuity Paylists, 1884–94.
*'Other relatives' were generally parents and grandparents of the family head receiving annuities.
**Percentage change between the 1884 figures and the 1894 figures.

ley he acted in his own interests as missionary, government agent, and land owner.[118] The Stoney were the first to feel the pinch of Vankough- net's 1883 cutbacks. They received the cattle promised in the treaty only in 1880, and their land in the foothills was not conducive to agriculture because of killing frosts in both spring and fall. As early as 1883, it was being recommended that no more attempts at farming be made. When they were told they would no longer receive any government rations, they had little choice but to continue to hunt and trap.[119] Predictably, after a season without rations and a failed hunt, sickness increased. In the winter of 1885–86, measles broke out on the reserve, with especially high mortality among the children and the elderly. As with whooping cough, influenza, and tuberculosis, the severity of measles is directly linked to the state of the patient's environment, and especially to nutri- tion. Measles is a highly communicable virus spread mainly through droplet infection. Closed and crowded living conditions greatly increase the likelihood of contracting it. The complications that lead to death are a result of viral replication or secondary bacterial infections such as pneumonia, diarrhoea, and encephalitis. Among malnourished chil- dren in the developing world, the fatality rate can be more than 10 per cent.[120] Agent William deBalinhard claimed that the Stoney people suf- fered a 3 per cent loss due to measles in 1886, but their death rate for that year was 104.2 per thousand, or 10.5 per cent of the population (Tables 1.11 and 1.12). Especially among the children, the death rate was very high for the next three years – 153 per cent of live births in 1887, 128 per cent in 1888, and 138 per cent in 1889. Agent deBalin- hard admitted there was a large loss of life and added that everything possible was being done for the people, but he assumed that the high death rate was the result of the people leaving the house where a death had taken place and moving into lodges: 'It has been observed that the Stonies have always seemed to have less power of resistance to attacks of sickness of every kind ... although no satisfactory explanation of this unfortunate peculiarity has been discovered.'[121] Fresh beef was issued to relieve some of the misery. A doctor from Calgary visited monthly and found that many of the people also suffered from consumption, which had caused the death of Chief Jacob Goodstoney in 1885.

By the winter of 1886–7, measles had spread to the Blackfoot people. The previous autumn, Reed had instructed that rations of beef and flour be cut back because the people had grown their own potatoes. And beef and flour rations had always been reduced in winter, even though that is when they were needed most, because there was little work to do and it was therefore difficult to work for rations. For example, the beef ration was nearly 40 per cent lower in January 1886 than in May, when spring farm work began.[122] By February, agent Magnus Begg was reporting that 'a good many had died amongst the youngest ones.' The people charged that the cuts in rations were killing the children, but according to Begg, 'of course that has nothing to do with children having measles, but Indians do not look at it in that light.'[123] He was relieved, however, when he was authorized to increase flour rations for the spring work.

The relationship between hunger, destitution, and disease remained constant throughout the Native communities of the plains. But the destructive results of the government's policy of treading the middle ground between provoking violent reaction by hungry people on the one hand, and keeping treaty and relief supplies at an absolute minimum to forestall pauperism on the other, were most evident on the Treaty Seven reserves. Events between 1883 and 1894 on the Treaty Seven reserves unfolded somewhat differently than on the other prairie reserves. Certainly, some things were the same. Departmental cutbacks meant fewer farm instructors and a cut in rations. Clothing shortages left the people vulnerable to exposure. There was a housing shortage, which was especially acute among the Blackfoot because of the great distance from any usable timber for building materials. And as with other plains people, complaints were made that items promised in the treaty had not been delivered. But at the same time, there were plans afoot by influential friends of the government to develop a prime cattle ranching industry in the area. The presence of the NWMP and five reserves in the region assured the nascent cattle industry of both security for their herds and a ready market.[124] So attempts were made to keep the people of Treaty Seven more content and less likely to cause trouble for the cattle ranchers. Doing so would also to ease the way for the transcontinental railway that was running through their territory.

Between 1884 and 1887, the people of Treaty Seven received more rations and supplies than the Treaty Four and Treaty Six people combined. In 1884, for example, the yearly per capita expenditure in Treaty Four for rations and supplies for the destitute was $11.26, and in Treaty Six it was $7.49; but in Treaty Seven it was $53.53. By 1886 the expenditure for Treaty Four had risen to $11.99, in Treaty Six to $15.62, and in Treaty Seven to $61.08. The discrepancies cannot be accounted for by price differentials, because the beef and flour in Treaty Seven, purchased from the I.G. Baker company in Montana, actually cost less per pound than the bacon and flour purchased from the Hudson's Bay Company in Treaties Four and Six.[125] However, agricultural progress in Treaty Seven may have been slower, and as a result ration expenditures may have been much higher than in the other treaty areas.[126] Nevertheless, in the years 1884–8, the Treaty Seven people received between 50 and 70 per cent of the total expenditures for supplies and rations, even though their population never exceeded 35 per cent of the total population.

This is not to suggest that the Treaty Seven people lived in any sort of government-sponsored affluence, for the department continued to practise the strictest economy regarding Native people. The per diem ration in Treaty Seven was still considerably less than Dr Kittson's estimate for minimum rations.[127] But the department judged it unwise to reduce expenditures in Treaty Seven by cutting rations and supplies, as was done in the other prairie treaties. According to William Pocklington, 'it has afforded me much pleasure to find that [a cut in rations] is not the present intention of the Department; if it were, very serious trouble would be the result, as these Indians are a powerful tribe, rich in horses, with many warriors well armed, and a large supply of ammunition.'[128] The higher levels of rations and relief were reflected in the Blackfoot birth and death rates. At the Battleford reserves between 1884 and 1890, there was not one year when the birth rate exceeded the death rate (Table 1.5). At the Blackfoot reserve, the birth rate was higher than the death rate in 1884, 1889, and 1890 (Table 1.9). Perhaps more significant, at the Blackfoot reserve the child death rate exceeded the birth rate in only one year, 1885 (Table 1.9). In contrast, at Battleford the child death rate exceeded the birth rate every year with the exception of 1890 (Table 1.5). The File Hills and Crooked Lakes reserves in Treaty Four experienced roughly the same ratio of child deaths to births as the Battleford reserves (Tables 1.1 and 1.3). The relative political strength of the Treaty Seven people, on their reserves in the heart of a growing cattle industry with intimate links to government, provided the people with better chances of surviving the first years of government administration.

Nevertheless, the department had to control costs, and at the Treaty Seven reserves it did so by reducing the number of people receiving annuities and rations. People were simply struck off the treaty paylist. Between 1881 and 1883 the number of Native people receiving annuities was reduced by 21.8 per cent.[129] Of course, there may have been losses due to an excess of deaths over births. But if the average birth

and death rates prevailing in the next five years are applied to the
1881–3 period, the population loss would have been in the order of
thirty-six people, or 1.3 per cent.[130] The interpreter to the Blackfoot,
Jean L'Heureux, was given a salary increase of $15.00 for his work in
helping the government reduce the numbers receiving payments and
rations, and thus saving the government 'thousands of dollars.' People
were also struck off the lists on the Blood reserve in 1882 and 1883,
until in 1884 agent Pocklington advised that it would be unwise to
reduce the numbers further or there would be trouble. Reed admitted
that most of the population losses were accounted for by the department's policy of striking names off the paylists. He claimed that people
had fraudulently received payment for relatives who never existed.
According to him, it was not until agencies were subdivided and the
people came under closer scrutiny that the department discovered the
practice. When questioned, the people would say that the relative had
died or was on the plains.[131] The department, then, struck many names
off the paylists. Oral history supports the charge of 'trickery' at payment time: 'George Manshot's father ... was called "Accounted With."
Those women would ask the mother of that baby, "Let me count you as
my own." So they just changed his clothes and claimed treaty money for
him.'[132] This charge of fraudulently receiving payments was also suggested by instructor Jefferson in Treaty Six. But Jefferson indicated that
the suspected fraud ended in about 1881, when the people were settled
on reserves and in frequent contact with instructors.[133] It is difficult to
ascertain the truth of the matter because in the early years of the treaties the paylists only recorded the chief's name – all others were simply
entered as 'Indian.' Nevertheless, it seems clear that while there were
negotiations over who was entitled to annuities, ultimately the department had the last say.

By the 1890s, rations and expenditures in Treaty Seven had been
reduced. The railway and the cattle industry were more secure. As well,
the people had been given a vivid reminder in 1885 of the strength of
the Canadian government. Despite the relatively better conditions, the
people of the Blackfoot and Stoney reserves were becoming weaker and
weaker. Dr Neville Lindsay of Calgary listed in order of importance the
most prevalent diseases affecting the people: scrofula, phthisis (tuberculosis), sore eyes (trachoma), syphilis, rheumatism, and pneumonia. He
noted that 'poverty induces scrofula and numerous diseases resulting in
death.' The doctor prescribed cod liver oil, syrup of iodine iron, and
maltine 'together with plenty of nutritious food, comfortable clothing,

physical labour or exercise in the open air in good weather, and roomy dwellings for winter, well ventilated.'[134] That prescription was unfortunately beyond the reach of most of the people.

Yet another ugly incident on the ration house steps indicated the extent of the people's frustration. In early April 1895, ration issuer and one-time NWMP corporal Frank Skynner, known as 'Owls Eyes,' was shot and killed on the South Blackfoot reserve by Ajawana, who was later killed by the NWMP.[135] Earlier that day, Ajawana had approached Skynner at the ration house requesting food for his sick son. The boy, renamed Ellis when he entered the Rev. John Tims's Anglican boarding school at Old Sun's camp, had just been released from school because of open scrofula sores on his neck. The sores – tuberculosis with abscess of the cervical lymph glands – had become a disturbingly familiar sight at the school. Ajawana threatened Skynner's life if his son died. When the boy died, Ajawana made good on his promise. The other employees were not at all surprised to learn of Skynner's fate, for he had been threatened on a number of occasions. The elders had requested Skynner's removal two years earlier. They had also requested the removal of the dictatorial and inflexible Tims, who refused to allow children to leave Old Sun's school for short holidays even when future good relations with the people might have suggested he do so. According to Skynner's fellow employees, he was 'thoroughly unqualified' for his position. He had made a practice of cutting rations to those who were ill, and he gave the old people their rations in bones instead of beef. After Skynner assaulted Little Calf's wife, pregnant women feared they would be injured in the ration house. R.G. MacDonell, a local trader among the Blackfoot, stated that Ajawana had asked him for work because the department's practice of paying wages in rations instead of cash was not right. At Reed's suggestion that Ajawana was insane, MacDonell stated that there was no stronger proof of Ajawana's sanity than his refusal to work under such conditions. According to the farmer on the reserve, Ajawana was not insane, and the direct cause of Skynner's murder was Skynner's own practice of refusing rations to sick people. The Skynner incident suggests how department policies were actually applied by some local employees, although most department employees showed genuine concern for the welfare of the people they served. It also indicates high levels of stress and dissatisfaction with reserve conditions. Privately, Reed confided to the assistant commissioner that if the man was not crazy, 'it would suggest the existence of a state of feeling between the wards and employees of the Department which would be most deplorable, and point to something radically wrong about their mutual relations.'[136]

Relations between the government and the people were indeed deplorable, and were unlikely to improve. In its rush to make treaties with Native people and prepare the west for agricultural and economic development, the government had not foreseen the enormous costs that it would be incurring.[137] Annuity payments increased yearly after 1875 as more and more people joined the treaties and settled on reserves. Moreover, relief payments for rations and clothing continued to climb as the severity of the economic crisis became clear. Each year between 1882 and 1887, the department's appropriation had to be supplemented. For example, in 1883 the department exceeded its original appropriation by 63 per cent; in 1884 by 40 per cent; in 1885 by 66 per cent; in 1886 by 151 per cent, and in 1887 by 49 per cent. Clearly, when the department promised 'the Queen's generosity,' it had little idea what it would mean to make good on the promise. By 1888, the department's appropriations were closer in line with its spending. Throughout the period, the costs for relief alone were close to or exceeded $500,000 annually.[138] Even so, the 'Queen's kindness' was never enough to prevent hunger, disease, and death. Confrontations between desperate young men and frightened employees were a direct result of the conditions on reserves, and the violence was aimed at the real site of government power on the reserves – the ration house.

The department was underfunded because the House of Commons (and the Canadian public) balked at the rising costs of administering the west. The government was bound legally and by common humanity to aid the people. Yet a segment of opinion (not limited to the Liberal opposition in the House) worried that aid would create a class of permanent paupers. David Mills, former superintendent of Indian Affairs in the Mackenzie government, charged that the government had turned the Native people into 'pensioners upon the Public Treasury' who were fed and clothed by the government and 'are doing little or nothing for themselves.' Macdonald's Conservative government had committed itself to providing relief, yet was determined to provide as little as possible. The moral reformism of the age held that the poor – and by extension Native people generally – were to be treated with a firm hand to help them avoid pauperism and to cultivate habits of industry and self-reliance. In answer to Mills's charge, Macdonald replied that matters of famine relief were handled by Commissioner Dewdney, but when the people were starving they were helped because 'we cannot allow them to die for want of food.' He went on to assure the House that Dewdney and the agents 'are doing all they can, by refusing food until the Indians are on the verge of starvation, to reduce the expense.'[139]

The economic disaster on the prairies in the first years of the treaties was ultimately the result of the rapid destruction of the bison herds. But the hunger/disease nexus that was thereby created cannot be explained by arguing that the government acted in good faith but was overwhelmed by circumstances. That the treaties were land surrenders was rarely discussed; instead, Aboriginal people were led to believe that the treaties were expressions of good faith on both sides. Yet the government had already determined the political status of the people as wards of the government in the Indian Act, which was revised in 1880 and amended as the need arose. It was only in the years after the treaties were signed that the people learned of its existence. What they had agreed to in the treaties was that they would allow settlers to share the land in return for an enduring relationship with the government and aid to begin farming. Speaker after speaker at treaty discussions asked the commissioners whether they understood the depth of the commitment. Morris had replied in 1876, 'We cannot foresee these things [calamities], and all I can promise you is that you will be treated kindly, and that in extraordinary circumstances you must trust to the generosity of the Queen.'[140] Aboriginal people might be excused for thinking that they were in the midst of 'extraordinary circumstances' in the 1880s, but the government's response was limited by its desire to force its understanding of the treaties. Violence on the ration house steps was a reaction to the much greater assault on the health and vitality of communities – the daily humiliations, and the agony of watching yet another child slowly die. The erosion of health on reserves would continue for many years. Insidious poverty replaced the earlier turbulence as chronic diseases became entrenched. But Aboriginal people were not without their own inspiration and strength. The women 'set to work with a will that impressed everybody.'[141] The wisdom of the ages, the spiritual connections to the land, and the knowledge and experience of the healers survived. Dreams still counted.

Chapter Two

'Help Me Manitou': Medicine and Healing in Plains Cultures

Years ago my first born was sick. I tried many medicines and gave away many horses but he was no better. Then one night I dreamed that I was to make a Sun Dance. When I awoke I promised Manitou (the Creator) that I would make one next summer. That morning it seemed as though the boy improved and by next morning he [was] definitely better.

Fine Day, 1934.[1]

The medical/healing complex of plains Aboriginal peoples functioned within a world view that saw the world and its inhabitants as part of a Great Circle of Life. The Creator was aided by the Grandfather Spirits of Fire, Thunder, Wind, Sun, and Water, as well as the animal and plant Spirits. People exist within this context as worthy creatures, but no more worthy than any other being. To live a secure, healthy life was to acknowledge and respect the spiritual as well as the physical world, because there was little distinction between the two. Medical therapeutics in plains cultures recognized that illness was a manifestation of the body and spirit searching for harmony or balance. The healer's art was to seek out the cause and provide treatment to restore the patient to equilibrium. Depending on the diagnosis, treatments ranged from the application of herbs and roots, to spiritual intervention, to community-wide ritual and ceremony. Throughout the process healers, like wise doctors everywhere, trusted in the body's natural inclination to recover from all illnesses, save one. This viable and culturally appropriate medical/healing complex was not abandoned when the people settled on reserves. Indeed, the experience and wisdom of the herbalist and midwife were generously shared with the non-Native immigrant community

struggling to survive on the prairies. The people's healing complex continued to change and adapt to altered circumstances and evolving needs
despite the best efforts of missionaries, physicians, and the government
to discredit healers and repress their practice.

Past medical therapeutics are most often judged by modern assess-
ments of their effectiveness: Did they work according to our understanding of science and medicine? Therapeutics that are considered
effective are retained; the rest are ignored as quaintly outdated or
offered as evidence of medical progress. But therapeutics are much
more than chemical formulae and responses. Therapeutics imply a relationship between healer and patient – a relationship that must be
viewed within a particular cultural context. Therapeutics 'involves emo-
tions and personal relationships and incorporates all of those cultural
factors which determine belief, identity and status ... Individuals
become sick, demand care, and reassurance, and are treated by designated healers. Both physician and patient must share a common framework of explanation.'[2] If illness could be sent by a malevolent shaman,
then it was imperative to have a healer who could both understand and
treat the condition. Herbal remedies, sweat lodges, spirit helpers, and
dances 'worked' as therapies because patient and healer shared a sense
of how the body functioned and what caused illness. That therapies may
be judged ineffective in another time and place does not limit their significance. For instance, today's cancer patients share their physician's
faith in science to such a degree that they willingly undergo near fatal
doses of chemotherapy that are for a time much worse than the disease.
Therapeutics are culturally relative and must be studied within the
framework of explanations, relationships, and world view.

At the risk of crude oversimplification, the Cree and Assiniboine and
the Blackfoot people (Blackfoot proper, Blood, and Peigan) shared a
world view or spirituality that positioned humans as but one part of the
Great Circle of Life, which they shared with the spirits of the animate
and inanimate alike. Indeed, according to some a blade of grass might
be more worthy to communicate with the Great Spirit or Creator
because unlike people it had done no wrong.[3] Animals and plants were
available for people to use, but respect for their spirits, through gift or
ceremony, had to be shown or they simply would not make themselves
available. For example, it was necessary to place tobacco where medicinal plants grew if they were expected to have the power to cure. Such
spiritualism was the stuff of everyday life and ensured individual well-
being. Fasting, prayer, and daily ablutions in rivers or streams were com-

mon practices that ensured good health.[4] Just as important was the well-
being of the collective. Illness was not necessarily a private matter, but
a misfortune that often involved the entire community and required
a community-wide response. The collective required ceremony and
prayer to confirm its strength and vitality. The soaring disease and death
rates of the reserve period did not shatter this world view. The healer's
remedies and the well-being that flowed from the sacred ceremonies
continued to make medical and spiritual sense, even if the people's economic and political lives no longer did.

The English word 'medicine' is often used by North American
Aboriginal peoples to refer to objects and people involved in healing
and magico-religious ceremonies. It is not a perfect translation. In Cree,
for example, there are two terms that refer to healers. *Mamaxtawiyiuu* is
translated as 'medicine man' and denotes a supernatural gift for healing
that cannot be taught; while *maskikiwiyiuu* is translated as 'herb doctor'
and refers to knowledge that is handed down from generation to generation.[5] There were also midwife-healers who may or may not have used
spirit helpers. Non-Native therapeutics tend to be concerned almost
exclusively with the individual physical treatment of illness. In plains
Aboriginal cultures, treatment of minor and common ailments might
follow that model. However, another level of therapeutics that might be
better termed in English as religious or spiritual in nature, also held significant regenerative and healing power.

The ceremonial life of the plains peoples – the songs, dances, bundles, and sacred rites – is a subject so complex that the most learned
elders may spend a lifetime understanding it. There was no priest class
in plains cultures, and almost anyone could experience the supernatural through dreams. But certain individuals had much stronger spiritual
connections than others. This ability to communicate with the spiritual
world – to divine the location of bison herds or the enemy, or to seek a
cure for illness – was a valuable community asset. In the post-treaty
period when neither the bison nor the enemy held much importance,
the spiritualist's gifts were turned to other things. In what may have
been an adaptation to the smallpox epidemics and later the high mortality rates on the reserves, most of the rites and dances performed by
the Blackfoot and Cree were used to aid the sick.[6] Many of the ceremonial dances begin with an individual making a vow or pledge, very often
to seek a cure for the illness of a loved one. The noted Blood holy
woman Mrs Rides At The Door made her first vow in the 1940s when
her daughter was very ill in hospital: 'I was there with her, and the

nurses said that she was dead. They started to cover her, but my old mother and I wouldn't let them. Instead we began to doctor her in our Indian way, and we revived her. The nurses were Catholic nuns, and they just stood and watched. If one of them had revived my daughter's life in that way, I think they would have written about it in the newspapers.'[7]

The Plains Cree pledge to make a dance, while the Blackfoot pledge to buy a bundle or medicine pipe. A bundle is a sacred object comprising a pipe and skins, feathers, or bones that represent powerful spirits. To buy a bundle is to learn and perform (or have performed) the dances and songs that accompany it. Considerable preparation and expense is involved in taking a bundle or making a vow, and it is never undertaken lightly. At one time the payment for a pipe bundle was horses and blankets; by the 1930s automobiles were acceptable payment. The owner of the bundle is expected to take special care of it, putting it outside in the morning before sunrise and taking it inside before dark. Rose Ayoungman explained that if there is sickness one vows, 'If I get better I'll take a certain pipe.' She quickly learned the need to follow protocol as a pipe owner when she inadvertently caused days of rain by washing the blanket that covered the pipe.[8] The Sun Dance, or Thirst Dance among the Cree, attracted the attention of non-Aboriginal observers because of its size and duration, but many other ceremonies and rituals were used in curing and healing. For instance, the Shaking Tent ceremony, variously practised by the Blackfoot, Assiniboine, and Cree, invoked the power of the spirit world through a clairvoyant to aid the living in any number of ways, from divining the location of enemies to diagnosing illness.[9] The Blackfoot, Assiniboine, and Cree ceremonies all observed a strict protocol and an exacting attention to detail. Although prayer, fasting, and songs and ritual characterized all sacred plains ceremonies, the rites were not performed only to maintain spiritual well-being: very tangible results were expected and often realized. It was this aspect of the healing complex that was most misunderstood and regularly dismissed by non-Aboriginal observers. Plains ceremonials did not pray for salvation in the next life; instead, they enlisted the direction and aid of the spirit world to control and influence *this* life.

The ability to heal began with a vision quest, which was common among many North American Native peoples, often as a part of the puberty ritual. Removed from society for a period of time to fast and pray and receive a vision, the young person might acquire a guardian spirit, in Cree a *pawakan*. The vision quest held significant risk, both from the elements and from the spirit world; this was especially true among the Blackfoot, with their notion of Night People or 'ghosts.' In earlier times the young person would consult the spiritualists in camp, who would perform the Ghost Dance and thereby protect the novice from the Night People.[10] The vision quest was intended to test strength and fortitude. Poundmaker's deputy Fine Day, a noted healer, once stared at the sun for four days. Although many might embark on a vision quest, not all became healers; only those with particularly strong powers because of the good results were called on to invoke their spirit helpers in aid of others. The ultimate blessing that could be granted in a vision was the ability to cure. Healers were as often women as men, but women generally learned of their spirit helper in dreams rather than vision quests; and among the Blackfoot at least, the dream would recur four times. For example, the spirit helper might pronounce: 'I will have compassion upon you, my son. Your request shall be granted. I will endow you with abundant wisdom. You shall be a great doctor among your people. Many ponies and much property will come your way.'[11] Spirit helpers were often in animal form, such as the bear spirit or the horse spirit, but they could also be in the form of the thunder or stone spirits. Healers were instructed by their spirit helpers in the songs, ritual, and construction of the curing bundles. The bundles usually contained a sucking tube, sharp blades for bleeding, bags of plant material, and objects such as the skins of the animal spirits that aided the healer.[12] The spirit helper did not protect against all eventualities, but only in specific circumstances, and the new-found ability to heal was not announced until needed. At present far fewer spiritual healers are practising, but the ability and power to heal is still readily recognized. Blood elders maintain that 'in our community we never doubt when someone is going into healing that the person is gifted and has supernatural powers from a spirit entity.'[13]

When a person fell ill, relatives sent gifts of clothing or (in earlier times) horses to the healer to be offered as sacrifices to the spirit helpers who had bestowed their power.[14] If the gifts were accepted, the healer went to the patient. The healer publicly made a pipe offering, called upon the spirit helper, asserted his right to undertake the cure, and reminded the spirits that they must keep their promises. The songs given by the spirit helpers were sung, and a whistle might appear and disappear, further establishing the healer's connection with the supernatural. Singing was performed throughout the healing process (the Blackfoot also pounded drums). Healers also might blow on the patient or suck out the cause of illness. The intrusive object was shown to the spectators while the healer explained how a malevolent shaman had sent the object out of resentment or jealousy. Healers also administered herbal medicines, which were kept wrapped in small packets and stored in an animal hide. Medical treatments, learned through practical experience, were used together with the shamanistic procedures of singing, sucking, and blowing. At times a number of healers would assemble and 'doctor' a patient in succession.[15] For each patient there could be only one illness that ended fatally, and the healer's task was to assure the patient, family, and friends that the present illness was not the one. Accounts of supernatural curing are rare because healers claimed that to reveal the source of spirit power would be to weaken it. At times even family members were excluded from knowing. The following account, prepared by a non-Native, suggests how the process may have unfolded.

In the 1890s Walter McClintock, one of many Americans who hoped to record Aboriginal ways before they disappeared, was allowed to spend time with the Montana branch of the Blackfoot. Mad Wolf, the Blackfoot leader, 'adopted' McClintock and gave him a Blackfoot name, which was a fairly common strategy. Mad Wolf may have been hoping that McClintock would act as an advocate for the Blackfoot, besides recording their way of life.[16] McClintock was permitted to observe and photograph a healing ritual. Stuyimi had been ill for some time, weak and emaciated and growing worse. McClintock states that Awunna was the healer and his wife Ekitowaki the assistant; however, the two worked together using different spirit helpers. They removed Stuyimi's clothes to the waist. Ekitowaki began to brew herbs from her medicine pouch, and while purifying herself with incense, beseeched the bison spirit to help her find the source of the disease. Her fingers danced over Stuyimi's body until she announced that the illness was in his chest. She prayed: 'Hear us, Great Spirit in the Sun! Pity us and help us! Listen and grant us life! Look down in pity on this sick man! Grant us power to drive out the Evil Spirit and give him health!' Awunna (and McClintock) chanted and drummed while Ekitowaki produced a small patch of bison hide and danced in imitation of the bison. She placed the patch on a hot stone and then placed it on Stuyimi's chest while sprinkling herbal tonic on the stones. She repeated this, applying three stones to his chest and three more on his back. Awunna then knelt and, beating on his medicine drum, chanted his eagle prayer. He blew yellow paint through his medicine whistle over Stuyimi's body and with an eagle wing imitated an eagle's flight.[17] No two healers performed the same rites, since they used the medicines, dances, and songs they had received from their spirit helpers. The healers then left their patient to prepare for the Sun Dance that was about to begin. Stuyimi's fate was not recorded.

Peigan elders continue to enlist the aid of spirit helpers to cure, even though this sort of supernatural healing is not as widely used as it once was. A group of elders will gather to build a sweat lodge to cleanse the soul and spirit for divination and to pray for cures. A sweat lodge is a small hut made of willow saplings bent to form a dome and covered with robes or pine boughs. Inside it, sweetgrass is burned, tobacco is offered, and water is sprinkled on hot stones to create steam. Prayers rise up with the steam. Sweat lodges are also constructed for their therapeutic value to treat specific ills. Herbs and roots such as sage and vetch, when sprinkled on the stones create a healing steam. The heat also releases the active ingredients in the willow saplings and pine boughs to create a soothing mist that is especially beneficial for respiratory problems. Very recently, a group of Peigan elders were asked to make a medicine pipe sweat for a non-Native man who was suffering from cancer. The elders did not know the patient, but the protocol of non-refusal when approached for help left them with no choice but to perform the sweat. Although he was too ill to attend, the elders performed the sweat and prayed for the recovery of the sick man. The following day the patient telephoned the elders to announce that he was declared healthy and cancer-free. The Creator had heard their prayer. Not all ceremonies go as smoothly. In the 1940s a Peigan healer was asked to attend an elderly man who was mortally ill. In the dying man's lodge the healer began his song to invoke the aid of the spirit helper, the squirrel. He tossed the squirrel hide on the man's bed. The animal hide had to come to life for the cure to succeed. Just as he released the skin, a dog burst into the lodge, leapt over the dying man, snatched the hide, and ran off. Unfortunately the patient died. This story serves to remind everyone of the limits of human control.[18]

As members of a relatively small society, healers had personal knowledge of the patient's medical history, family history, and vices and virtues. Trust and a personal relationship would naturally build between patient and healer. Today some healers are trusted more than others, and older healers are often seen as more experienced or knowledgeable than younger ones. An Assiniboine elder maintains that 'if I need to go to a medicine man ... the one I always go to is —— because he could blow that whistle – not whistle, that bone, eagle bone. And he could see right inside you like an X-ray, and he'll know what's wrong.'[19] However, when presented with a dangerously ill patient, the healer might announce that the patient's transgression was so serious that the spirit helpers were powerless, or that the malevolent influences had been allowed to work for too long. Family and friends left with the certain knowledge that all had been done that could be done: the patient or the disease, not the therapy, was at fault. Despite the apparent failure, the community's faith in both the healer and the therapeutics was strengthened. [20]

After death the souls of the Plains Cree travel the Milky Way and then on to the Green Grass World, where all souls live together in freedom. Blackfoot souls travel eastward to the Sand Hills, a dry alkali area on the plains. The bodies are prepared for the afterlife dressed in their finest clothes. The Cree interred their dead in a five-foot-deep grave lined with robes, and in winter the corpse was placed on a raised platform in a large tree. The Blackfoot wrapped the body in robes and secured the corpse to a tree platform with a leather thong. During the smallpox epidemics whole villages were abandoned with the dead inside their lodges. Understandably, these 'ghost villages' held particular terror for the Blackfoot, and for anyone else who came upon them. Sometimes a lodge was erected on a hill with the corpse reclining against a willow backrest. Burial sites might become rather crowded with backrests and burial lodges. In 1927, to celebrate the fiftieth anniversary of the signing of Treaty Seven, a monument and dedication ceremony was planned at Blackfoot Crossing. So as not to offend the sensibilities of the distinguished guests, agent George Gooderham planned to 'clean up' the area, which had long been used as a burial site. When no one on the reserve would take part in the destruction of the sacred site, a non-Aboriginal man, William Parker from Cluny, was hired to bulldoze the area. Grave houses and mortuary relics were shoved over the cliff and burned.[21] Such was the legacy of the first fifty years of the treaty.

Mourning was often a protracted affair, and women were expected to mourn longer than men. Relatives of the deceased unbound their hair, walked barefoot, and cut gashes in their forearms and legs to make their mourning public and unmistakable. At one time women would cut off the end of a finger, but in the reserve period the people understood that this custom was against the law and might result in jail or a fine.[22] The lodge or house where a death occurred was abandoned and often burned, which may have been a practical adaptation to the smallpox epidemics of the eighteenth and nineteenth centuries. Ghosts of the deceased might visit the house, thus forcing the family to make a long journey to help them forget their loss. This practice was severely curtailed by the restrictions on travel imposed by the government. The Cree offered a four-day mourning period; after this, a feast was held, during which a braid was cut from the deceased and placed in the 'Carried on the Back Bundle,' which became a sacred family possession.[23] But as Fine Day explained, 'The priests are putting a stop to this custom by cutting short the hair of the children so that we can't make up a braid.'[24] When a very close relative died (i.e., a parent or child), the survivors cropped their hair very short. Assaults on the people's customs were incessant and often had cruel consequences. Schoolchildren, their heads shaved when enrolled, cried themselves to sleep in the belief that their parents had died.

Of all the curing ceremonies, the most demanding to pledge and therefore the most likely to bring successful results was the Cree Thirst Dance, or Blackfoot Sun Dance.[25] The pledge or vow was made during a time of extreme duress, often to seek a cure for illness or to offer thanks for a cure received. The Cree conducted the Thirst Dance to enhance their relationships with the cosmic forces and their own *pawakan* or spirit helper. The core idea behind the Thirst Dance was regeneration to ensure abundant food and good health. Because of the demands made on the sponsor, the pledge was never made lightly, and other options were tried first. When his son was very ill, Cree healer Fine Day stepped out of his lodge: 'I stretched my arms up. "Now, Manitou my father, you have given the sun dance lodge for people to pray to you that all will be well. I am afraid of losing my son. But I will put up a sun dance lodge when it is convenient for you ... So help me Manitou to finish this sun dance that I am promising" ... My boy began to get better.'[26] Fine Day vowed eight Thirst Dances in his lifetime. The Thirst Dance sponsor either had his own songs or induced a ritualist to conduct the ceremony. The dance took place in an enlarged lodge; the centre pole was brought ceremoniously into the camp. The altar was erected on the north side of the lodge. Dancing, fasting, and prayers lasted for several days or up to two weeks. Cloth and smoke offerings were made, and acts of self-torture – piercing the breast or severing a finger – were inflicted. For government officials, this self-sacrifice was the most repugnant aspect of the dance, and they attempted to legislate it away. It was seen, inaccurately, as a barbaric torture test intended to 'make braves.' Actually, the self-mortification was intended to show sacrifice of oneself to the

Creator, the ultimate gift. On the final day of the ceremony a general gift exchange took place, which lent prestige to the sponsor and allowed for the redistribution of wealth.[27]

The Blackfoot, Blood, and Peigan celebrated the Sun Dance. The many age-graded societies met to dance and renew their bonds with one another. Positions in the societies were bought and sold, medicine bundles were transferred, and songs, rituals, and rites were learned. Women joined in their *ma'toki* society. Those who had made a vow or pledge during the year, for the return of health perhaps, provided a feast of saskatoon berry soup for the *ma'toki*.[28] Membership fees included horses, guns, and other property. The Sun Dance itself was pledged by a virtuous woman, often when a member of her family was dangerously ill. She raised her eyes to the sun and called upon it that health might be restored: 'I will officiate and put up a Sun Dance lodge next summer as a request to the Divine Powers for a quick recovery from illness of my relative.'[29] She offered gifts to the sun, such as cloth and tools. When the illness passed, these were hung in trees or deposited on a hill. Perhaps she also vowed to be the medicine woman at the next Sun Dance; this was literally a vow to purchase a *natoas* bundle and perform its ritual. After a four-day fast and the ceremonial cutting and raising of the centre pole for the Sun Dance lodge, ceremonial bison tongues (or cattle tongues in later years) were cut and chosen by women who had vowed to openly declare their virtue. Holy Fox Woman was a renowned Peigan healer and bundle owner in the nineteenth century. Her holy headdress or bundle spoke to her, telling her that if she ate meat from cattle she would die. Later in life she took part in a Sun Dance ceremony at which beef tongues had been substituted for bison; after unwittingly eating the beef, she immediately began haemorrhaging and died on the spot.[30] The power of the sacred was thus demonstrated for all to see.

Specific herbal or botanical cures were sometimes received in dreams or visions by individuals and later entered therapeutic practice. A Blackfoot woman, Last Calf, was suffering terribly from the hacking cough of tuberculosis. She and her husband were camped near a beaver lodge when she noticed tracks and left food for the beaver family. The beaver appeared to her in a vision and returned her kindness by giving her a cure for tuberculosis. She was instructed to boil the pitch of the lodge-pole pine in water and drink the infusion while singing a special song. Over the vigorous protests of her husband, Last Calf drank the infusion, which made her violently ill. She vomited profusely and felt she would die, but the following morning her chest was clear. Thereafter, the infusion was widely used to treat tubercular cough.[31] More often, people learned about botanicals and their preparation from older members of the community. Assiniboine healer Mrs Walker was raised by her grandparents Four Eagle Woman and Chief Take the Coat, who had taken treaty in 1877 and originally selected reserve land at Cypress Hills; five years later, however, they were forced to move to southern Saskatchewan. Her grandparents taught her about medicinal roots and plants.[32] It was not enough for a healer to know which plants treated which ailments. Healers also had to learn which season a plant or root should be harvested, how to prepare it, how the medicine should be administered (decoction, infusion, poultice, or by ingestion), how it should be stored, and how it was to be mixed. Some plant materials had to be collected in a precise manner to preserve the active ingredients. After harvesting roots and plants for healing, a gift of tobacco was left at the site in order to show respect.[33] Cree elder Abbie Burnstick recalled that there was much to learn to become an effective healer: 'It's a big lesson. You have to learn which ones are mated together. Like ratroot [wild ginger], it goes with another plant to make a medicine. Sometimes, you need a whole bunch of things to put together to make one medicine.'[34]

While specialized knowledge was required for healing, there were also medicines – spring tonics, for instance – that most community members would collect and administer for themselves. For example, an infusion of wild onion and horsemint, or Oswego tea (*monarda*), was taken as an emetic. Saskatoon berry juice, an infusion of the phlox plant, and Rocky Mountain maple were all used as cathartics.[35] As a general spring tonic, children were given a brew made from rushes. A powerful diuretic was made from the stems of the horsetail rush (*Equisetum arvense*). Herbal tonics collected in the wild are still very much a part of everyday life. Assiniboine elders speak of using the sweet-tasting cambium layer of white poplar trees: 'You cut ... like a U this way and you lift it up ... to get rid of your bile. You ... peel that and you hold it up and you see all that juice in there ... and you take – you get rid of all the bile that's in you that you can't get rid of when you're taking pills or something. I always do that. We always call it ice cream trees, because they're sweet and they're juicy. Let's go and eat ice cream juice we'd say.' Sage is still used regularly as a tonic and 'blood purifier.' For yarrow, 'each of the flowers all ready set for a human person. And they're in branches, so you can take a branch ... and it's good for you. The hockey players use that – and they eat that – and they keep it in their mouth, they drink the juice in the middle of the game, and they don't feel tired. They just play right through.'[36]

Clearly, the plains medical/healing complex functioned on a number of levels from the purely physical to the sublimely spiritual. It reflected a world-view that was remarkably well adapted to prairie existence, and it sought to make the physical and spiritual worlds both knowable and predictable. Not every illness had a spiritual component or required spiritual intervention. Nosebleeds and backache were treated in a perfunctory manner, with medicines and techniques that were widely available and passed down from parent to child. More serious illness was treated using the full spectrum of therapeutic approaches depending on the diagnosis. The sheer tenacity of plains medical therapeutics suggests that it 'worked'; and it continues to work for those who share the system of belief that body, mind, and environment must be brought into harmony.[37]

Christian missionaries were the most vehement advocates for repressing ceremonial dancing and the 'medicine man' because they recognized, as the secular officials perhaps did not, the clear link between healing and faith. Indeed, the missionaries, especially the medical missionaries in Treaty Seven, were attempting to establish an identical (Christian) paradigm. The people prayed to the Creator and spirits for good health, and put their faith in the therapeutics of the healer; the missionaries hoped to substitute prayers to the Trinity, faith in the next world, and bottled emetics and cathartics. John MacLean, a Methodist missionary on the Blood reserve in the 1880s, quickly discovered that the people shared with the Native healer an understanding of the body and disease that was completely foreign to his own. He watched a healer pierce a sick child's arm with a sharp flint, extract a small amount of blood, and then wash the child with warm water: 'I told the father that it was wrong and would do no good ... The mother and other members of the family were quite sincere in all they did, thinking it was for the good of the sick child.'[38] Missionaries had been living among Native people since before the settlement period, but with the advent of reserves, police, and the Indian Act, they found themselves more influential than ever before. As representatives of the various Christian faiths, they were interested mainly in saving the people's souls from everlasting perdition. Their aggressive struggle for souls, both with Native healers and with other denominations, suggests that they were sincere in their desire to bring the people to the light of true Christian salvation. For instance, the Catholic Oblate order alleged that Native cultures and traditions harboured Satan and had to be eradicated. There could be no other way.[39] In their efforts to win the people from the spell of the medicine man, missionaries focused initially on what they presumed was the source of his power – the Sun and Thirst Dances.

The terrible conditions in the early reserve period gave impetus to the dances and added to the burden of overworked healers. At the same time, officials of the Department of Indian Affairs had little desire to disrupt the people's dances. In 1884 Indian commissioner Edgar Dewdney was attempting to control the plains peoples and was unwilling to create new conflict by forcefully repressing the dances, at least not yet. 'I have never known any trouble brought about by the holding of [the Sun Dance],' Dewdney advised, 'I am in hopes that the ceremony will gradually die out; and it will be better to allow it to do so, without using strong measures to prevent its celebration as many of the old Indians, who generally inaugurate the dance, attach great importance to it.'[40] But the Anglican and Catholic missionaries in Treaty Seven advocated the use of police to stop the dances. Father Albert Lacombe demanded that the department stamp out the great obstacle to his work: 'It is to be regretted that the government doesn't stop that demonstration altogether ... You are strong enough by your moral influence and your mounted police to make the Sun Dance die out.'[41] Reverend John Tims, dubbed 'Long Knife' by the Blackfoot, suggested that the department engage the police to 'protect' those people who chose not to attend.[42] Father Joseph Hugonnard of the Qu'Appelle school was one of the most persistent advocates of repression. In his view, arrest and punishment were the only means to completely root out dancing: 'Clemency in their eyes [is] a sign of weakness.'[43]

Initially the department proceeded with caution in its attempts to repress the Sun and Thirst Dances. There was no force of law behind their efforts. It was clear that the Sun and Thirst Dances were important and valued ceremonies, and the department feared that any use of force would lead to reprisals. Moreover, department officials hoped that the superiority of Christianity would in time become evident and that the people would allow the dances to die from neglect. In defence of the policy, one agent noted that Queen Victoria herself was purported to have said, in reference to the people of India, that the rites and ceremonies of indigenous people were not to be interfered with if their religion comforted them as hers comforted her, or until they got a better one.[44]

Moral suasion was not successful. The policy was ambiguous. Agents were given responsibility for repressing the ceremonies but were allowed to choose their own methods.[45] The power of the Sun Dance camp to renew the people's spiritual and temporal ties to their culture and one another was recognized by department officers in the field. They recognized as well that to use anything stronger than moral suasion was to invite conflict. So agents and inspectors regularly reassured their superiors that the present year's Sun Dance was sure to be the last. In 1885, agent William Pocklington on the Blood reserve reported that the Sun Dance, if left alone, 'will soon have ceased to be the great festival of the year.' Two years later he reported that the festival was losing its importance and 'a few years more will probably see the end of it.' In the winter of 1888–9 whooping cough and tuberculosis killed 148 Blood children and adults. Pocklington reported that the people had held a Sun Dance, but added that the dance was losing its importance. Agent Magnus Begg on the Blackfoot reserve reported that the most recent Sun Dance lacked candidates for the torture ceremony and that the people were losing interest in the ceremony 'and I should be glad if they were disgusted as it is an unmitigated nuisance, always occurring at the time they should be working at the crops. I am continually trying to get them to do away with it.' On the Assiniboine and File Hills reserves, the agents commented that the Sun Dance was quickly dying out and that the people were assuring him it was their last dance.[46] Agents were frustrated by the continued celebration of the dances despite all their efforts.

The stated rationale for repressing the dances was that they interfered with farm work and 'unsettled' the people. In truth, the Native people's special knowledge of healing, which they gained through visions and experience and passed on through the transfer of bundles at ceremonial dance camps, was being actively suppressed. That this repression came at a time when disease and premature death pervaded the reserves was not a coincidence. The clash of therapies, Aboriginal versus Euro-Canadian, was part of a wider struggle to divorce the people from their own culture and marry them to Christianity and the associated political economy of capitalism. The notion that healers were dangerous quacks who duped the people out of their possessions, and who succeeded only by the power of suggestion, and who probably hastened death, took root within this larger struggle and has enjoyed remarkable longevity.[47] The construction of the healer as quack and the dances as a barbaric waste of time served to justify repression of both. The department insisted that it was the people's customs and their preference for the medicine man that had led to their continuing misery, not their economic circumstances and the department's policy of repression. The inconsistency of the government's position was noted by Dr George Orton, medical officer of health for the Manitoba superintendency. He pointed out that the department and the missionaries had done everything possible to discourage and discredit the Native healers, 'who by experience in the use of vegetables and other remedies in the treatment of wounds and disease handed down from generation to generation doubtless have been the means of saving many lives and relieving much suffering.' Dr Orton was told that while it was never department policy to discourage Aboriginal healers, the missionaries could do as they wished.[48] Agents, pushed by department policy and the missionaries, resorted to increasingly oppressive measures to end ceremonial dancing. Although they had no legal power, they did have access to the real source of power on most reserves – rations. In the summer of 1890 at Poundmaker reserve, a Thirst Dance camp was broken up when the agent threatened to have the ringleaders arrested and the annuities stopped. The farm instructor was ordered to stop all rations. On the Ermineskin reserve in Treaty Six, agent Samuel B. Lucas reported that the Thirst Dance was shortened because 'the rations [were] greatly reduced, and in many cases cut off.'[49] People were presented with a stark choice: they could shed their culturally appropriate response to illness, or they could eat.

It was more than coincidence that the Sun Dance season, June or early July when the saskatoon berries were ripe, was followed by a general improvement in the people's health. Summer allowed the people to move out of crowded and stuffy log huts and into well-ventilated lodges. These lodges were now built of canvas rather than hide, but they were still practical and inexpensive and easily cleaned, and they were regularly moved to prevent the collection of debris. People could camp next to their fields and fresh water. Considering the nature of their diseases – tuberculosis, whooping cough, measles, and influenza – it is obvious that their health improved whenever their living conditions did. Summer provided easier access to the many varieties of berries and wild plants that grew on reserves, and clothing shortages were not as serious a problem in summer. A yearly cycle of illness quickly became apparent. Agents consistently reported that the people's health improved in late spring, remained good through the summer and fall, and then deteriorated in winter. For example, at the Blackfoot reserve in 1888 the people's health was good in summer and fall until January, when agent

Magnus Begg reported the 'usual colds.' By the beginning of March there was 'considerable sickness.' In May of the following year, Begg reported that the people's health was not good 'but will improve by moving around.' By June they had moved into lodges 'and I consider it a good thing, as it gives their houses a chance to get ventilated and they are the healthier for the moving around.'[50] Likewise at the Battleford reserve in March 1888, agent Peter Williams reported 'more deaths in this month than in any preceding month for the last year but most of them were men and women with old standing diseases.' The death rate in 1888 was 54.4 per thousand, and the birth rate 25.8 per thousand. Thirty-nine children died, while only thirty-six were born. By May there was 'little or no sickness,' and by June the health of the people was 'fairly good.' In the winter of 1889, whooping cough reappeared and forty-two children died while only forty-one were born.[51] Levels of stress were greater in winter because of clothing shortages and because rations were always reduced in winter. The log houses, small, overcrowded, and poorly ventilated, aided the spread of infection and ensured a good supply of victims.

Sun Dances, vowed in the midst of winter's death, disease, and hunger, were celebrated in the warmth of early summer. Healers promised good health, and sure enough, the people's health improved. The pageantry, drama, and opportunity to renew friendships were also a wonderful balm after another hungry winter. But the real significance of the dance was its power to renew the people's ties to one another and to the Creator. The living conditions on the reserves ensured high morbidity, and perhaps resulted in more Sun Dances being vowed. And those sacred vows, made in fear, had to be honoured. The agent at the Peigan reserve, resigned to the obvious, noted: 'It not infrequently happens that in cases of severe illness an Indian's relations will promise, in case of his recovery, a dance to the sun. This occurred last winter, and the sun dance [sic] just about to take place is the result.'[52] In the summer of 1888 at least five dances were reported across the prairies, and surely many covert or unreported dances.

Some winters were worse than others. In the winter of 1890, epidemic influenza – 'la grippe' as it was called – reached the prairies. It was a worldwide epidemic that foreshadowed the even deadlier 1918–19 epidemic. Influenza is a highly contagious viral disease characterized by sore throat, cough, chills, and fever. It is spread by droplet infection and usually appears in winter when people congregate in poorly ventilated buildings. The mortality from the 1890 epidemic was generally confined to the elderly and the very young. The most common cause of death in the 1890 epidemic was bacterial pneumonia; to avoid it, bed rest and good nutrition were necessary. Chief Piapot was desperate: 'I have lost 26 people by sickness, one of them my Headman whom I raised from a boy.' He pleaded with Dewdney for help 'to get beef for my sick.'[53] Agents across the prairies reported increased mortality from the epidemic. In Treaty Four at Touchwood Hills, influenza 'carried off many of the consumptive people.' At File Hills nearly everyone was affected and the agent treated the people himself with cod liver oil. At Duck Lake in Treaty Six the death rate from influenza was 115 per thousand. In January at Edmonton a sympathetic instructor named O'Donnell exceeded the maximum daily issue of beef and flour. He was admonished for it and told that a material reduction was necessary since the circumstances did not warrant the issue of rations. In Treaty Seven all the reserves were affected.[54] At Battleford there 'was scarcely a soul free from it.' The elderly were the most severely affected. Chief Mosquito died in January. Agent Peter Williams reported that although there had been a number of deaths, there was no need to call in the doctor because the deaths were caused by 'long standing disease.' But in February and March, when Williams feared that the cattle were also dying of influenza, a veterinary surgeon was promptly called. In the midst of the epidemic, in the severely cold and stormy March weather, Williams stopped the rations to a number of families at the Sweet Grass and Thunderchild reserves after they refused to send their children to school. He reported that the storehouses on those reserves had been broken into and that bacon, biscuits, and beef had been taken. The death rate on the Sweet Grass reserve that year was 88 deaths per thousand, and on Thunderchild's 46 per thousand.[55]

Influenza reduced the influence of certain recalcitrant chiefs and elders – by killing them. When ex-chief Beardy at Duck Lake died, Inspector Thomas Wadsworth noted that his death was 'hardly to be regretted, as he remained to the last a heathen, a strict observer of old-time heathen rites.' Ebenezer McColl of the Manitoba superintendency hoped that the deaths of prominent chiefs would destroy the influence of traditional 'pagan observances' and help the department to inculcate the people with the enlightened habits of civilization. Regardless, at least eight Sun or Thirst Dances were reported the following summer at the File Hills, Piapot, Moose Mountain, Battleford, Onion Lake, Blackfoot, Blood, and Peigan reserves. Many more dances may have been held without the department's knowledge.[56]

When neither moral suasion, nor disruption, nor intimidation dissuaded the people from dancing, the department turned to the force of law. In 1895 the Indian Act was amended by section 114, which made it illegal to give away money or goods at a festival or dance. As well, anyone who assisted in a celebration 'of which the wounding or mutilation of the dead or living body of any human being or animal forms a part or is a feature' was guilty of an indictable offence and liable to two to six months' imprisonment. In July 1896, Kahpeechapees of the Ochapowace reserve was sentenced to two months' hard labour for sponsoring a Thirst Dance. In his own defence, Kahpeechapees contended that it was a religious matter, and 'God himself had given him these rites with a view of saving his own soul.' For fear of reprisals, the police in Treaty Seven were unwilling to take such harsh measures. If the people agreed to discontinue the torture ceremony, the police were willing to allow the dances to continue. At Touchwood Hills the agent had the dance leader arrested for breach of peace, 'and I do not think that they will ever attempt to hold another in this agency.'[57] As if to suggest that legislation had actually put an end to the dances, deputy superintendent Hayter Reed gloated in 1896: 'The "medicine men," the guiders of thought and action and the inspirers of fear in all but the very boldest, had to be fought. To win Indians from such a thraldom, and to get them to disregard the influences of generations, required no small amount of courage and skill in management.'[58] Yet, resistance continued, along various avenues: petitions, judicial test cases, modification of the ceremonies, and covert ceremonies. Piapot was arrested and later deposed for sponsoring a Sun Dance. Ever the dissident, however, he died in late April 1902 on the very day the Order-in-Council was passed deposing him.[59] Dance houses were torn down and issued back to the people as firewood. The agent at the Moose Mountain reserve, intending to disrupt a dance, was firmly made to sit down and watch until the people were finished. Although he was not injured, he was made to understand that he had neither the right nor the power to stop the dances.[60]

In 1896, assistant commissioner Amédée Forget suggested that the dances were losing support in the Native communities. While aged medicine men continued to practice the Native religion, the 'industrious owners of good farms, herds of cattle and comfortable homes perceiving the unsettling influences of these ceremonies and their inconsistency with the teachings of the Christian faith which they have adopted, hold entirely aloof therefrom.' Acceptance of the tenets of Christianity and the new economic order was a reasonable accommodation to the changed realities. Yet resistance did continue. Agent Allan MacDonald at Crooked Lakes did not share Forget's optimism: 'Considering the amount of persuasion employed by the different denominations at work, as in this agency, paganism is dying hard.'[61] The continued efforts to undermine and ridicule the people's world view resulted in an ever-deepening suspicion of the government's motives. After 1885, once the ration policy and the pass and permit systems were in place, the smothering paternalism of the past took on a sharp edge. Robert Jefferson, farm instructor at Poundmaker's reserve, contended that his efforts to enforce departmental policy regarding the Thirst Dance through ridicule, pity, and disgust only undermined any trust that might have grown up between himself and Poundmaker's people.[62]

The government did not formally legislate against Aboriginal medicine, but there was a consistent informal policy to repress and undermine Native healers. Elders consistently assert that it was department policy to fine or jail healers. Assiniboine elders recall that shortly after the people signed the Treaties, 'they were told to throw away the herbs and healing roots ... They were afraid that if they got caught they would go to jail or get a $500 fine.' However, the reserve's healers and midwives continued to practice covertly.[63] In his memoirs, agent and later commissioner William Graham recalled that 'every effort was made by those who were in charge of Indians to discourage most of the methods used by the Medicine Man, but it took time to do this.'[64] Despite the commissioner's wishful thinking, healers continued to practise, but they did so under very real threats. Assiniboine elders recall that 'the old medicine men used to gather here [at the reserve].' As late as the 1950s a healer treated a woman for gallstones: 'He gave her a drink and then he performed his ceremonies and then he said she will either throw it up or pee it out. And she peed it out. And they knew in Fort Qu'Appelle Indian hospital that she had gallstones. But when the ambulance finally did come out for her she had got rid of all her stones. And when she went over there, they wanted to know what had happened, because she didn't have any more. And they wanted to know who doctored her. And [the healer] said don't tell, because at that time they could have jailed him for that.'[65]

By the early twentieth century, officials' perceptions of the people's healing rites had changed: those rites were no longer demonstrations of savagery and indolence, but rather manifestations of the people's disregard for human health. It was realized by that time that tuberculosis was a contagious disease with the capacity to spread from reserves to towns;

this discovery offered new opportunities for the department to interfere with the dances. According to deputy superintendent Frank Pedley in 1907, one of the greatest threats to health was 'the practice of continual dancing, which stirs up the dust which the promiscuous expectoration of the affected has charged with germs, and at the same time stimulates respiration.' Pedley also referred to the longstanding departmental perception that people's ill-health was the result of 'ignorance of nursing, inattention to the directions of medical advisors ... defective preparation of food and premature marriages.'[66] These perceptions were thus made to fit the new imperative, which was to stop the dancing. Once seen as a threat to the peaceful acquisition of the prairies for settlement, the plains people had come to be seen as a disease menace to the burgeoning settler society.

Despite ongoing repression, disruption, and arrests, the dances continued. They were adapted to changed circumstances, but their healing power remained. In the 1930s at the Crooked Lakes reserves, a modified form of the Sun Dance was still being held each year.[67] The complex world-view of the prairie Native peoples, with the Creator at the centre and the deities of the Sun, the Moon, and natural phenomena, was not abandoned in favour of Christianity in the face of disease and oppression, as some have contended.[68] Fine Day told anthropologist David Mandelbaum in 1934 that the spirits continued to have relevance. The North Wind, *atayohkau.kiwetin*, was the strongest and most powerful. 'He is looking after us every day and that is the one we breathe. You drive with the wind every day – he is in your [car] tires.'[69] But plains Aboriginal people were forced to develop an ideology of resistance and accommodation: resistance to assimilation, and at the same time accommodation to changed economic and political realities.[70] Meanwhile they combated their own dehumanization by continuing to hold their ceremonies. Religious syncretism was often the result. For example, in 1885 missionary John Maclean on the Blood reserve was frustrated when he learned why the people refused to attend his Sunday services at Bull Back Fat's camp: 'The Catholic priest had held service early in the morning and the people said that they did not care to pray anymore today. I tried to urge them, but they had prayed to the sun and attended the popish service, so they would not come out.'[71] There was nothing inherently incompatible in the people attending Mass on their way home from Sun Dance camp. Perhaps adding to Maclean's frustration was his realization that no one could be certain whose god the people were directing their prayers to. Many years later, in the 1930s at

Crooked Lake, a Sun Dance included a brief interlude during which missionaries brought Aboriginal girls from the nearby school dressed in their school uniforms of 'blue shirts, brown stockings, brown sneakers, and faded middy blouses.' The singing and dancing of the Sun Dance stopped, and the spectators and dancers went outside, where the missionary Mr Ross conducted a service. The sermon was based on the Forty-Fifth Psalm, and the school girls sang 'Jesus Loves Me This I Know.' The Sun Dance then resumed. Asked if the interruption was resented by the people, the interpreter stated emphatically that it was not. Nevertheless, because of repression or cultural change, or both, some dances and ceremonies were no longer celebrated, while other dances gained popularity. The Thirst or Sun Dance was one that persisted, and was considered an 'active force' in Plains Cree life well into the 1930s.[72] It continues today on many prairie reserves.

The healing practices of the plains people were incompletely understood by those who administered their lives. What *was* understood was that the people needed to embrace Christianity and capitalism as quickly as possible. Healers, their spirit helpers, Native botanical knowledge, and the regenerative power of ceremonial dancing had no place in this new plains society. That the people were hungry and surrounded by disease was presented as proof that assimilation was necessary. As deputy superintendent Hayter Reed put it, the people were making the difficult transition from 'savagery to civilization.' Since civilization was not easily won, disease and death were a natural part of that process.[73] Nevertheless, the healers continued their work, and dances continued to be vowed, for the need for individual treatment and community regeneration was more urgent than ever.

An aspect of the plains people's medical/healing complex that has received little attention from either historians or department officials is the culture of childbirth and the role of the midwife. Perhaps because of the almost exclusive focus on death in Aboriginal communities, birth has gone relatively unnoticed. But the midwife-healer was a powerful figure in plains cultures, and an examination of her work adds a new dimension to our understanding of how Native life was lived. Also, it was through the services of Aboriginal midwives that immigrants were afforded a glimpse of the medical knowledge and experience of plains peoples.

Many women healers were also midwives to their communities. They were empirically trained, and some also received their ability to heal through communication with the spirit world. Children were brought into the world through the care and experience of the midwife and her helpers. The mother kneeled with her back against a chest-high support and was attended by three other women. The primary midwife stood behind the mother and supported her; another received the newborn and cut the umbilical cord; the third assisted the other two. To speed the birth of the placenta, hot water was placed under the woman as she knelt. The umbilical cord was cut 'at a point one hand grip and one thumb's breadth' from the abdomen. A light dressing made from the powdery centre of the prairie puffball (*Lycoperdon gemmatum batsch*) was applied to the infant's navel; this acted as a styptic.[74] Blackfoot elder Russell Wright explains the importance of the culture of childbirth: 'When a child was born, it was traditional for the midwife to cut the umbilical cord and the child's aunt or older sister would clean and dry it. Then she made a hide pouch in the form of a turtle or some other animal, beaded it, and sewed the cord inside. The child wore it for the first five years of life at special occasions when people gathered together. The pouch reminded people the child had many parents and everybody was responsible to help the child grow to become worthy to the tribe.'[75] (In later years, when more children were born in hospital, staff threw the cord away.) The newborn was placed in a soft leather bag stuffed with moss, which acted as an absorbent diaper. Then the child's parents prepared a feast and the naming ceremony began.

As with most cultural rites in Aboriginal communities, the naming of a newborn child was a public affair. Fine Day described a Cree naming ceremony:

> When a child is born its parents prepare food, get some cloth, fill a pipe, and call in an old man. Many people come to watch. They tell the old man what they want and give him the cloth and pipe. The old man lights the pipe then puts it down and talks to God and to the Spirit that taught him to give names. After he has talked he sings one song. Then he says 'Bring the baby here.' He takes the child in his arms and gives it the name and begs God to give it good luck so that it may grow up and become old. He asks the Spirit that gave him the power to give that name to be the guardian of that child. Then the child is passed around the people until it reaches its mother. The men and women, as they hold the child, express a wish for the baby.[76]

And so the life cycle began again. Despite the people's crushing poverty, the cycle never stopped. Lives were becoming shorter, and many who received names never lived to become old as was the wish, but those who did protected and celebrated the received wisdom. The naming ceremony reflected the people's world-view, which rested in the child's understanding that the group would provide, protect, and right wrongs. The collective was all; without one another, none could go on.

In their narratives, adventures and traders made note of childbirth among plains women, but their accounts tend to be distorted by economic, gender, and ethnocentric biases. The prevailing view was that Aboriginal women gave birth painlessly and without effort. Male observers had few opportunities to observe the process, and this must have influenced their conclusions. But accounts were also distorted by the fur trade itself. Women on long trading voyages far from the aid of a midwife had no choice but to make do either without help or with the help of only their husbands. In the early nineteenth century, trader Daniel Harmon noted that a Native woman in his travelling party walked all day through snow and water and in the evening gave birth to a son. The next day 'she continued her march, as though nothing unusual had occurred!'[77] Traders confused women's self-sufficiency in childbirth for painless childbirth, and their observations were distorted by the nature of their contact with plains women. Traders could not help but contrast the seeming self-sufficiency of Aboriginal women with the apparent frailty of non-Native women. The experience of Letitia Hargrave, who lived at York Factory in the mid-nineteenth century, offers a clear contrast between cultures of childbirth. At the birth of her first child, Hargrave was attended by a doctor, and she was thankful for his presence because she was completely inexperienced. The doctor even made the bed. As for the Native women, Hargrave noted that 'they never have a doctor, nor do they go to their bed, but sit on their knees.' Hargrave's Native companion encouraged her to move about during labour, and 'I will never forget the look of astonishment and incredulity that she stared at him [the doctor] when he congratulated me on my good behaviour. She must have thought him easily pleased.'[78]

There was no substitute for a capable midwife. Besides having experience and knowledge, she was a reassuring presence, especially for young women. Midwives often lived with the family for some time after the child was born to nurse both mother and child, and to perform the mother's work. Ellen Smallboy, a Cree woman from Moose Factory in the late nineteenth century, recalled that her husband's grandmother helped her prepare for the birth of her children by gathering moss in summertime. She also recalled that it was not always possible to have a midwife present and that her husband had to assist her in the birth of her fourth child. Alone with her husband, Simon, in the dead of winter, she instructed him to prepare boiling water and to tie and cut the umbilical cord. She assumed the kneeling position and pulled on a line looped around the pole of the lodge. Although Simon was careful and competent, she washed the baby herself.[79] Smallboy recalled her experience as an expression of her own competence and strength, much as non-Native pioneer women prided themselves on their strength and self-sufficiency after giving birth with the help of only a husband or older child.[80] Moreover, among Aboriginal women it was culturally inappropriate for them to mention that they were in labour until just before the birth. The cultural imperatives of self-reliance and non-interference with others prevented women from calling for the midwife until the last moment. They were expected to prepare in advance for the birth of their child and to retain their calm and composure in the face of distress.[81] It was considered improper to cry out or lose control. In this way, composure and self-reliance were mistaken for painless and effortless childbirth. Given the isolated nature of reserves and the kinds of work women did, it was not uncommon that a woman had to act as her own midwife. Elders who recall childbirth without attendants stress that they had no choice but to be strong. Mrs Blackbird of Ahtahkakoop's reserve in Treaty Six noted that when necessary, women were 'midwife to ourselves ... We would even simply go off into the bush, giving birth to the children there and then bringing them back from there ... We never used to lie down ... The children had no sooner been born when we were back to work; so long as we would have a support tied around here, around our abdomen, and at the same time we also drank medicine, Cree medicine.'[82] This account suggests that the process was neither painless nor effortless, and that plains women learned to control pain and ease postpartum recovery through abdominal girding and herbal tonics.

In the nineteenth century the presumption grew that Native people were savages, and this led traders and adventurers to distort the culture of childbirth. As studies of colonialism have shown, charges of barbarism were used to justify the theft of Aboriginal lands. Native women were represented as drudges and as mere chattel in their own cultures; Native men were represented as slothful and as forcing women to perform the most difficult tasks. And there was no clearer proof of Aboriginal savagery than the supposed indolence of men and their brutal treatment of women.[83] Daniel Harmon noted: 'All the Indians consider women as far inferior in every respect, to men; and, among many tribes, they treat their wives much as they do their dogs ... When they decamp, the women transport the baggage; and when they stop, while the men are quietly smoking their pipes, the women are required to pitch the tents, and to set the encampment in order.' It was perhaps a short step from this to representing plains women as neither needing nor wanting aid in childbirth. Harmon married a Cree woman, Elizabeth Duval, and eventually had fourteen children with her, although he never once mentioned her by name in his narrative.[84] Perhaps because of his personal relationship, Harmon conceded that the Cree shared responsibility and work between husband and wife: 'The husband shares the labour with his wife; and the women govern every thing in their tents, so that the husband presumes not to dispose of the most trifling article, without the consent of his wife.'[85] Perceptions of Native women were rooted in the contemporary views of women, and Native women's experience was noteworthy when it deviated from that norm. Harmon's account suggests that the sexual division of labour accorded more equality and autonomy to Native women than was enjoyed by their non-Native counterparts. The 'ideal' nineteenth-century woman was frail and idle, in sharp contrast to the self-sufficiency of Native women. The ethnocentric and class biases of male observers thus distorted the roles of Native women.[86] The perception of Native women as particularly at ease with childbirth was a more romantic view of Native women than the one that would follow. As conditions deteriorated on reserves in the late nineteenth century, Native people were increasingly seen as racially inferior. Small infant head size, not women's self-sufficiency, was touted as the reason for painless childbirth.[87] Small head size of course was seen as prime indicator of lower intelligence. In any case, the role of the midwife was discounted in this supposedly effortless process.

Settlement on reserves and increased European immigration did not diminish the role of the midwife. Assiniboine elders recall that Mrs Walker was a midwife and 'medicine woman' or healer. She was called upon to deliver babies on the reserve, including her own grandchildren. She was not the only midwife on the reserve, but throughout the time she practised she never lost a baby. In the 1930s she at times enlisted the aid of her daughter: 'I had to boil water and sterilized the scissors and string. I remember helping her deliver my sister's baby. I was very scared. I was scared that I would drop him ... When my mother helped women she would make them kneel down because she said the baby came faster. It was better than lying down. She had a special medicine for the mother.' As Mrs Walker aged, she developed arthritis in her fingers and feared she could no longer safely help women. Her half- sister took on the work. The culture of childbirth survived well into the reserve period, albeit with adaptations. Native midwives survived the arrival of Euro-Canadian doctors, and worked alongside their male counterparts, like other prairie midwives early in the century. Mrs Walker was called by families on the reserve to help with childbirth, but Dr Isman from the nearby village of Wolseley was also called: 'He would have to come from Wolseley by buggy and sometimes he couldn't come. She would go though. He told her to go.' Mrs Walker did not charge for her services 'but she was given things like material or blankets, but she never asked for anything.'[88]

On reserves where medical missionaries had established hospitals, Native midwives were seen as unwelcome competition. In 1893 the Oblate missionary on the Blood reserve in Treaty Seven, Father Emile Legal, secured department funds to build a cottage hospital staffed by the Catholic order Sisters of Charity. The fourteen-bed hospital was built near the mission school and was originally intended to serve the schoolchildren. Only reserve residents who had no one to care for them presented themselves at the hospital. In 1908 the department's medical officer, Dr Peter Bryce, admitted that the people rarely used the hospital.[89] In 1912, in an effort to create a relationship between the hospital (and doctor) and the people, the hospital began to accept maternity cases. But as agent Hyde explained, the Native midwives had all but cornered the practice: 'Maternity cases have been almost entirely attended to by the native Indian doctors who I must say have been remarkably successful in that class of patient, and in that way have proved quite a thorn in Dr. Edwards' side although everything is done to discourage the so-called Indian doctor in his work, which is pretty hard to do seeing we have no proper place to offer them to come to, but when such cases begin to come to the hospital they will have to be exceptionally successful to overcome this handicap and become popular with the Indians.'[90] The agent called for the Indian Act to be amended to force people into the hospital, and for all children to be born with a Euro-Canadian doctor present. He did not make clear just how the department was to enforce this, but in his opinion the 'Indian mid-wife' was the root of the problem.[91]

By 1923 admissions were beginning to increase at the hospital, for a number of reasons. First, the hospital was now allowing women to stay with their sick children, and children to stay with their sick mothers. Second, midwifery was on the decline generally in North America, for various economic, social, and political reasons.[92] Third, the churches and schools were gaining influence in Aboriginal communities, especially among ex-pupils. Fourth, the efforts (both formal and informal) of department officials to discredit, ridicule, and restrict midwives and Native medicine in general were having a deleterious effect on women's choices. An Assiniboine elder recalls that although a midwife helped with the births of her first children, after 1930 she went to hospital to have her children: 'Most women went to the hospital for their babies by then because there were no more midwives on the reserve.' She suggested that women wanted to have their babies 'in the new way.'[93]

The experience and special knowledge of Native midwives and healers was valued by immigrant and Native communities alike. Until the 1920s, immigrant women on homesteads were rarely attended in childbirth by a physician. Children were born at home, and were most often delivered by the father or a neighbourhood midwife. Even when a physician lived nearby, the fees were prohibitive. Moreover, male physicians were not necessarily seen as competent, and many women preferred the services of an experienced midwife. An early immigrant woman recalled that the doctor at Indian Head, Saskatchewan, was an elderly man and not particularly competent; he always worked with a midwife 'whom mother thought knew as much as he.' At Grenfell in southern Saskatchewan at the turn of the century there were three doctors: an 'army doctor and not patient with women; a deaf old doctor, and a good doctor who often drank too much.'[94] The services of an experienced midwife were invaluable on the prairies, and very often Aboriginal women were the only midwives in newly formed immigrant communities. They willingly shared their knowledge with the newcomers. Mrs McDougall, the 'second white woman in the foothills' and the wife of Methodist missionary David McDougall, recalled that her Native midwife, Mary Cecil, assisted her in the birth of her child in 1871. As McDougall put it, she was a servant and a friend.[95] A Cree woman, Mrs Bastien, cared for immigrants in the Rocanville district of Saskatchewan, acting as both doctor and midwife. According to one immigrant she was the 'nearest thing to an angel on earth.' And although the family brought a 'doctor book' of home remedies to the prairies, 'Mrs. Bastien was no doubt better.' Another settler in the same district recalled that a Native woman acted as a general nurse to the family and was called in to attend all of the family births.[96] Most homesteaders were young, with growing families, and were far from the reassuring presence of older, experienced women. Native women healers and midwives were a welcome and often a life-saving presence in immigrant communities on the prairies, and were seen as the most competent. Non-Native women did not want 'to go to the hospital because [they] knew Indians could deliver babies.' During the Great Depression of the 1930s, immigrant women engaged Aboriginal midwives when there was no money to pay for doctors and hospitals. An Assiniboine elder recalled that her mother and aunt were called to help a non-Native woman in labour, and that 'they were just as poor as we were.'[97]

Homesteaders also accessed Native healers' knowledge of the healing botanicals of the plains. One homesteader recalled that when his wife's baby sister was suffering from dysentery, the local doctor could not help her and they were afraid she would die. A Blackfoot woman 'brought in a bunch of white prairie flowers to steep into a tea and this cured it up promptly. I think the flowers were yarrow.' He also recalled that the Native people used the white berries of the red willow for a spring tonic and 'blood cleaner or purifier.'[98] Most early settlers relied on the old European spring tonic of sulphur and molasses, but some preferred the indigenous remedies. One such spring tonic was the sweet-tasting inner bark of the white poplar, the 'ice-cream tree,' which acted as a mild purgative.[99] Immigrants' recollections of Native women's knowledge of the plains pharmacopoeia stressed the practicality, the simplicity, and (most importantly) the effectiveness of their cures. Cuts on the foot from rusty wire or nails were a common occurrence, with serious complications if not treated. A poultice made from the broad leaf of the poplar was an effective treatment: 'It was good, also gentle, and cleaned the wound absolutely.' Settlers made their own Balm of Gilead just as the Native people did, by boiling poplar buds. One homesteader recalled that in her district there were two Native women 'who were wonderful when it came to illness,' and who brewed herbs for fever and colds, and mixed the prairie puff-ball fungus with lard to make a salve: 'It was a quick cure for impetigo and ringworm, etc.' A settler in the Baljennie district of Saskatchewan recalled, 'I once had a touch of lumbago and an Indian woman of the Cree nation told me to get some twigs of ground cedar [and] to boil them for half a day and then to drink the liquid. I did this and the lumbago cleared away.' Even physicians referred patients to Native treatments: 'I remember in cases of erysipelas the Doctor telling us that Indians used cranberry poultice and he found it very effective.'[100] The knowledge and experience of Native healers and midwives seems to have always been given as a gift, with no payment expected. As in Mrs Walker's case, goods might be received in payment, but they were never demanded.

Plant medicines were quickly 'discovered' by immigrants and became part of the capitalist economy. For example, seneca or senega root (*Polygala senega*) was intensively harvested by non-Native settlers. This root was used by the Woods Cree to treat toothache, and in powdered form was used in a mixture of many herbs to treat various ailments. An Assiniboine healer used it to treat sore eyes.[101] By the 1880s, immigrant families were rushing onto the prairie to harvest the root. While the men dug it out, the women and children pulled off the green tops and washed and dried the roots. Harvesters could earn from eight to ten dollars a day. James Clinskill, a merchant in Battleford who traded heavily in the root, noted that 'the work was surer pay, less labourious, and more profitable than washing gravel for gold.' Senega root was highly valued by the patent medicine industry as a powerful diuretic and expectorant, and had a slightly astringent flavour similar to wintergreen. According to Clinskill, so much root was harvested that it brought down the world's price. Clinskill had established himself in Battleford hoping to take advantage of the proposed northern railway route through the Battleford and Prince Albert districts. He served on the Territorial Council as member from Battleford in 1888–9, but he grew tired of waiting for the railway that never arrived and moved his store to Saskatoon in 1899. His firm alone shipped 10,000 pounds of senega root in one summer. But, he said, 'our [Battleford] Indians would not dig it or allow anyone to dig for it on the reserves' because they would not disturb a 'medicine plant.'[102]

Despite the prohibition by some groups, in Treaty Four by the 1890s women were collecting the root to sell at nearby immigrant villages. Agent Allan MacDonald at Crooked Lakes reckoned that senega root was the chief article produced for sale in 1894. Agent J.B. Lash at Muscowpetung's reserve reported that the people had earned a large amount of money gathering senega root, which should have been welcome news during 'a very bad year with a general depression and a crop failure.' But Lash worried that 'this work takes them off the reserves for weeks at a time, and keeps up the old habit of roaming the prairies.' Senega root continued to be a valuable resource and one of the few means for women to earn cash. The Assiniboine healer Mrs Walker used senega root in her practice, but she also 'would dig senega root and would sell it in Sintaluta to buy groceries.' The appropriate sacrifice of tobacco was left at the harvest site only when the plant was needed for medicine. Glecia Bear recalls that as a young mother she would fashion a swing in the trees to hold her baby while she dug senega root for ten cents a pound. She would spend the cash on food. Alpha Lafond recalled that she took along a lunch and would spend the whole day digging using special handmade sticks.[103] Harvesting senega root for cash is one example of the adaptations Native people made during the reserve period.

During the early reserve period, Native women forged vital links between the Aboriginal and settler communities, much like those formed during the fur trade era, between Native and newcomer.[104] Their knowledge and experience were welcomed by the immigrants, who were attempting to sink roots in a strange and often dangerous country. Immigrants had much more respect for reserve women than was shown by officials in the Department of Indian Affairs. Department officials perceived the home as the field where Euro-Canadians would win the battle between barbarism and civilization. And in their Victorian conception, the home was the exclusive purview of women. They resorted to the supposed indolence and carelessness of Native women to explain the high death rates and especially the high infant mortality in households on the reserves. As Hayter Reed explained in 1896, 'The mortality among the young is ... greatly due to the too early marriages on the part of the girls.' Reed also suggested that Native mothers lacked experience; for example, they allowed children 'after an attack of measles, too much freedom, resulting in cold, this being followed by fatal results.' Reed's comments also implied that there was a certain immorality or at least impropriety in allowing young girls to marry and become mothers. Children were seen to suffer in other ways at the hands of their mothers; because they experienced too much freedom at home, 'consequently, they grow up self-willed, stubborn, and easily provoked.'[105] Images of Native people as incompetent parents also served to justify sending children off to schools far from home.

Aboriginal women quickly adapted to the cash economy in the reserve period. Agents reported that besides caring for their own families and homes, and for their own livestock, crops, and gardens, Native women tanned hides to make moccasins and mitts to sell to immigrants. They also sewed beads, made baskets, and gathered wood, wild fruit, and senega root to sell at neighbouring villages. Many also worked as domestics for immigrant families.[106] The work women did was often the only source of cash for the family, yet negative images of Native women as unrestrained and lewd were used to try to keep them on reserves. Agent William S. Grant of the Assiniboine agency reported that 'they [women] are kept out of the small towns as much as possible.' Grant feared that women were frequenting the towns to prostitute themselves – a characterization that served to legitimize the restraints placed on reserve residents, especially after 1885.[107]

In the reserve period, the medical/healing complex continued to provide for the needs of the sick. The healer and midwife were kept busy despite efforts to suppress their work. Although the prairie settlers may not have shared the Aboriginal people's world-view, their medical knowledge was readily appreciated and gratefully received. (The immigrant community must have seemed particularly in need of harmony, arriving on the plains as they did with neither elders nor medicines.) Native people's search for well-being and harmony was made increasingly difficult by economic and political conditions on reserves. The persistence of their faith in ceremonial dancing and the medicine bundle suggests that they did not forsake their search, and that the therapeutic regime continued to make sense to them in a way that little else on the reserve did. But much was lost. As an Assiniboine elder sadly observed, her mother, who was a healer, did not teach anyone on the reserve how to prepare the roots and herbs: 'She kept it secret, she couldn't teach anyone. They took away our culture. The dances were important. The people were afraid to dance.'[108] Blood elders today suggest that the change from supernatural or spirit-inspired cures to primarily herb-based treatments occurred after the people signed the 'peace' treaty with the government. The forms of sickness had changed, so the treatments had to as well. Healers were no longer treating wounds from hunting and battle; instead, they were combating diseases induced by the living conditions on reserves. The people have assimilated Euro-Canadian medicine into their healing complex, but the use of sweat lodges, face-painting, smudges, and herbal 'brews' is still widespread and has been incorporated into the treatments offered at the recently opened Kainai Hospital.[109] Therapeutics have changed with the times.

Representations of Aboriginal people as indolent, dirty, and without regard for human life were constructed to serve a bureaucracy that perceived plains cultures as in need of fundamental change if they were to accept Christianity and capitalism. Culturally appropriate responses to illness – the healer and the dance – were actively suppressed to serve this end. The high death and disease rates that coincided with the establishment of the reserve system confirmed for officials that the Aboriginal people were likely a 'vanishing race.' The solution was rapid and complete assimilation. But it was clear that the 'tribal system' was not going to quietly disappear. So government and missionaries focused their attention and resources on the children, who once separated from their parents' world could be indoctrinated with Christianity and sent back to the reserves like Trojan horses to change them from within. If they made it home alive – and many did not – they often brought disease.

Chapter Three

'I Was in Darkness': Schools and Missions

Aboriginal people had pressed for education provisions in the treaties; specifically they wanted schools on the reserves. What they received was schools that reflected the paternalism of the 'white man's burden' – that were established to 'elevate' Aboriginal students and replace their world view with the tenets of Christian capitalism. The system would be financed largely by the federal government and administered by ecclesiastics. The government left the management of the schools to the religious orders because a number of schools in the west were already being run by various Christian denominations, and were considered successful. As well, it was thought that Christian education would provide Native people with the necessary moral instruction. Finally, missionary teachers would provide the right mix of enthusiasm and patience for the work, and would be cheaper to employ than qualified teachers.[1] Not coincidentally, as soon as schools were established the need arose for medical care for students. Cottage hospitals, little more than infirmaries for students, were seen as necessary if sick children were to remain at the schools. They were also designed to attract the parents to the schools, where they might learn to place their faith and trust in Christianity. The medical staff, usually the teachers themselves, were often women who were religious and who provided care for little more than the cost of their room and board. The Department of Indian Affairs attempted, unsuccessfully, to remain removed from the actual operating of the institutions; it preferred to grant funds to missionaries rather than involve itself directly. Denominational education and medical care were the norm in nineteenth-century Canada and not the purview of government, notwithstanding treaty obligations to provide schools and teachers, and 'medicine chests' at least to Treaty Six agencies. The real work of assimilation was left in the hands of the Christian churches, while the government ensured that at all times its expenses were foreseeable and limited. For the children, life at school was a struggle for survival that very many of them lost. The survivors rarely remember any good times at school; instead, their stories are a painful record of abuse, loneliness, and hard work.

The various Christian denominations were already established in the west when the treaties were signed. In the 1820s the Anglican Church Missionary Society and the Methodists were invited to Red River by the Hudson's Bay Company to teach the Aboriginal trappers the habits of industry and morality. Catholic missionaries, especially the Oblates, joined the Protestants in the west, and by the 1850s there were missions throughout the North-West. Often alone, with few resources, and vastly outnumbered, they set themselves the huge task of converting the Aboriginal people. At times their very survival depended on the Aboriginal people they had been sent to save. For instance, in the early 1860s Methodist missionary Thomas Woolsey was labouring alone with few resources among the Cree of Smoking Lake near Edmonton. Seriously ill with fever, convulsions, and a badly swollen throat, he was nursed back to health by the local Cree healer, who gave him a powder mixed with beef broth and applied a paste to his throat; this, even though the patient had 'a deep prejudice against all Indian medicines, a feeling that was shared with most white men.'[2] Through patience and perseverance, the missionaries were able to make friendships if not converts. Missionary influence among Native people had more to do with their status as 'holy people' than with the validity of their religious doctrine. Priests presented themselves to Native people as spiritual people deserving of respect, and they were generally accepted as such.[3] Oblate priests such as Fr Constantine Scollen and Fr Albert Lacombe, and Methodist John McDougall, were recruited by the government to influence and interpret in the treaty-making process, and they quickly became natural allies of the Department of Indian affairs in the shared goal of 'Christianizing' Aboriginal people. Missionaries were often vigorous critics of government policy, especially departmental parsimony, but they shared with the department the fundamental goal of assimilation, as well as the understanding that they knew what was best for Native people.

Throughout the world, education and ministering to the sick were hallmarks of missionary activity. Medical care was seen as an essential first step toward winning the people's trust, and perhaps their souls, and on the Canadian reserves there were plenty of opportunities to dispense medical treatment. In the 1880s, Methodist missionary John Maclean established himself on the Blood reserve at Blackfoot Old Woman's camp. Maclean was born in Scotland in 1851, arrived in Canada in 1873, and was ordained seven years later. The people would not come to him for medical treatment, so he patiently made rounds from lodge to lodge, seeking out the sick. The most frequent medical complaint heard by Maclean in the first month of 1885 was what he termed 'biliousness.'[4] The prevalence of stomach and bowel complaints was no doubt related to the poor quality of the rations. Maclean also gave out salves and carbolic washes for 'sores' – perhaps erysipelas, which was also prevalent on the Blackfoot reserve. Erysipelas is a skin infection caused by the same streptococci that produce scarlet fever. It is age-specific, with adults usually contracting erysipelas and children contracting scarlet fever. When left untreated, the condition is serious if it is secondary to some other wound or infection – especially puerperal sepsis (childbed fever). In early 1885, Maclean described a seriously ill man who had three rifle balls still in his leg from an earlier war with the Sioux. According to Maclean, although they could only communicate in sign language, 'he finally expressed his faith in God and hoped to meet me in the final abode of the just and pure.' Although his patient died the next day, Maclean was elated to have claimed a convert. Unfortunately for their patients, death did not necessarily spell failure for medical missionaries. But events soon overtook Maclean's small successes. He found that during the Riel Rebellion people were unwilling to have any missionary treat them. On 24 May 1885, Maclean confided in his diary that 'some of the Indians spoke strongly against the missionaries and argued that they were bad, as the Indians who favoured the Christian religion soon sickened and died.'[5] Most medical missionaries established themselves at schools, among the children, whose opinions were not so difficult to contend with.

In all likelihood, the Native leaders who negotiated the treaties had been hoping for schools that would teach students spoken and written English, to augment parental teachings. What they received was far different. Following the American experience in education for Aboriginal children, day schools were eschewed because parents remained too much a part of their children's lives. Industrial schools, where children were completely removed from the influence of parents and the community, were seen as far superior. Students were to receive a basic academic education as well as instruction in the trades. Three new industrial schools were opened in 1883–4 to augment the boarding schools already existing. The Catholic Oblate order managed the Qu'Appelle school at Lebret in Treaty Four and the Dunbow school in Treaty Seven, while the Anglicans opened the Battleford school in Treaty Six. The industrial schools were established off the reserves to sever the children's links to their culture, and enrolled children over fourteen years old. Boarding schools were usually located on or near reserves and catered to younger students, from eight to fourteen. Day schools on reserves were given much less financial support. Eventually, thirty-two residential schools (as they were later called) were established in Saskatchewan and Alberta. Catholic-run schools dominated, with twenty-one schools; the Protestant denominations established eleven. At first the industrial schools were financed completely by the government, but by 1892 they were deemed to be too expensive. A new funding arrangement was established whereby a grant was paid to each institution based on the number of students enrolled. All operating costs – food, clothing, salaries, heating costs, and so on – were to be paid from the grants. The funding arrangement shifted the burden of operating the schools onto the missionaries and ultimately the students, who soon began spending half-days in the classroom and half-days labouring in the fields and kitchens to support the school. Work, prayers, and harsh discipline defined the school experience.[6] Remembered one survivor: 'I went to Brandon [residential school]. I was so lonely. I did not know one word of English, just the Assiniboine language ... I couldn't talk in my language. Who could I talk to? I was in darkness. Outside, where they couldn't hear us I would talk Assiniboine with the Sioux children, it is very similar.'[7] The Blackfoot had no word for formal education or school and called it 'going to sit': 'When the old-time people visited with each other they would say, "He has gone to make his children sit," meaning some father went and enrolled his kids at the boarding school.'[8] This was clearly a misunderstanding that likely was based on the school recruiter's explanation of the experience. Children worked hard. 'I worked in the laundry when I got older – 15 or 16 years old. We washed sheets, pillow cases and towels, all the bedding. We worked all day. There was a big tub washer, a spinner and a dryer. Monday was wash day. Tuesday we folded and ironed everything. We only used dryers in wintertime. There was a big room with lines where the bedding dried. We worked in the kitchen too.' Alan Pard at the Peigan Sacred Heart residential school recalled that he was often slapped in the head by the nuns, and called 'Chien!' Only years later did he realize what they were saying to him.[9]

Medical care for schoolchildren was left to the missionaries. In 1885, Dr Maurice Seymour offered to supply medical attendance for the Qu'Appelle industrial school and surrounding reserves; Edgar Dewdney replied that medical services were unnecessary, since medicines had been sent to the school and the Roman Catholic nuns were expert in handling the sick. As well, the reserves were being supplied with medicines, and the agents had been instructed in their use.[10] Dewdney believed strongly that Native people should attain self-sufficiency as soon as possible. He reasoned that if they were freely provided with services that ought to be paid for, the people would become paupers and the road to self-sufficiency would only be made longer. Although Aboriginal communities might never advance to the level of non-Native Canadians, they could certainly become self-reliant, and then they could provide for their own medical needs. That they were attempting to do just that, but were constrained by the department, seems not to have occurred to Dewdney. Nevertheless, he insisted that the missionaries and schools could handle any medical care necessary.

The same desperate conditions found on the reserves – dirty, overcrowded living quarters, poor diet, inadequate clothing, and constant exposure to disease – prevailed at the schools. At the Qu'Appelle school in 1886, five children died of 'consumption' out of a total enrolment of fifty-five. The next year, three children died from consumption because, according to missionary Fr Hugonnard, they were admitted with 'weak constitutions.' Dr Seymour, who had finally secured an attending position over Dewdney's objections, visited the school twice a week, while insisting that the 103 children needed his services more often. Seymour worked for the department until 1904. In 1909 he became provincial commissioner of public health and in 1923 deputy minister. Seymour was instrumental in establishing a sanatorium in Saskatchewan after his son became ill with tuberculosis. In its first decade of operation, the Qu'Appelle school had enrolled 344 children; of these, 174 had been discharged because of either age or illness. Of those 174 students, more than half died either at the school or shortly after leaving – most of tuberculosis.[11] It had become common practice to discharge seriously ill children to their homes rather than have them die at the school. Ironically, this practice caused parents and relatives to seek out healers at the Sun and Thirst Dances. By 1902, of the 1,700 students discharged, 40 per cent were dead or in poor health.[12] At the Battleford school, of fifteen students enrolled in 1887, two died from 'brain fever,' or tubercular meningitis, and one, Chief Thunderchild's nephew, died from exposure when he chose escape and an eighteen-mile walk back to the reserve in the frigid cold rather than life at the school. The school principal, Rev. Thomas Clarke, noted that the children's health was 'excellent' but that the children did not remain ill very long, 'either recovering immediately from indisposition or almost as rapidly passing away. Consumption is the bete noir and nothing arrests their rapid dissolution when this fell disease has once seized them.'[13]

Upon enrolment, children were often given new 'Christian' and surnames that administrators could pronounce and spell. In 1886, when twelve-year-old Ochankuga'he was enrolled at Qu'Appelle, Fr Hugonnard suggested that there were 'no letters in the alphabet to spell this little heathen's name and no civilized tongue could pronounce it. "We are going to civilize him, so we will give him a civilized name."' He was renamed Dan Kennedy.[14] In May 1889 at Dunbow school, six-year-old 'Kate McGibbon' was examined by a visiting physician and diagnosed with scrofula (tubercular abscess of the cervical lymph nodes). Her painfully swollen neck was lanced and 'painted' with iodine, and she was given iodide of iron syrup three times a day. In June the dose was increased; in July it was increased again and coupled with regular doses of cod liver oil. On 9 August, Kate was admitted to the school's hospital, where she was given cod liver oil and treated with poultices for the ulcerating sores on her neck. By February 1890 a milk and meat diet was recommended. Cod liver oil and iodide of iron syrup was continued for the rest of the year. By January 1891, Kate McGibbon was dead. Unfortunately, Kate's short life was not unusual. 'Joseph Slattery,' age fourteen, was examined in December 1888 and diagnosed with ulceration of the eyes, but no prescription was noted. In March of the following year he was treated for pneumonia, but appeared to be recovering. By May there was consolidation of his lungs, and he was given a cough mixture and cod liver oil. In June he was diagnosed with bronchitis and given linseed and mustard poultices, but by October he still had not recovered. In December, his diagnosis was changed to consumption, and by January 1890 he was dead.[15] Dunbow, like many of the other schools, had a very poor health record. Farther north at the Stoney reserve, the principal of the McDougall orphanage (in fact a Methodist boarding school) reported matter-of-factly 'a great deal of sickness and death.' Government per capita grants were paid according to the number of students registered, and principals were regularly admonished when they failed to report promptly the death of students: 'I hear for the first time that no. 56 and no. 63 being absent without leave died at home.

These are matters which should be reported in due time ... no. 86 is dead and this should have been reported.'[16] Administrators had abandoned names entirely and referred to children by number alone.

Medical opinion was in agreement that poor diet, overcrowding, inadequate clothing, and exposure to disease were the chief causes of the high morbidity and mortality in the schools. Dr Seymour at the Qu'Appelle school reported that 'overcrowding and breathing vitiated air are the two best recognized causes [of tuberculosis].' Dr Neville Lindsay of Calgary agreed that the schools needed better ventilation. He also pointed out that the schools were unclean, the food was poor and inadequate, and the children's clothing and bedding needed to be replaced.[17] Parents were objecting to the poor conditions, harsh discipline, and overwork at the schools, and this was making it harder and harder to secure recruits; as a result, students were retained at the schools for as long as possible. When Tom Many Feathers at St Mary's school on the Blood reserve turned eighteen, he requested his discharge. His grandfather, Running Wolf, had agreed that Tom would attend school, but only for four years until he turned eighteen. But the principal, Fr Jacques Riou, understood that when Tom was discharged his younger brother would be sent to replace him. When Running Wolf refused to send another child to the school, Riou dispatched the police to Tom's home on the reserve to arrest him for desertion. To his grandfather's outrage, Tom was taken back to the school and put to work at 'hard labour' with no lessons. Agent R.N. Wilson suggested that given such an incident, 'it is not surprising that Indians prefer keeping their children within their own control.'[18] Per capita grant funding also meant that if healthy students could not be found, then ill students were admitted. And lagging enrolment meant that the institution's fixed costs had to be met by the labour of fewer children, who were fed less and were therefore that much more prone to illness. When parents sent a healthy child to school and that child was returned to them ill or dead, they were unlikely to perceive that the schools were in their remaining children's best interests, and this made it increasingly difficult for schools to recruit students. In 1895 the government, pressured by the missionaries, legislated compulsory school attendance.[19]

The burden was becoming onerous – not least to the children – but the educational policy and its funding system were fundamental to the department's efforts to Christianize and civilize. Explanations for the atrocious death rates at the schools were looked for elsewhere – for example, in the 'hereditary taint' of tuberculosis among Native people.

Dr S.E. Macadam at the Battleford school reiterated the argument that the chief cause of death was the rough transition from 'savagery to civilization.' The transition from the free outdoor life to confinement in the schoolhouse hastened the children's innate tendency to develop tuberculosis. Dr A.W. Allingham, who attended at the Round Lake school near Qu'Appelle, noted that the children were more susceptible to tuberculosis at school because their resistance was lowered through homesickness and worry.[20] Allingham went on to suggest that the practice of gathering together the 'pure and tainted' created new victims. Children should be examined by a medical doctor upon admission, and the schools disinfected periodically. Medical opinion notwithstanding, commissioner Hayter Reed concluded that the schools were clearly not responsible for the deaths of the students. The conditions on reserves were to blame: 'food, exposure to cold, dampness, scanty clothing, wet feet, etc. are more conducive to the generation of the disease.' The superior advantages of the schools were 'more than counter-balanced by the comparative loss of open air exercise which the children get so freely on the reserve.'[21] Efforts were made to improve ventilation and increase school production of vegetables and dairy products. But the department's frugal per capita grant system squeezed the churches to admit more and more pupils, feed them less, and keep windows sealed shut to reduce heating costs. Fundamental criticisms could not be countenanced because the mission-run schools were the expensive showcase of the department's efforts to Christianize and civilize.

Yet the very real health problems in the schools demanded some response. When missionaries expressed an interest in establishing hospitals in conjunction with the schools, they were actively encouraged by the department.[22] The connection between the schools and the mission hospitals was intimate by design. Children who became ill in school would not have to be sent home and could remain on the school rolls. Hospitals might also slow down the spread of disease in schools by isolating the very ill; and it was hoped that the civilizing mission of the hospital might touch the parents as well. The government provided buildings because the missionaries, with no clear title to the land, were unwilling to invest in the structures themselves. Building maintenance and rations – items that could be easily controlled – were also provided by the government. The mission hospitals typified the nineteenth-century notion of hospital as almshouse. They were directed by boards whose members would never have entered them for treatment, and existed to uplift and convert patients as much as to cure them. In 1893 at the Blood Reserve the Oblate missionary Fr Emile Legal received department funds to build a cottage hospital. These early buildings were more cottage than hospital, usually rough log structures with straw-filled mattresses. Legal undertook to supply the nursing staff, three Sisters of Charity who also taught at the school. According to department inspector Alex McGibbon, the fourteen-bed hospital was clean and comfortable. By the middle of its second year the hospital had admitted fifty-four patients, fourteen of whom died either at the hospital or shortly after discharge. McGibbon noted the poor record and explained that there were just too many serious cases of consumption, which had been admitted too late for proper treatment. The hospital's Sister Superior Eusebe conceded that on average they were treating only five patients at any one time, and that they were the poor (comparatively) who had no one to care for them. Until people were forced to seek hospital treatment, she continued, the situation was unlikely to change.[23]

To the north on the Blackfoot reserve, Anglican missionary John Tims began agitating for a hospital as soon as the Catholics were granted their hospital on the Blood reserve. John William Tims was born in England and trained in London at the Church Missionary Training College. In 1883, directly after being ordained, he was sent to the Blackfoot reserve, where he immediately squared off with the Catholics in the struggle for souls. When he attempted to set up a mission near the Catholics in Crowfoot's camp, Crowfoot refused to let him: 'Since one church had been built all the old men and women and children had died and if another Church was built, all would die. They had too much church.'[24] Tims built the mission at Old Sun's camp instead, and was joined in 1885 by Harry Gibbon Stocken, who had just arrived from England. Together they distributed medicines freely from a wooden medicine chest (containing medicine bottles and an eye dropper, hypodermic needle, knife, mortar and pestle, and needles and thread) that Tims had brought with him from England, even though they had only 'a modicum of instruction.' By 1888 Gibbon Stocken had moved west on his own to the Sarcee mission south of Calgary. He was clearly out of his depth when he attempted to treat a woman suffering from 'twitching.' Recalling a conversation he had had with a homeopathic doctor in England regarding the principle of 'like cures like,' Gibbon Stocken reasoned that since strychnine caused twitching, it might also cure it. He administered the strychnine tablets three times daily, and the woman recovered temporarily.[25] Deaths caused by treatment rather than disease often went unrecorded. Tims at the Blackfoot reserve was not content merely to dispense medicines. In 1894 he built a hospital in conjunction with Old Sun's boarding school.

The department agreed to supply the rations for the hospital provided Tims employed a nurse. Agent Magnus Begg reported that the one-storey, eight-bed hospital was the 'best building on the reserve.'[26] Nevertheless, three years later the hospital was still not open because the church could neither furnish the hospital nor provide the staff. The building's foundation was sinking, and the plaster was cracked and breaking. In the meantime, in 1895, Tims was driven from the reserve by the Blackfoot, who had come to despise him for his dogmatism and intransigence. The health record at Old Sun's school was particularly poor (and never did improve), and when Tims refused to release a very sick child to her parents he was threatened with death. Tims was reassigned to the Sarcee missions, while Gibbon Stocken returned to the Blackfoot mission. In February 1896, Gibbon Stocken and his wife decided to accept their first patient in the unfinished hospital, even though no trained staff were available. He later explained that a missionary rarely leaves training college without 'at least a moderate and practical knowledge of medicine.' They nursed their tubercular patient for six weeks before he died, but 'his Christian deathbed was a source of much pleasure.'[27] In early 1897 the department furnished a hot air furnace, a cooking range, and a bathtub; the rest of the furnishings, as well as wages for the staff (missionaries Henry Turner and his daughters Isabel and Alice) were eventually provided by the Toronto Women's Auxiliary. The eight-bed hospital sat next to the boarding school on a bank of the Bow River.

Henry Turner was seventy years old and in retirement and considered an 'honourary physician.'[28] In their letters to the hospital's benefactors, the Women's Auxiliary, he and his daughters typified the missionary spirit. Alice Turner's role was to teach the school's forty-three 'inmates ... I have a great time endeavouring to teach them civilised life. They are quite as intelligent as our own children I think.' Her letters were designed to tug at the hearts and wallets of the congregation. There were now so many children in the school that the kitchen could no longer be used as a laundry, and at the very least the mission needed another washtub. Their sole tub was used by the laundress, 'an Indian woman [who] washes pretty well, but does not half get the soap out;' the tub was also used for hauling drinking water from the river and for cooking.[29] With such conditions at the school, the children's health was certainly compromised. Alice also aided her father in their hospital work, which, she enthused, '*must* go right with so many of one mind to push it along.'[30] As a missionary, Turner's role was to bring his patients to the light of Christian faith through humanitarian aid and basic medicine. The mission hospital was content to provide meals to the hungry, used clothing to the naked, and a warm bed to the ill and alone. Given the crude facilities, Turner wisely avoided any surgical or medical procedures that might, if they failed, cast the mission in a negative light. He treated the children's scrofula with lancing and poultices. Although some advocated surgical removal, Turner refused to perform surgery on a condition that appeared to resolve itself, albeit temporarily. The credit for cures might be shared between Turner and the Lord, but failures must be borne by the Lord alone. The missionaries might have contented themselves with leaving cures in the hands of the Lord; but the new, Liberal-appointed medical officer for the reserve, Dr James D. Lafferty, harboured no such intentions. Lafferty charged that Turner was 'a retired medical man well advanced in years' who could not even undertake simple surgery on his Blackfoot patients. Lafferty continued to rely on the surgical treatment of scrofula and began to admit his patients to Calgary's Holy Cross hospital. The department quickly advised Lafferty to use 'the utmost discretion' in admitting Native patients. Only the most seriously ill patients who could not be treated elsewhere were to be admitted to non-reserve hospitals: 'The department considers that too many Indian patients are being sent to the hospital and that the cost for their maintenance will exceed the funds at the disposal of the department.'[31] It was later conceded that most scrofula patients treated surgically died in a short time, but Lafferty supposed it was the people's peculiar reaction to the chloroform anaesthetic that killed them, and not the surgery! The mission hospital had run up against a new kind of westerner – one who shared none of the missionary's protective impulse toward Aboriginal people. At forty-eight, Lafferty was not a young man, but he epitomized the attitude that the west was ripe for development and that Aboriginal people must quickly assimilate or be left behind. Likewise, he was a brash representative of the new, 'scientific' medicine, which placed its faith in antiseptic procedures and bacteriological discoveries. Turner's stoicism, perhaps well-suited to the cottage hospital, contrasted sharply with Lafferty's aggressive character.

James Delamere Lafferty was born in Perth, Ontario, in 1849 and in 1870 graduated with a medical degree from Queen's University. In 1876, after a brief stint at the sprawling, thousand-bed Bellevue hospital in

New York City, he married Jessie Gray, the daughter of a prominent Presbyterian minister. Lafferty signed on as medical superintendent of construction for the CPR, moving west with the railway construction and, like many Ontarians, quickly recognizing the bounty the North-West Territories had to offer. His association with the railway probably did not hurt his real estate speculations, and by 1882 he had acquired property and a string of private banks in Portage la Prairie, Emerson, Brandon, Regina, and Moosomin. His family remained in Ontario until he was sure the Riel Rebellion was over, and in 1885 settled in Calgary.

Calgary may have been created by the CPR, but it was owned by ranchers. Ranch money built the public utilities and underpinned the newspaper. Along with businessmen and professionals, the ranchers created an elitist society that had more in common with eastern cities than the frontier. Lafferty apparently had little trouble breaking into this social structure and was elected mayor in 1890. Still engaged in the banking business, he opened branches in Edmonton, Moose Jaw, Lethbridge, and Calgary. The west welcomed him, and he welcomed the west.[32] But by the early 1890s his banks were being pushed out of the financial marketplace by the incoming Canadian chartered banks. He may have subsequently fallen out with the ranch crowd, which would have been providing him with wealthy clients; or perhaps his association with the Liberals made him an unlikely choice for the ranch families, who tended to be linked to the Conservatives. In any case, he made use of his personal friendship with the newly elected prime minister, Wilfrid Laurier, to win a government contract as the medical officer for the Blackfoot, Sarcee, and Stoney reserves near Calgary.

Lafferty demanded control over admissions to the Anglican mission hospital on the Blackfoot reserve as well as control over all medical care on the reserve. The missionaries, he charged, were running the hospital to conduct their church work, which ran contrary to his medical work 'and must operate against my influence with the Indians.' Hospitals, in his estimation, were 'not required for soup kitchen work.'[33] The department equivocated. Yes, he should have the authority to remove incurable and infectious patients from mission schools, and he should have control over hospital admissions.[34] But Turner and the missionaries were not ready to cede control over 'their' hospital, and the department agreed that the Anglicans should control the building, as well as the ration and drug accounts. Gibbon Stocken correctly assessed the department's position toward mission hospitals: 'Every encouragement was given to us to proceed with our work and we were assured more than once that it had the hearty approval of the department.' If the department wanted control of the institution, it would also have to staff it and provide hospital accommodation for all reserves, and 'they were not disposed to undertake such an institution themselves.'[35] Lafferty assumed that once he had wrested control from the missionaries, he and the hospital might 'fulfill its mission and be a very useful and civilizing institution and do a good work in educating the Indians as to the advantages and superiority of the white man's treatment of injuries and disease over their own pagan system.'[36] Of course, neither he nor the missionaries had consulted the people, who obviously preferred to be treated by their own healers. In 1899, while Lafferty and the missionaries were squabbling over a hospital that almost everyone on the reserve avoided, there were, in a population of 1,060, 31 births and 84 deaths (47 of whom were children). The hospital had treated only 51 patients in the year, and claimed that 20 had 'improved' and only 3 died.[37] Clearly, neither the medical officer nor the missionaries were being consulted in most cases of illness. However, healers could not mitigate the effects of overwhelming poverty on the reserve. In order to pay for new schools, the department had chopped another $140,000 from its expenditures for the people, who were still struggling with the loss of their bison economy.[38]

The hospital never did make much of an impression on residents of the Blackfoot reserve. Years later it was described as a 'realy [sic] lonely place.' Nurse Jane Megarry was born in Ireland and arrived in Canada about 1901; she trained at the Galt Hospital in Lethbridge, and worked at the Anglican St Paul's school on the Blood reserve and later at the Anglicans' Blackfoot hospital. Megarry recognized that the people simply did not care for the hospital 'as they had very little faith in the white doctor or his medicine.' The 'old time Indians,' as Megarry called them, relied on their own healers, who made medicines from herbs and roots. She did, however, treat a number of people who presented themselves at the dispensary with tuberculosis sores, rheumatic pains, and 'eye trouble.' When a family member was brought to the hospital, the whole family including the children went along and refused to leave their loved one alone. Megarry fed the family members and in return 'got odd jobs out of them,' which helped with the upkeep of the hospital.[39] Neither 'superior' Euro-Canadian medicine, nor the medical personnel themselves, could offer any real challenge to the Blackfoot healers. True to form, the department suggested that since there was the 'greatest difficulty' in keeping patients in hospital, agents should have the authority to force hospitalization.[40] Compulsion and coercion were familiar department approaches and collided with the people's cultural and social imperatives. As Megarry recalled, when a patient died at the hospital, the other patients were taken away by their families, fearing the consequences of remaining in a building where a death had taken place.[41]

While Lafferty was agitating for control of the Blackfoot hospital in 1899, he was also lobbying for funds to establish a hospital on the Stoney reserve in conjunction with the Methodist McDougall orphanage (boarding school). As a surgeon, he needed the facilities only a hospital could provide, and he also needed the 'surgical cases' the reserve schools could provide. He had been admonished at least once for admitting Native people to municipal hospitals, and now complained that 'to leave them unrelieved and suffering has a demoralizing effect on the Indians and lessens my influence so much among them.' The Methodist missionary, Rev. John McDougall, promised to supply a nurse and furnish the hospital, and the Stoney people agreed to get out the logs, if the government would provide $200 for lumber, flooring, and windows. Lafferty assured his superiors that the expenditure would not be wasted because the people had forsaken 'Indian' medicine and would accept a doctor's help, 'which could be rendered with so much more virtue if they were away from their close houses and kept clean and were given their medicine regularly.' In July 1900 the scheme was given departmental approval and a budget of $500. But as with the Blackfoot hospital, the Stoney hospital remained unoccupied for another five years because the missionary could provide neither nurse nor furnishings. Catholic missionaries had more success providing medical and hospital care because they had access to the trained nurses of the Quebec order the Sisters of Charity (or Grey Nuns, as they were popularly called). By 1905, department inspector J.A. Markle was advising that the plans for the hospital on the Stoney reserve be shelved. The Methodists, he explained, will consider the hospital their own private institution, and other religious denominations will not send their patients there. Instead they will request like institutions on other reserves, 'particularly when they learn that the only expense to them will be, vide precedent, the salary of one nurse.'[42] The trend toward providing assistance to missionary hospitals was setting an expensive precedent for the department. Moreover, competition between Christian denominations on the reserves tended to waste the meagre departmental resources that were available, as costs and buildings were duplicated on reserves in the struggle for souls. The Anglicans on the Blackfoot reserve had always felt threatened by the Catholics in Crowfoot's camp, who were now agitating for their own hospital. As Gibbon Stocken warned church supporters, it was more important than ever to fight to maintain control of the hospital, 'owing to the aggressive attitude of the church of Rome.'[43]

By 1904 the Anglican Blackfoot hospital under the guidance of the new missionary, Dr William Rose, was hugely successful – that is, according to Gibbon Stocken: 'The work done here has materially helped in setting the gospel before these people.' Unfortunately, the church of Rome was hindering its work, as were the 'evil lives of our own countrymen,' and as were the Sun Dances. In a rather dubious statement to his eastern benefactors, Gibbon Stocken reported that even the 'medicine men' were presenting themselves for treatment: 'Some ... are talking of giving up their heathen practices as such, with a view to embracing Christianity.'[44] The work of the hospital was aimed primarily at the people's souls, and thus deaths might still be viewed as successes – albeit in the next world. The hospital's 'excellent work,' however, had little impact on the death rates on the reserve. In 1900 it had a population of 985, and there were 39 births and 97 deaths (69 of whom were children), for a death rate of 98.4 deaths per thousand.[45] In 1902 the reserve's population was only 896, and there were 34 births and 100 deaths – a death rate of 111.6 per thousand.[46]

In 1912, Old Sun's boarding school was moved to a new location away from the banks of the Bow River. The hospital now stood alone on the river bank, which was acknowledged to be 'unsanitary.' The hospital, mostly irrelevant in any case, could not survive at all without its close physical connection with the school. It was not used by the reserve residents; 90 per cent of the patients were schoolchildren and the other 10 per cent were their parents.[47] Gibbon Stocken lobbied the department to pay to have the hospital moved, but when pressed for monthly reports showing the number of patients treated there, he admitted that there were none because of staff shortages. He also complained that the people refused to come to the hospital, because the staff were all strangers and no one could speak their language. The hospital building was isolated 'and the Indian is superstitious of isolated buildings as being the abode of ghosts.' If the hospital were moved to the mission site, Gibbon Stocken later added, nurses of the 'right stamp' could be hired, and 'the Indians assure me they would patronize it much more generally than they do.' The department's medical inspector called it a 'so-called hospital,' and recommended the establishment of a non-denominational government-run hospital at the agency headquarters. But agent John H. Gooderham, demonstrating a good understanding of the department's position, added that 'the whole care and expense would fall upon the department and it is a question if it would be more successful than a mission hospital ... also I doubt if it would be patronized by the Catholic patients.'[48] The hospital remained at its original site until 1923, when the band council, using its own funds, built a sixteen-bed brick hospital. The project succeeded only after the local Native healers were assured they could continue to practise their medicine. At the band's insistence, it remained a strictly non-denominational hospital.[49] In 1930 it was renovated to accommodate forty patients, and in 1947 it was transferred to the Department of Health and Welfare.

In 1896, Canadians elected Wilfrid Laurier's Liberals, ousting the Conservatives, who had designed and implemented Indian policy for nearly twenty years. Laurier placed westerner Clifford Sifton in charge of western development. Sifton, a Brandon lawyer who had gained experience as a member of the Manitoba government, was appointed both minister of the interior and superintendent general of Indian Affairs, and at the age of thirty-five was the youngest member of Laurier's cabinet. By placing him at the head of both departments, Laurier was making it clear that Sifton's role was to manage western development. Unfortunately, the needs of Indian Affairs ran a poor second to the work of filling the west with earnest farmers. Sifton and his deputy James Smart, an old associate from Brandon, ran both departments and began an aggressive policy of western development.[50] In 1902 Indian Affairs again received its own deputy, Toronto lawyer Frank Pedley, but only because of the sheer volume of work in the Interior Department. Indian Affairs had been notorious for patronage appointments, and many employees were fired, to be replaced in due time with Liberal appointments. The budget was slashed, and administration was centralized in Ottawa. Few of these new officials had any experience with Aboriginal people, and they tended to be completely unsympathetic to the people's struggle. The focus was on western progress and development.

The new bureaucracy embraced what had become a stereotypical view of the 'race' and their health. James Smart in his first report stated that the high death rates among the people were primarily the result of 'pulmonary phthisis and scrofula.' According to Smart, the cause was obvious: 'the herding together in small and ill-ventilated houses ... Even

TABLE 3.1
Selected Treaty Four, Six, and Seven Agencies: Population, 1895–1920

	Battleford	Blackfoot	Crooked Lakes	Edmonton	Hobbema	Stoney
1895	861	1267	616	729	522	535
1896	860	1226	637	732	697	581
1897	928	1145	601	698	666	581
1898	857	1099	587	681	617	593
1899	828	1096	588	679	601	614
1900	807	985	577	673	617	627
1901	754	942	563	703	607	661
1902	766	896	558	690	645	647
1903	767	845	558	694	645	641
1904	869	842	520	712	655	652
1905	886	803	534	694	691	660
1906	886	824	547	694	750	648
1907	875	817	544	689	745	640
1908	911	795	552	677	770	661
1909	920	768	562	683	785	667
1910	925	767	573	643	789	665
1911	954	763	578	649	766	659
1912	971	752	576	673	783	647
1913	911	737	585	680	776	659
1914	882	734	591	678	781	654
1915	917	731	595	708	795	659
1916	954	726	613	718	817	670
1917	968	719	620	731	827	673
1918	998	718	629	742	839	678
1919	1026	690	637	754	819	657
1920	1054	695	646	769	832	663

Note: Population figures for 1917–20 are estimates only. The Sessional Papers stopped publishing population statistics in 1917. The estimates were arrived at using a moving five-year average. Where populations were on the rise, that rise continued at the same rate, likewise if they were falling. The 1919 figures also take into account an average 4 per cent loss due to the influenza epidemic in the autumn of 1918.
Source: NA, RG 10, vols. 9428–33, Annuity Paylists, 1895–1900; CHC, Sessional Papers, 1902–22.

after more commodious dwellings have been erected, the tendency is to huddle together during the winter season.' Their lung conditions were aggravated by dust raised by dancing. The high incidence of scrofula was 'no doubt largely the result of intermarriage ... and the ever narrowing degree of consanguinity.' Infant mortality remained high because Native mothers were 'mere girls.' But, Smart reported, the population was increasing, which was further proof of the 'wise and humane policies of the government.' Populations in some agencies were increasing, while others were continuing to decline (Table 3.1.) Since the race did not seem to be vanishing, the Liberals began to reconsider the expense and supposed benefits of the industrial school system: 'To educate children above the possibilities of their station, and create a distaste for what is certain to be their environment in life would be not only a waste of money but doing them an injury instead of conferring a benefit upon them.'[51] The 'injury' referred to had nothing to do with the real dangers to health in the schools; rather, it was deemed dangerous to create unrealistic expectations in children that they might rise 'above their station.' The new bureaucracy certainly shared its predecessor's concern for economy and efficiency.

The industrial schools, suggested (recycled) commissioner David Laird in 1901, might be put to better use if they employed a few nurses to train suitable older girls in the art and skill of nursing the sick. The training would benefit the girls when they began their own families, but more importantly it would eventually lessen the costs of medical services on reserves. However, once home, young women would hardly be seen as qualified to treat the ill, just as the male school graduates would not be seen as able or fit to direct the affairs of their communities. That the school system placed their faith in these measures points to the gulf that existed between those who directed the department and those who were to benefit from it. Nevertheless, the industrial school principals generally agreed that the nurse training scheme was desirable – but only, they quickly added, if the department paid the salaries of the nurses, since the per capita grants were already insufficient. T. Ferrier, principal of the (Anglican) Brandon school, advised that the school would pay the nurse's salary if the department allowed him to enrol 125 pupils instead of the present 100. The department declined Ferrier's offer. Several principals noted that nearby hospitals would send a nurse to the schools to provide training at reasonable rates. James Dagg of the Episcopalian Middlechurch school suggested that the Deaconess Order of Nurses would send a nurse for less than the estimated $25–35 monthly salary of a lay nurse. Father Joseph Hugonnard at the Qu'Appelle school pointed out that his school already had a hospital staffed by Grey Nuns, who worked for $12.50 per month. A lay nurse would be expensive and isolated. He added, however, that a scheme to train girls would benefit the settlers, who often asked him to send out girls who could nurse for a short time. In the summer of 1901, Laird decided to implement a program whereby the department would pay the salaries of three nurses, outside the per capita grant, to visit the schools in turn. Every three months the nurses would move; thus, each would cover four schools in a year.[52] Eventually the department decided to pay the nurses $25 a month.

Dr M.S. Fraser of Brandon was put in charge of the program, and to reflect the proprietorship of the schools it was suggested that one Catholic nurse and two Anglican nurses be appointed. Fraser, a Baptist, appointed a nun and two Baptist nurses. The role of the nurses was never clearly stated. Were they teachers or nurses for the school? Did they answer to the principal or to the commissioner? No curriculum was prepared, and within a month of their appointments two of the nurses had resigned. They complained that it was impossible to teach nursing in three months, and besides their salaries were far below the current salaries of trained nurses, and they wanted their own rooms. The tubercular children should be removed from the schools, but there was no place for them. Dr James Lafferty in Calgary thought the program was a failure because of the innate unsuitability of Native women for the task of nursing: 'The absence of initiative and prompt decision in the Indian character will always stand in the way of any practical application of the limited training they can get.' By 1906, Laird was conceding that the program had been an ill-conceived failure. If it took four years to train a nurse, he wondered, how could school girls learn the skills in three months? Because the nurses were teaching in the schools but were not staff members, there was friction and conflict with the principals. 'I have come to the conclusion,' Laird wrote, 'that the practical results of the system we have hitherto pursued are almost nil.'[53] Such poorly conceived efforts that were virtually destined to fail only reinforced the perception that Native people were possessed of a peculiar constitution that made them resistant to treatment.

Education was the department's single greatest expense, and the industrial schools especially were its greatest financial drain. The huge expenditure, the low enrolments, the high death and disease rates in the schools, and the lack of concrete results led many to question their efficacy. Sifton remarked in the House of Commons that the industrial schools were a waste of time and money: 'I have no hesitation in saying – we may as well be frank – that the Indian cannot go out from school, making his own way and compete with the white man ... He has not the physical, mental or moral get-up to enable him to compete. He cannot do it.'[54] The department was ready to move away from the industrial schools toward an emphasis on the much cheaper boarding and day schools. In February 1907, Dr Peter Bryce, the department's chief medical officer, was ordered to investigate and report on the health conditions in industrial and boarding schools on the prairies. Although appointed in 1904, he had devoted most of his time to the medical inspection of immigrants for the Department of the Interior. Peter Henderson Bryce was an energetic and dynamic personality. Born in 1853 in Mount Pleasant, Ontario, he studied natural science and geology, earned his medical degree at the University of Toronto, studied neurology in Paris, and lectured in science and applied chemistry at Guelph's Agricultural College. From 1882 to 1904, he was the secretary of Ontario's Provincial Board of Health and the health officer for Ontario in charge of vital statistics. In 1889 he chaired an Ontario Royal Commission to investigate venereal diseases in horses. He was elected president of the American Public Health Association in 1900, was the vice-president of the American Congress on Tuberculosis in 1904, and was a member of the executive committee of the Canadian Association for the Prevention of Consumption. In 1904, as well as chief medical inspector for the immigration service, he was chief medical officer for the Department of Indian Affairs. On top of which, he was a well-known lecturer and writer on subjects from hypnotism, sewage disposal, and malaria, to milk supply, house atmospheres, and the influence of forests on rainfall and health. Bryce was a very busy administrator and bureaucrat. In his capacity as medical inspector of immigrants for the Department of the Interior, and in his involvement in the many reform movements that sought to maintain the 'racial purity' of Canada, he exerted some influence on immigration. He was also influential in transforming the Canadian public health movement into a scientific medical specialty firmly grounded in the germ theory of disease.[55]

Bryce's *Report on the Indian Schools of Manitoba and the North-West Territories* appeared in June 1907. It detailed the poor conditions of the church-run schools and the even worse conditions of the students in boarding and industrial schools on the prairies. It was a rather quick look. His inspection of thirty-five schools began in March, and by June he had submitted his report. Bryce made clear the links between health and sanitation and the impact of tuberculosis infection on overcrowded, undernourished children: 'General ill health from the continued inspiration of an air of increasing foulness is inevitable; but when sometimes consumptive pupils and, very frequently, others with discharging scrofulous glands, are present to add an infective quality to the atmosphere we have created a situation ... dangerous to health.' The report focused on the ventilation, sanitation, and physical state of the buildings; he did not examine the children, instead asking school officials for student health records. Of the 1,537 students with records, 35 per cent were either sick or dead. At the File Hills school, 69 per cent of all ex-pupils were dead. Working from these returns, Bryce found an 'intimate relationship between the health of the pupils while in the schools and that of their early death subsequent to discharge.' In all cases the reported cause of death was tuberculosis. Bryce found that the medical condition of the children upon admission to school was rarely inquired into, and that principals and physicians ignored or minimized the danger of accepting tubercular students. No attempt was made to ventilate the dormitories or classrooms. For seven months of the year the windows were sealed shut to save fuel; for ten hours a day the children were confined in the dormitories. Bryce was surprised that the morbidity and mortality statistics were not worse, and declared that the schools should be made to understand the 'modern gospel of fresh air.' Martin Benson, head of the department's education branch, called the report 'damnatory ... If boarding and industrial schools are breeding places for consumption, the sooner they are closed the better.'[56] The Bryce Report fit conveniently into department plans to close the expensive and inefficient industrial schools and focus on the day schools. It is also apparent that Bryce was also working in conjunction with Sam Blake, a Toronto lawyer and lay member of the Anglican Missionary Society of the Church in Canada.[57]

Blake was growing more and more disillusioned with Canadian Aboriginal missions and schools, and was urging that the society spend its time and money on more exotic missions in the Far East. His plans met with considerable opposition from western Anglican missionaries such as John Tims, who had spent his life in mission work in Alberta. Tims, after being forced from the Blackfoot reserve in 1895, had been appointed Archdeacon of Macleod and director of missions. He resented Blake's attacks on his work but worried most that to desert the western missions would be to admit defeat and give up the whole field to the Catholics: 'Of one thing we may be certain. Rome will be our residuary legatee. If we withdraw from Schools and Missions our Roman brethren will not be slow to profit by our neglect and desertion.'[58] Bryce and Blake worked together to bring the health problems in the schools to light. Seen in that context, the Bryce Report seemed to be blaming the churches for the condition of the schools.

Bryce, however, also submitted eleven recommendations that were never made public.[59] In them, he clearly blamed the government for the appalling conditions in the schools. The per capita grants given to the schools were too small to provide both education *and* good health for the children. The funding arrangement had forced the churches into making decisions that were detrimental to the children's well-being. He urged the government to take over the financial management and control of education, as the Protestant churches had recently proposed. Since only 50 per cent of Native children could be accommodated in the industrial schools, there should be an expansion of day schools and boarding schools, and the industrial schools should be eliminated. According to Bryce, of the eight industrial schools, 'several are expensive successes, but most are expensive failures and ought not longer to be continued.' Bryce recommended that radical improvements be made in the school buildings. A medical officer, trained in public health, should inspect the schools biannually, and small tents should be erected alongside schools to isolate patients. The tent hospitals could be used for scrofulous and tubercular patients, 'where, instead of being sent home to die, they may in most cases, when dealt with early, be nursed back to health without jeopardizing the health of other pupils.'[60] His recommendations made the case for closing the industrial schools, but in calling for non-denominational schools wholly financed and managed by the department, they also went far beyond what the department was willing to undertake to rectify the problem. The Bryce Report (without his recommendations) received the kind of publicity that Blake and Dr Bryce had hoped for. The press was outraged. The editor of *Saturday Night* magazine asked, 'What is Canada Trying to do with her Indian Wards? Indian boys and girls are dying like flies in these institutions or shortly after leaving them.' A headline in the *Montreal Star* shouted, 'Death Rate among Indians Abnormal'; the *Ottawa Citizen* led with 'Schools and White Plague.' Public indignation at the conditions in the schools was rather disingenuous, given the long-standing state of affairs in Native communities generally; it also testifies to the department's skill in keeping that state of affairs from the public view.

The Bryce Report was distributed to agents, inspectors, and school principals for comment. Department employees were aware of the government's desire to restructure the education system, and suggested that the schools themselves (and by extension, the churches) were to blame. The agent at Duck Lake, James Macarthur, blamed the situation at the Catholic Duck Lake boarding school on the 'divided authority' for the schools between church and state. The building was completely unsuitable, and the children should have been having a monthly medical examination and not what he called a perfunctory line-up. Had this been done there would have been no unseemly 'scramble for pupils' by the churches, and the 'worse than brutal practice' of discharging very ill students would not have arisen. Macarthur reckoned that the death rate at the school was 4 per cent per year. Inspector William Chisholm noted that when children were sent home, 'they usually show a steady improvement,' and he called for a greater emphasis on reserve-based day schools or boarding schools. The only solution to the problem of tuberculosis in the schools was the 'fresh air treatment' employed in sanatoria; since that was not possible, the next best thing was 'the open air life and freedom that is enjoyed by all Indian children at home.' David Laird countered that the sanitation in the schools was probably as good as in most public buildings in the west. He thought the report should have remained confidential because the headlines 'brought our schools into undeserved disrepute.' The disrepute was not all that undeserved, according to T.E. Jackson, acting agent at Carlton. He noted that at Prince Albert's Emmanuel College the mortality had been 'deplorably large' and had contributed to the reluctance of parents to send their children to boarding and industrial schools. Although their homes were humble, many ill children recovered at home.[61] Conditions at the schools were nothing new to employees. As part of their employment they were expected to help recruit students and return runaways. They knew only too well how negatively the schools were viewed by parents.

While department employees blamed the high mortality on school conditions, school principals blamed the high death rates on reserve conditions. In their view, the department, not the schools, was the source of the problem. Principal George Hogbin at the Anglican Calgary industrial school suggested that the food children received at home, which was 'often very badly and indigestibly cooked,' the poor housing on the reserve, and the transition from a hunting to a sedentary life had all combined to cause the high death rates at the schools. Why blame the schools? he asked. Principal W.R. Haynes at the Anglican Pincher Creek boarding school agreed. His school was always fresh and airy, so much so that 'you need an overcoat and hat on to come into these dormitories.' Haynes did note, however, that the people were 'full of tuberculosis ... If every pupil were rejected on the grounds of tuberculosis in their families, I am afraid you might as well close the schools altogether.' Principal E. Matheson at the Battleford industrial school, referring to the prevalence of tuberculosis on the reserves, asked 'Why not begin at the beginning and strike at the root of the thing?'[62] The reserves, not the schools, were the reservoirs of tuberculosis.

A few took offence to Bryce's report. Principal Dodds of the Cecilia Jeffrey boarding school suggested that since the 'seed or germ' of tuberculosis was contracted at home, the schools could hardly be blamed. It would have been more productive, he noted, had Bryce made some concrete recommendations. Those recommendations were never circulated, however. Dodds continued, 'The open window was well known as a means of ventilation long before the wise men [Bryce] came from the east ... Is this all that modern science has done or can do?' Inspector S. Swinford of the Manitoba inspectorate sarcastically pointed out that 'it is a difficult matter for a person with only a practical knowledge of Indians and Indian schools to criticize statements on scientific questions made by medical faddists of the day.' He concluded by saying that the children in schools in his inspectorate were 'jolly healthy' and 'fairly bubbling over with vitality.' The principal of one of the schools in Swinford's inspectorate, the Birtle boarding school, disagreed. He noted that of ninety-one graduates, forty-four were living and forty-seven were dead. According to him, the fault lay not with the schools but with conditions on reserves, where most children had the 'hereditary taint' of tuberculosis with 'scrofulous tendencies.' Moreover, the per capita grant system made it difficult to maintain healthy conditions in the schools, because children with scrofula and tuberculosis were admitted for two reasons, one mercenary and one humanitarian. The per capita grant was a temptation to retain pupils, regardless of their health, and for humanitarian reasons it was cruel to send sick children home to a certain death. He also regretted the publicity given the Bryce Report, because many Native people were literate and knew of the report, and that would make it even more difficult to get new pupils.[63] Principals of the Anglican-run schools argued that it was not so much the schools that were killing the children, but the parents, the government, and the government's newest medical inspector.

Principals of the Catholic schools, which enrolled by far the most students, simply dismissed the Bryce Report. To them, the schools were providing a valuable humanitarian service and should be continued despite their problems. Father Leo Balter of the Sacred Heart boarding school at Saddle Lake in Alberta refused to acknowledge that the schools were in any way responsible for the death of students; the principal cause of tuberculosis infection, he boldly announced, was heredity. Balter stressed the inhumanity of denying access to school to sick children: 'It is also a duty of charity and humanity to procure the intellectual development and the salvation of his soul to a weak child whose sojourn here below will not be very long.' According to Father George Hallam of Muscowequan boarding school, Bryce's ideas were 'new fangled' and his insistence on good ventilation for the schools was a 'white elephant.' The chief medical officer 'shouldn't expect palaces for children and for us to feed and clothe them.' Joseph Hugonnard of the Qu'Appelle school also took the high road. Since according to Bryce and the press, everything seemed a failure, would it be better not to educate the children at all? The death rates in the schools were the result of poor health inherited from their parents: 'There are some here who have no better place to be sent, and who have regular medical attendance and sanitary conditions.'[64] The missionaries saw themselves as providing a humane service – education and instruction in the Christian faith was a public service undertaken with the purest motives. For those missionaries directly involved in the school system, the Bryce Report was a direct and unwarranted attack on their efforts. If the children who came to them were sick, better to provide them with Christian instruction in this world than have their souls wander aimlessly in the next.

For all the justifications and rationalizations put forward by the missionaries, the discussion ultimately revolved around whether tuberculosis originated in the schools or on the reserves. While it was a burning question for the department, for the children the point was moot: regardless of where a student contracted the disease, the future was not bright. Parents strongly suspected the schools were at fault, hence their continued resistance. And the department, although it had consistently denied responsibility for the health care of reserve residents as such, did admit a responsibility for the health of schoolchildren. So the question of where tuberculosis originated was significant. In then-commissioner Hayter Reed's 1896 survey of school principals, agents, and medical officers, the prevailing opinion was that poor living conditions on reserves, and the equally poor conditions in the schools, caused the high incidence of tuberculosis. It was recommended at that time that children be screened before admission, the proper ventilation of the schools be attempted, and that an adequate diet be implemented; essentially, these were Bryce's recommendations. Despite the evidence at the time, Reed had decided that the people on reserves had a hereditary disposition to tuberculosis; the schools were not to blame. Note that in the 1890s the industrial schools were the showpiece of the department. Reed was highly supportive of the 'civilizing' aspects of the industrial schools and was committed to their success. But by 1907 the costs of the schools and their nearly negligible results made many doubt their efficacy. The Bryce Report was without question a valuable ally in the fight to have the education system reorganized. But western Protestant missionaries, and the Catholic Oblate order that managed most of the Catholic schools, resisted any fundamental change.

Lafferty joined the attack on the schools in late 1908 when he reported that fully 80 per cent of the students in the five Alberta schools he inspected were afflicted with pulmonary tuberculosis, while some had scrofula and tuberculosis of the bones as well. At Old Sun's school on the Blackfoot reserve, thirty-four of the thirty-five students were suffering from pulmonary tuberculosis. The Catholic Crowfoot school on the same reserve did not fare much better, with twenty-two of thirty-nine children so afflicted. At both the McDougall orphanage on the Stoney reserve, and the Sarcee boarding school on the Sarcee reserve, 100 per cent of the children were reportedly ill with pulmonary tuberculosis, and at Dunbow (St Joseph's) industrial school at High River, forty-six of seventy students were sick. Lafferty observed that if the diseased children were discharged, the schools would lose nearly all their pupils and it would be financially impossible for the churches to run the schools under the per capita grant system. According to Lafferty, the Native children were more disposed to tuberculosis infection because they possessed little resistance to disease due to the change from the outdoor life to school. The only way to maintain the school system would be to accept only healthy children and to discharge immediately any infected students. This had not been done in the past, Lafferty argued, because the physicians examining the children had been pressured by the principals to admit students. The physicians reasoned that there was so much tuberculosis in the schools already that there was no point in excluding students. Lafferty urged the department to hire 'non-sectarian and impartial' physicians to examine the children, but as was noted earlier, he was involved at this time in a struggle with the Anglican missionaries at the Blackfoot reserve over access to the hospital and control over admissions. This may have influenced his recommendations. Nevertheless, the implication in Lafferty's report was that it was indeed the schools, and not the reserves, where tuberculosis was spreading, and that the government should administer them.[65]

In reaction to Lafferty's report, Frank Pedley, the deputy superintendent, repeated his concerns about the viability of the schools. He suggested that the high disease rates in the schools 'rendered useless [the]
large expenditures on Indian education.' He informed the superintendent that the department should either find healthy students or shut
the schools down. As a first step, Pedley amended the admission forms
'so as to exclude students with tuberculosis.'[66] The amended forms were
only as good as the medical officers completing them, however, and
there were consistent problems with the diligence and dedication of
those officers. In the supplementary estimates for 1907–8, Pedley also
asked for an increase in expenditure of $20,000 specifically for tubercu-
losis control. By way of justification, he mentioned the 'peculiar constitution' of the people and the bad press the Bryce Report had
unleashed. He was able to increase the appropriations for 'supplies for
the destitute' and for day, boarding, and industrial schools. Unfortunately, to do so he had had to cut $14,466 from the budget for imple-
ments and livestock. The next year, 1908–9, a new general
appropriation of $5,000 appeared under the category 'to prevent the
spread of tuberculosis,' but only $2,568.39 was spent. To put that in per-
spective, in the same year the department spent $8,000 for printing and
stationery. Mindful of the growing public awareness of the dangers of
tuberculosis and its spread, Pedley recognized the need for a policy that
'may be seen as humane and enlightened.' According to Pedley, the
increase was necessary 'to grapple with tuberculosis amongst Indians, to
lessen its dangerous features and to *prevent as far as possible its spread*
[emphasis added].' Tuberculosis on the reserves was, in his words, a
'menace to white populations.'[67]

Yet the menace to the Native population continued. In May 1909, Lafferty and Bryce were ordered to undertake yet another school medical
inspection. Medical inspections had become the weapon of choice in
the public health movement, and the department's focus on tuberculosis investigation made action unnecessary in the meantime. Six months
later, Bryce and Lafferty had finished their inspection of 243 students in
seven residential and boarding schools in the Calgary district. In their
investigation the two doctors dismissed the accepted methods of tuberculosis diagnosis. The tuberculin test, where Koch's tuberculin was
either instilled in the eye or rubbed on the skin, was rejected as too
expensive. The use of Roentgen rays and a fluorescent screen was-
considered too time-consuming. And an examination of the sputum
for the presence of bacilli was judged both too expensive *and* too time-

consuming. So instead they proceeded with clinical methods, available to every medical officer to Indians, 'which for years have proved adequate for diagnosing most cases of tuberculosis.'[68] Their diagnosis, then, relied on a number of factors: temperature, pulse, respiration, height and weight, general appearance, the number of years in school, and the condition of the throat and nose and lungs and chest. Though both doctors conducted the examinations, Bryce alone wrote the report. Lafferty was uncharacteristically silent regarding any recommendations for improvement. As a long-time Indian Affairs employee, he was perhaps more in tune with what the department expected from its medical officers. He would not commit himself to making suggestions until he was aware of the department's wishes. In a letter to Bryce, he wondered whether the department wanted to take over the schools to prevent and cure tuberculosis, and to dispense with religious training. Or did the department want to equip and manage the schools but allow religious training? Or did the department want to maintain the status quo but allow inspections by the department medical officer? The superintendent of education, Duncan Campbell Scott, explained, 'Dr. Lafferty does not join with Dr. Bryce in these recommendations and finds himself at a loss to offer any suggestions unless he is aware of the views of the department.'[69] Scott, better known to many Canadians as a poet and man of letters, had risen through the ranks of the department, from a humble beginning in 1880 as a copy clerk, to chief clerk and accountant in 1893, to superintendent of education in 1909, and finally to superintendent general in 1913.[70] He saw Bryce's recommendations as far in excess of what the department was willing to accept. Lafferty wasted no time in distancing himself from the recommendations.

In his report, Bryce concluded that Native school children were exposed to tuberculosis mainly in their homes, and that all children who were awaiting admission to school showed signs of tuberculosis. He found that the death rate for Native schoolchildren was 80 per thousand population, while the average death rate for Canadian children was only 4.3 per thousand.[71] In this huge gap he saw hope for what might be accomplished by providing early and adequate medical supervision, with fresh air treatment, rest, adequate food, and graduated exercise. What he had in mind was a sanatorium. But knowing that his superiors would balk at the idea of Native children basking in the sunshine, gorging themselves on cream and eggs, he suggested that new methods of sanatorium treatment be introduced. Marcus Paterson of the Brompton sanatorium in Frimley, England, had shown that absolute bed rest was not necessary. Instead, the 'Frimley method' stressed graduated labour and the idea of 'auto-inoculation.' Patients were put to work once their temperature was normal because work caused an inoculation of the patients by their own bacteriological products. According to Paterson: 'The aim of the physician is to keep the blood well garrisoned and well armed, swarming with its protective sentinels the anti-bodies so that all invading forces may be overcome at once ... If we allow our patient to exert himself, we make him liberate a certain amount of tuberculin (the poison) or toxin, to overcome which the body immediately re-acts and produces anti-toxin, which at once neutralises or kills the tuberculous poison ... Exercise or work, in graduated amounts is therefore, in every sense of the term, scientific.'[72] The Frimley method was also appealing because it included strict regulations and manual labour, which would have been seen as highly instructive for Native children. Moreover, as Bryce pointed out in his report, the Brompton Sanatorium was cost-efficient. Through graduated exercise and labour, it had treated 50 per cent more patients in 1908 than in 1907. This 'pick-axe cure' was similar to labour colonies for the unemployed.[73]

In his recommendations, Bryce suggested that certain schools be selected to incorporate the Frimley method. Each student would be considered an 'individual case of probable tuberculosis.' Bryce would have complete control and supervision without interference from church authorities. He would control the appointment and training of nurses and sanitary directors. Bryce also recommended that the school buildings be improved to allow open-air work rooms and dormitories. Expenditures would have to be increased to provide extra clothing, a special diet, and an improved water supply. His recommendations again called for increased government expenditure and a commitment to the health of Native people. Needless to say Bryce's report and recommendations were not well received. Even while he and Lafferty were in the initial stages of their examinations, the Catholic church was bringing considerable pressure to bear on the department to leave the school system fundamentally unchanged. As for Bryce's recommendations, Scott stated, 'While they may be scientific [they] are quite inapplicable to the system under which these schools are conducted.' The department argued that even if it was prepared to take over the management of the schools, the churches would never relinquish their share of control.[74] The western missionaries, Protestant and Catholic, had fought Bryce and Blake to a standstill. There was to be no fundamental change in the education system, and Bryce's struggle to have the department create proper facilities for isolating and treating ill students met the same fate.

Lafferty submitted his own recommendations once he understood the views of the department. As he explained to Pedley, his recommendations were premised first on the understanding that the department would not alter the status quo, and second on the assumption that every child of school age was afflicted with tuberculosis. If those contentions were correct, he continued, then it was incumbent upon the department to make 'reasonable effort, consistent with practicability and expense to improve the physical condition [of the children].' Lafferty recommended that sleeping galleries be added to the schools, that ventilation be improved, that open-air classrooms be built, that lavatories be provided for the sick and where possible for the whole school, and that isolation cottages be built. In this way the schools could continue to accept all children. He recommended further that full-time medical inspectors be appointed for each province, and that all schools be provided with milk, eggs, and adequate clothing. Lafferty also suggested that graduate nurses be appointed to every reserve to educate and improve health; this would do away with 'the necessity for much of the visiting which is now done by medical men and in nine cases out of ten are of very little service to the Indians.'[75] He closed by stating that although he agreed with Bryce's recommendations, he had been advised by the department that it was not in a position to carry out Bryce's suggestions in their entirety. Lafferty's suggestion that the department appoint additional medical officers and nurses was rejected. D.C. Scott pointed out that the appointments would be expensive and that nurses had the same effect on the Native people's health as hospitals – none. Schools, he added, were educational institutions, not hospitals, and while the department was prepared to deal with tuberculosis in its early stages, 'cases that develop rapidly and seriously are not to be allowed in residence.' The department did recognize the need to respond to the Bryce and Lafferty reports, but, as Scott stated, 'it is only necessary to carry out some common sense reforms to remove the imputation that the Department is careless of the interests of the children.'[76]

Eventually, the department reacted to the Bryce and Lafferty reports with a five-point plan of reforms: it would continue the system of refusing children admission if they were reported to be tubercular; it would build open-air dormitories; it would establish a minimum diet that the schools would be obliged to provide; it would increase the per capita grant to meet the increased expense; and finally, it would draw up a contract to be entered into with each school outlining the regulations regarding sanitation, diet, calisthenics, and breathing exercises. In Scott's estimation, these simple measures alone would meet the needs of the children, and do so without the 'enormous friction' that would result from any attempts to reform the medical and educational systems.[77] Years later, Bryce accused Scott of deliberately suppressing his report and recommendations, stating that it was only because of Scott's influence that his report on the medical condition of the Native school children was not raised at the annual meeting of the National Tuberculosis Association in 1910. According to Bryce, Dr George Adami, a pathologist at McGill University and president of the Tuberculosis Association, blocked any discussion of Bryce's report only because Scott had promised that the department would implement his recommendations.[78] In his annual report for 1910, Pedley noted that some progress had been made in lessening the effects of tuberculosis through improved living conditions, and that the removal of children from their homes to industrial and boarding schools 'where the utmost care is taken of them, can not fail of some effect.'[79]

Parents and children did not idly wait for action. The problem with the industrial schools was low enrolment, and enrolments were low because parents resisted sending their children to faraway schools where they would be exposed to abuse and disease. As Lafferty observed: 'There is no doubt that many of the Indians know that tuberculosis prevails greatly in the schools and that it influences a great many of them to refuse sending their children to school and can we blame them.'[80] Children resisted by trying to run away, or by simply refusing to learn. Sometimes schools burned to the ground. But with the combined weight and resources of the government, the police, and the Department of Indian Affairs arrayed against them, parents were rarely heard. They sent their children to school, or rather the children were taken from them to the school, and siblings were at times separated from one another. As Kaye Thompson recalled, 'My brothers went to Lebret because my father was a Catholic. My mother was Protestant so [we] girls went to Brandon. My parents had no choice. The agent went and told them, "Your child is of the age to go to school."'[81] Most schools discouraged or prohibited visits by parents, and as agent Robert N. Wilson of the Blood reserve remarked, 'as a matter of practice parents are kept ignorant of the illness of their children until they are dead or sent home to die.'[82] Because schools were often swarming with disease, they were often quarantined so that no children were allowed to leave and no out-siders were allowed to visit. Eleanor Brass recalled that at File Hills school 'they used to quarantine the school in the winter time and our parents weren't allowed to come and see us. This is when we went through a lot of abuse and torture.' She was locked in a room for a day with no food or bathroom – her punishment for passing notes in class. She was then beaten for wetting her pants and strapped over and over again. 'Finally I got so numb that I couldn't cry any more.' Young John, Chief Pasquah's son, tried to run away home. Everything was strange, no one would speak to him in his language, and he was desperately home-sick. John was brought back to school and beaten so badly that he was 'raw and bruised from the back of his neck to his ankles. He couldn't bear covers on his back for weeks. No doctor was called and no one but us children knew what went on.'[83] The department used other forms of coercion as well. In 1893, Star Blanket in Treaty Four had been deposed as chief by the department for killing a cow without permission. But, he explained, his people were very hungry and agency cattle were intended to be eaten. In 1895 the department offered to reinstate him, and his annual $25 salary, if he would agree to send the band's children to school. His son was eventually enrolled in File Hills school. Star Blanket did not object to education, but he would not allow children to be sent away: 'In the treaty we made then, the government promised to make a school for every band of Indians on their own reserve, but instead, little children are torn from their mothers' arms or homes by the police or government agents, and taken sometimes hundreds of miles away to large schools, perhaps to take sick and die when their family cannot see them. The little ants that live in the earth love their young ones, and wish to have them in their homes. Surely us red men are not smaller than those ants.'[84] His concerns were dismissed. But parental concern for the welfare of their children cannot be discounted when we analyse changes in the school system. Ultimately it was parental resistance to the schools that forced many reforms.[85]

The school system remained in place because it aimed to 'Christian-ize and civilize,' and that goal remained fundamental. Almost forgotten in all of the political machinations and the bureaucratic intransigence were the students themselves. Hundreds of children were dying as more inspections were carried out, more regulations were made and ignored, and more reports were filed. For instance, in 1909 Archdeacon Tims at the Sarcee school was ordered by the department to release seven stu-dents whose medical certificates noted the presence of tuberculosis.

Tims removed their names from the register but kept them in the school at the Church's expense because, he said, Bryce had advised that since all the children in the school were in the same condition, there was no harm in retaining them in the school! Four years later in 1913, Dr Harold McGill, who would eventually rise to become superintendent general, found one student with 'tubercular peritonitis' or tuberculosis of the stomach, and two or three students with infected glands. Since the only treatment given was 'hygienic measures and tonics,' he recommended that the children be isolated in tents on the school grounds. In 1917 Tims was reprimanded for allowing sick students to go home: 'You should deal firmly with the parents in this matter and not permit them to take their children home for treatment.' Tims, of course, had earlier been forced off the Blackfoot reserve for refusing to allow parents to take their sick children home. He informed the department that 'another pupil' had died and 'it has caused a great deal of dissatisfaction among the Indians that this boy was not allowed to go home and it is going to make it more difficult for us to obtain fresh pupils.' He also wanted to be reimbursed for the $45 spent on caskets in the month. In a memo, Tims admitted that the health of the thirty students in the school was becoming a concern. Three students had died the year before and another one recently. One student was on sick leave for a year and was unlikely to return because of 'running tuberculosis sores'; one was in hospital to have his finger amputated and his neck 'cleared of tubercular glands'; a student had haemorrhaged the previous week; and five children were developing gland trouble. 'The remainder of the pupils are all so sickly and look so weak.'[86] Tims urged the department to turn the school into a sanatorium with nursing care and a proper diet, because the church simply could not provide adequate care with its meagre grant. In April 1915 the department engaged an (Anglican) nurse to work at the school. By June she had resigned, to be replaced by nurse Agnes Hucomb, who was instructed to administer 'tubercular serum' or tuberculin to the children every week. Tuberculin was a preparation of tubercule bacilli that was believed to act in the same way as an anti-toxin or vaccination. It was purported to create immunity to the disease. Despite doubts about its worth and real concerns that it was in fact dangerous, American sanatoria employed it until the 1920s. The Canadian medical press considered it dangerous and experimental, and its use was never accepted in Canada.[87] As we shall see later, concerns about the spread of tuberculosis overrode any lingering doubts about the safety of anti-tuberculosis preparations for Aboriginal children.

With conditions so dire, the pay so low, and mismanagement so rife, the Sarcee school saw a veritable parade of nurses – eight in five years.

In November 1920, Dr F.A. Corbett examined the children. The findings of his report were now grotesquely familiar. The health of the students at the Sarcee boarding school was 'bad in the extreme.' All but four of the 33 students showed the presence of active tuberculosis; sixteen of them had open ulcers – 'foul sores' – and one child had haemorrhaged from the lungs. Corbett found a girl curled up on a filthy bed in a dirty, dilapidated room – the infirmary. The living conditions on the reserve itself were just as bad. In one house Corbett found an old man who was partially blind and suffering from chronic tuberculosis and a helpless woman lying on a dirty bed. In another house he found five children, all showing signs of tuberculosis. The mother had tuberculosis and the father had scrofula scars on his neck. Corbett urged that the school be closed and the building converted into a sanatorium with doctors and nurses in charge. Old Sun's school on the Blackfoot reserve was not much better. The children were 'below par in health and appearance,' and 70 per cent of the students had enlarged lymphatic glands of the neck. The building was overcrowded, with low ceilings and unvarnished floors. There was no infirmary, and although there were two small balconies, these were unavailable to students. Corbett recommended that the children sleep outdoors. The Sarcee and Old Sun's schools had been inspected in 1907, 1908, and 1909, and those inspections had found that all of the students in the Sarcee school, and thirty-four of thirty-five students at Old Sun's school, were suffering from tuberculosis. Six months before Corbett's inspection, the Anglican missionary society had alerted the department about the conditions at the Sarcee school and asked it to close the school and transfer the healthy children to another.[88] The missionary society suggested at that time that new heating systems be installed at the schools, and that the department consider the erection of a new residential school for the area reserves. Instead, the department renewed the grant to the missionary society. In light of Corbett's inspection, action was finally taken.

The school was renovated and part of it was converted into a small sanatorium. This had been Bryce's recommendation in 1909, but ever the accountant, superintendent Scott also proposed that more of the reserve be 'turned to cash' – that is, surrendered – to pay for the renovations. Corbett continued his annual inspection work and embarked on a wholesale removal of the children's tonsils and adenoids, which when infected were believed to be the precursor of scrofula. Indian commissioner William Graham reasoned that Corbett saved the department thousands of dollars every year, and 'we cannot be accused of neglecting the Indian children who are in our schools.' Graham, whose father had worked for the department, began as a clerk in 1885, became the agent at File Hills in 1897, and in 1918 was appointed commissioner for the prairie provinces. By the 1920s the Sarcee people were perceived as nearly beyond hope. A physician, Dr Thomas Murray, was appointed agent and doctor to the Sarcee reserve in 1921. In a sure sign that the department held out little hope for the people's recovery, Diamond Jenness, Canada's best-known anthropologist, was sent out to perform 'rescue anthropology' and document the Sarcee people's 'customs and beliefs' before they disappeared altogether. Jenness later stated that the Sarcee had lost their desire to 'recuperate, all ambition to stand on their feet in the economic world. So they are fast declining, and probably within another century this tribe will be no more.'[89] Finally, in 1921, the children with tuberculosis were isolated, given an improved diet, and provided with flush toilets: 'It was remarkable how quickly an improvement was visible.' After 1932, students no longer resided at the school, and with only a 'practical' nurse and cook in attendance, it was judged 'scarcely a hospital.'[90] The Sarcee school was not unusual, although the extent of disease may have been worse than at the Catholic schools, where medically trained nurses were available at little cost.

For nearly a century the Sarcee school and many others had been funded and encouraged by the department. That so many students did not survive the experiment was put down to their peculiar constitutions, the pagan influence of their homes, and their reluctance to embrace Christianity. Most of those who survived remember the schools with bitterness and pain.[91] The residential schools, a social experiment intended to 'Christianize and civilize,' succeeded only in incubating disease and spreading it throughout the reserves. While the Department of Indian Affairs did admit it had some responsibility for providing medical care to the schoolchildren, it refused to accept any obligation for the health of Aboriginal people on reserves. Nevertheless, a medical bureaucracy took root and grew.

Chapter Four

'Indifferent to Human Life and Suffering': Medical Care for Native People to 1920

The government may have agreed in Treaty Six to provide 'medicine chests,' but that promise was to be interpreted literally. The department consistently denied any obligation to provide medical care even while its own medical service grew. After 1880, almost in spite of itself, the department became increasingly involved in providing medical services to certain groups of Native people. The department's approach to deciding which groups should receive medical care changed over time, but general tendencies emerged. First, it was necessary to provide medical care in order to protect the department's pre-eminent institutions for social and cultural change, the government-funded schools; second, with increased immigration the department felt compelled to protect the non-Native community from disease; and third, the department recognized that by placing physicians near reserves it could accomplish its second objective while dispensing valuable government patronage. Thus, schoolchildren were given medical attention when rising death and disease rates threatened the effectiveness of the schools. And reserve residents received medical attention from carefully chosen physicians when contagious disease threatened to spread from reserves to towns. In keeping with the principle that the department was not responsible for the people's health, medical care was always given on an ad hoc basis. As late as 1946 the government was maintaining that 'neither law nor treaty imposes an obligation on the Dominion government to establish a health service for the Indians and Eskimos.'[1] That health status on reserves continued to decline despite a growing medical bureaucracy was variously explained by references to the people's race and their indifference to life. Government-funded medical care was largely ineffective because it was shaped and determined principally by the needs of non-Natives. For good reason, then, Aboriginal people approached the health care edifice cautiously and selectively.

Shortly after the western treaties were signed, a smallpox epidemic broke out in Manitoba that taught the department an important lesson: smallpox epidemics were expensive to control, dangerous to business, and preventable through vaccination. In November 1876, smallpox broke out at the recently founded Icelandic community at Gimli, on the western shore of Lake Winnipeg; from there it quickly spread to the Native communities at Sandy Bar. Dr J.S. Lynch was sent out to enforce a quarantine and stop any further spread. By February 1877 a Board of Health had been established. In hope of preventing a fresh outbreak in the spring, and the entire destruction for the year of the northern fur trade, the Hudson's Bay Company pushed for further measures. In October 1878 Dr D.W.J. Hagarty was appointed by Order-in-Council to the newly created position of medical superintendent of the Manitoba and North-West Superintendencies. Specifically, he had been hired to prevent another smallpox outbreak; if he failed, it would cost the government at least $13,000 for provisions, medicine, medical attendance, and quarantine. He was ordered to reside at Winnipeg and, for a salary of $1,800 per annum, to vaccinate all Native people in the Manitoba Superintendency. Hagarty's mission to vaccinate so many people scattered over such a large area was not successful. For instance, in the summer of 1879 he was able to vaccinate less than one-third of the people in the Qu'Appelle area because they were away hunting.[2] But a policy of vaccinating as many Native people as possible every spring continued well into the twentieth century.

Indian commissioner Edgar Dewdney could not justify the expense of a medical superintendent or the precedent of physicians on reserves. Dewdney was the most consistent advocate of the notion that Native people could and should become economically self-sufficient in three years after the treaties were signed.[3] Before 1885, Indian department policy had been grounded in the notion that once Native people embraced a sedentary agricultural life, 'civilization' would follow. Missionaries and schools would provide Christian instruction, and while Native people would always be a race apart, they might attain the lowest levels of Canadian national life. The department accepted that expenditures would be high initially, but also held that after two or three years of settled life on reserves bands should have attained self-sufficiency. The department's great fear was that by providing rations and materially aiding the people it might 'pauperize' them. Thus, the 'work for rations' policy was strictly enforced, even when many went hungry because there was little work to do. The work for rations policy meant also that there was little time or opportunity to acquire other necessities, such as clothing and housing. The policy was of course borne of parsimony; 'economy in all things' might have been the motto of the department. The justification was always that Native people must be brought to understand that self-sufficiency was the first step toward civilization. Self-sufficient Native communities could then provide their own medical care. Dewdney contended that the part-time services of NWMP surgeons Kittson, Miller, and Kennedy to vaccinate the people of Treaties Six and Seven at Fort Walsh and Cypress Hills were sufficient and that the position of medical superintendent was unnecessary. He added that if.it were not for the instructions he had seen inserted in some of the medicine chests, he would not have known of the existence of such an officer.[4]

Department policy created lethal living conditions and did more to prevent economic growth than to promote it. In 1881, chiefs from across the prairies had attempted to reach beyond the department to the governor general the Marquis of Lorne when he visited the west. Native representatives thought he must surely have the ear of the Queen, for he was married to one of her daughters. In careful presentations, the chiefs emphasized the need for food to keep their children alive, and for implements and oxen so they might grow their own food. Paksung, speaking for Chief Kakeesheeway from the Treaty Four area, stressed their desperation: 'The horses that have had the scab have been given to the children to eat. That is why there is sickness and they are weak and die ... Those chiefs here ask you to supply them with enough food. Those here wish that the Queen would open her storehouse to us.' Poundmaker urged the governor general to supply them with a reaper and mower: 'There is always much sickness on my reserve.' Red Pheasant admitted that he was unable to make his own living: 'I am too weak. I am like a child.' Button Chief of the Blood needed rations: 'Our children have been starving and many are dead.' The governor general listened to their requests and then, echoing the official line, lectured them on the virtues of hard work: 'I am sure that red men to the East when they work do well and do not starve and I have noticed that the men who talk most and ask most do not work.'[5] Native criticisms of the policy only confirmed for officials that they were correct in their estimation that Native people had to be forced to become self-sufficient.

After 1885, optimism began to fade. The protective, paternalistic

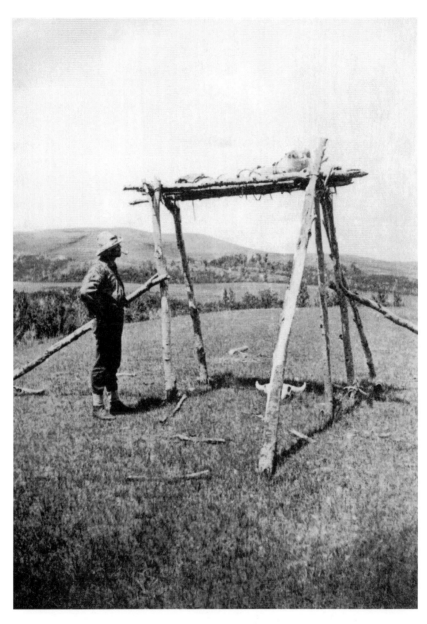

Blackfoot grave on a scaffold in the foothills, 1874. (Photo taken during international boundary survey.)

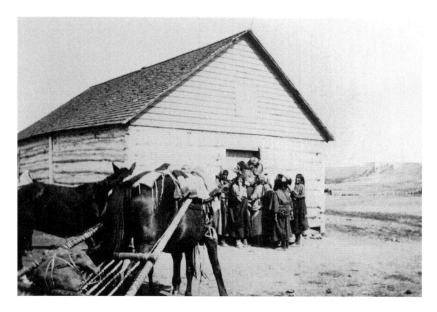

Women waiting at the Blood reserve ration house, 1897.

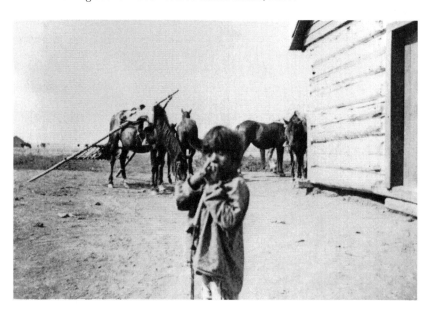

Young boy at the Blood reserve ration house, 1897.

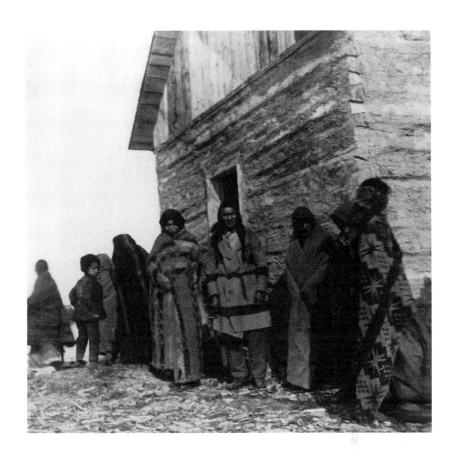

Stoney people at the reserve in Saskatchewan, c. 1900.

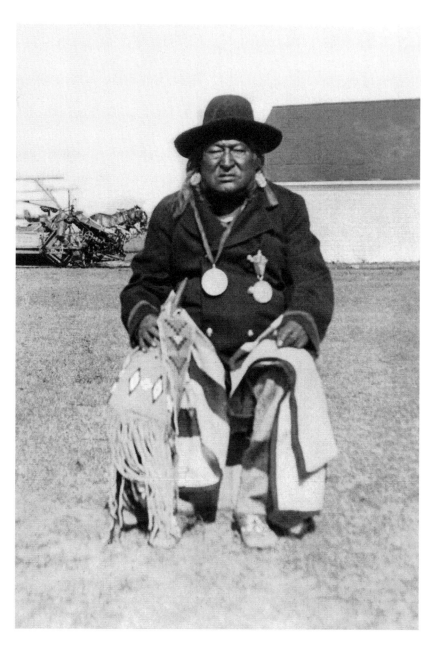

Blackfoot Old Woman, head chief, Blood reserve, c. 1905.

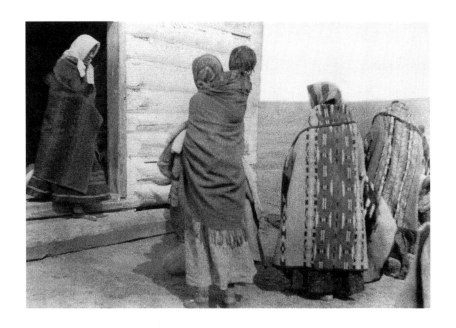

Ration issue (flour) at Upper Agency near Standoff, Alberta, Blood reserve, 1907.

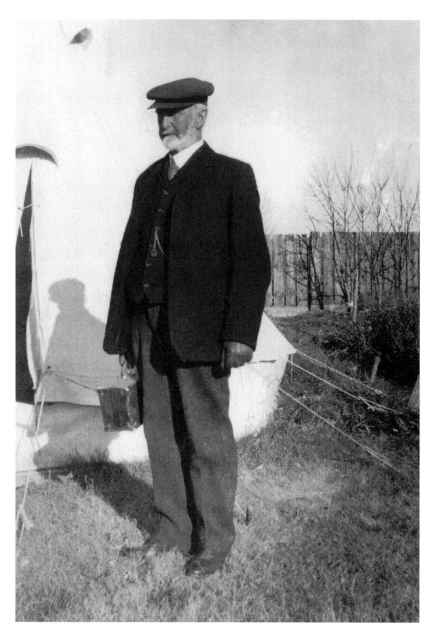

Dr O.C. Edwards at Standoff, Alberta, Blood reserve, October 1909.

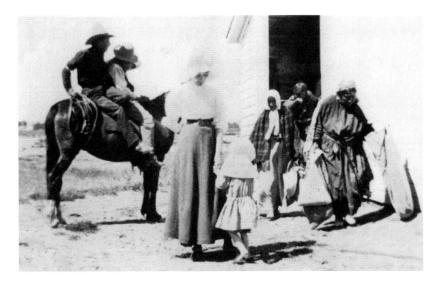

Claudia Gardiner (child, centre), who was Dr O.C. Edwards's granddaughter, and Miss Vaughan, the companion and household help, at Blood reserve ration house, 1911. Note the women's ration sacks.

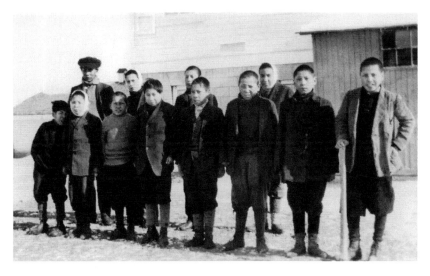

Boys on the Sarcee reserve, c. 1920. Note the bandages on some of the boys' heads, covering 'scrofula' sores.

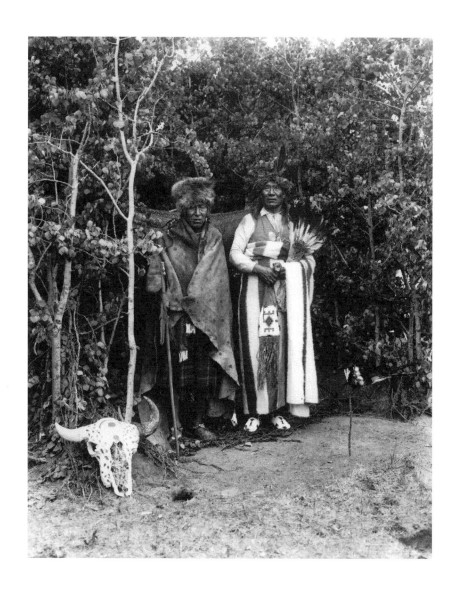

Blackfoot healers in the 1930s.

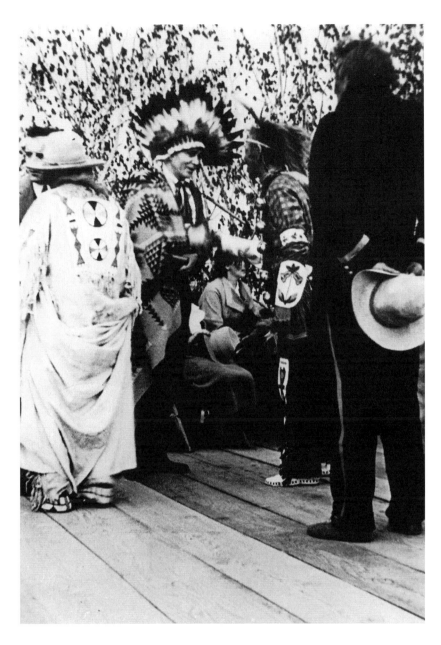

Dr R.G. Ferguson (centre) dressed in Aboriginal costume in the 1930s.

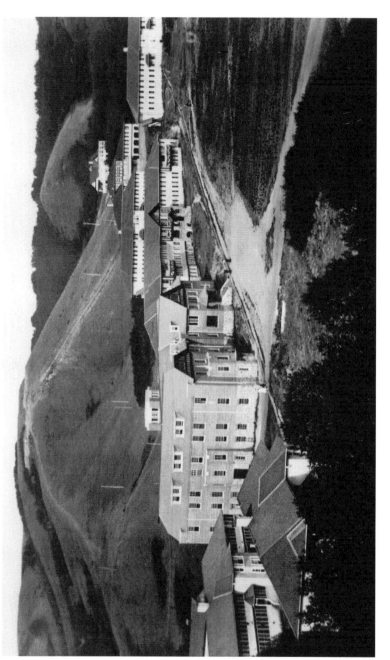

Provincial sanitorium (Fort San), Fort Qu'Appelle, Saskatchewan.

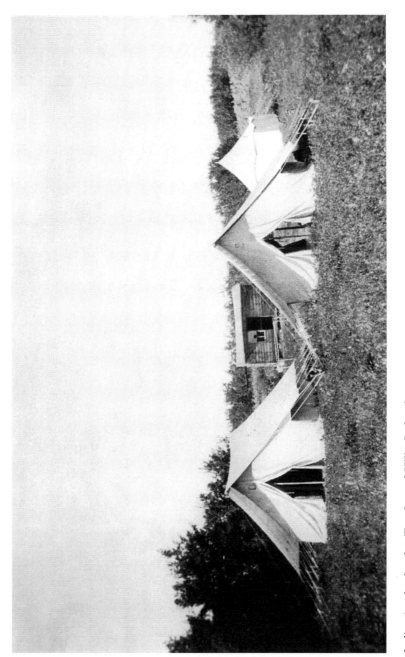

Indian 'sanitorium' at Touchwood Hills, Saskatchewan.

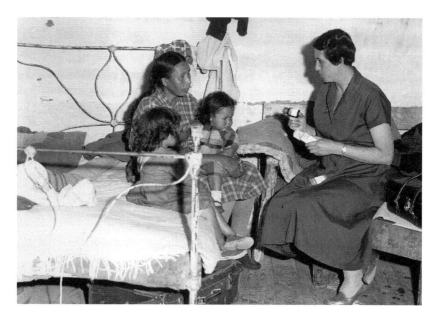

Native family with a public health nurse at Moosomin reserve, Saskatchewan, c. 1940s.

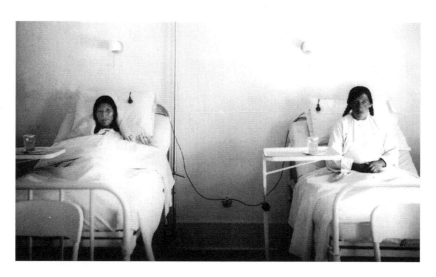

Patients in the new Blood hospital in the 1940s.

impulse of the 'white man's burden' quickly turned to coercion and repression as Aboriginal people generally were linked to the Riel Rebellion. Relations between department employees and the Native people grew strained. So-called rebels were denied rations and annuities. The people's poverty and poor health was no longer seen just as the benign working out of the evolutionary struggle; instead, it was a result of their own 'vicious practices.' In his annual report for 1886, Dewdney suggested that a large percentage of the sickness and death on reserves was 'directly due to hereditary disease, which had its origin at a time prior to that at which our responsibility began.' Agent J.J. Campbell of Treaty Four contended that the high death rates were the 'outcome of diseases, either inherited from their parents, or in the older ones brought with them from the Missouri as a result of former vicious practices. Their constitutions appear to be weakly and to have a consumptive tendency.' Later, Dewdney suggested that the death rate was perhaps not higher at all – it was just that better records were being kept.[6]

In 1886 the department was called to account in the House of Commons for its administrative record and to answer for the Riel Rebellion. In the always lively debate over supply, the Liberal MP from West Huron, Malcolm Cameron, strongly criticized the administration of the Indian department. He attacked all aspects of the department's administration and characterized the employees as a 'swarming army of carpet-baggers and camp followers.' Cameron charged that starvation on the reserves was the result of the government's cruel policy, which was intended to weaken the people into submission. His attack was certainly motivated by partisan concerns, as the department charged, but it also contained a few kernels of truth. Dewdney claimed that there was no starvation on reserves, when, as previously noted, there had been.[7] C.F. Ferguson, the Conservative MP from Leeds and a physician, rose in the House to defend the government.

Ferguson was perhaps typical of his kind: a loyal government member who hoped to benefit personally from territorial expansion. In order to settle the west in a rational way, the government had granted colonization companies the right to buy land in the west and encourage settlement. C.F. Ferguson and Associates was granted 30,720 acres and paid the initial instalment of $12,288 on land north and west of Fort Qu'Appelle. Among those who scrambled for the lucrative contracts were at least twenty-four other senators and elected representatives as well as several prominent businessmen. Companies paid as little as $1 an acre and could demand prices ranging from $3 to $15 per acre for the same lands when the colony's sections were fully occupied. Ferguson was also one of the directors of the Prince Albert Colonization Company, whose townships had been occupied for decades by the French-speaking Metis south of Prince Albert. The Prince Albert Colonization Company did not locate settlers on its lands, as it was required to do; instead it drove off existing settlers because it wanted to use its tracts for urban development in what was to be a major rail centre. The Prince Albert Colonization Company's methods have been linked to the outbreak of violence in the Riel Rebellion.[8] Ferguson's defence of the government continued. He informed the House that he had been present on the Blood reserve from June to October 1883 when Native people had indeed died (from contaminated rations); but, he argued, it was not the government rations that killed the people. Instead, Ferguson the physician explained that the people had a 'specially filthy habit' of placing their lodges too close together and not moving them to clean sites often enough. It was 'autumn fever or mountain fever' (he probably meant typhoid) that killed the people. Ferguson also noted that the adults suffered from chronic dyspepsia as a result of too much food and too little exercise. Dyspepsia, a synonym for indigestion, in the nineteenth century became a common diagnosis for patients who were guilty of some excessive behaviour, such as gluttony, or abusing alcohol, or masturbation. Ferguson also observed the children snaring gophers and assumed they did so for subsistence because their parents had starved them.[9] As a medical doctor, Ferguson's report carried some added influence, and his linking of typhoid to poor sanitation and living conditions pointed to some of the serious health risks on reserves. Notwithstanding all this, he personified the clear link between the ruling government party and the opportunities for personal profit in the new Canadian territories. His characterization of Aboriginal people as filthy and lazy and as unfit parents marked a significant retreat from the paternalistic optimism of treaty commissioners such as Alexander Morris.

While the Conservatives were defending themselves in Ottawa against charges that they had starved Aboriginal people, the NWMP had to deal with the half-starved people on the reserves, where rations and annuities had been suspended. Police inspector Cuthbert began distributing food and used clothing on Beardy's and One Arrow's reserves. He reported that one woman, without a coat, had walked ten miles to Duck Lake in below-zero weather to get a few pounds of flour from the farm instructor to feed her sick child. They had been subsisting on rabbits killed with a bow and arrow. Joseph Dion would recall that that same hungry winter, the women at the Frog Lake reserve raided mouse burrows for their caches of seeds and roots. Conditions improved when Indian department inspector Thomas Wadsworth arrived with a supply of food and clothing; but as Cuthbert noted to his superiors, the people were highly distrustful of department officials.[10]

The department was also receiving demands from immigrants in the west that something be done to protect their own health and safety. Petitioners from Prince Albert asked that Dr A.E. Porter of Prince Albert be appointed as a medical officer because the Native people 'often times [are] afflicted with very malignant diseases and not being able to procure for themselves proper medical attendance suffer great mortality in consequence ... Often, and at any time, they are afflicted with smallpox, scurvey [sic], typhus fever [sic] and other loathsome diseases owing to their domestic habits and manner of living.'[11] The petitioners especially feared the outbreak and spread of disease to their own settlements. For a number of reasons, the department was at first unwilling to entertain the notion of medical practitioners for reserves. It had provided medicine chests as stipulated in the treaty; the vaccination program was already in place to control smallpox; and diseases that could not be controlled by vaccination were not understood to be contagious, and therefore unlikely to spread.

Although the department insisted publicly that it bore no responsibility for medical services to Native people, it had already appointed a medical officer to Treaty Seven in present-day southern Alberta. Dr F.X. Girard was appointed in May 1883 to administer to the Blood, Blackfoot, Peigan, Stoney, and Sarcee people from his headquarters at Fort Macleod. By the late 1870s, Fort Macleod was recognized as the 'capital of the Canadian cattle kingdom.' The ranching industry and society that developed around Fort Macleod was led by a wealthy and politically powerful elite with close ties to Prime Minister John A. Macdonald's Conservatives, and in the early 1880s the town seemed destined to be a great metropolis.[12] Girard was most certainly a patronage appointment. Francis Xavier Girard, forty-two years old, was a resident of Longueuil, Quebec, and a friend of Hector Langevin, Minister of Public Works in Macdonald's cabinet. There were clear advantages to being the first, and only, physician in what was to become a hub of commerce. And it was made clear to deputy superintendent Lawrence Vankoughnet that Girard was to be employed by the department until he could establish a private practice. Dewdney objected to Girard's appointment immediately. His salary, $1,200 per annum plus expenses, was too high since it approached Hayter Reed's assistant commissioner's salary of $1,600. According to Dewdney, Girard should be required to reside on the Blood reserve to better serve the people; better yet, he should be dispensed with entirely. By 1885 Dewdney was arguing that since Treaty Seven had been divided into two distinct agencies, and farming instructors were in place to prescribe for the people, there was no need for a medical officer. Two years later Dewdney again pushed for Girard's dismissal on the grounds that he was 'very inefficient,' and that at the cost of $2,448 per annum for attendance at the Blood and Peigan reserves, he cost too much. Hector Langevin intervened, and Girard was kept on at a reduced salary of $800 per annum plus expenses.[13] Unfortunately, Fort Macleod did not live up to its early promise. Large-scale agricultural settlement was prevented by the exigencies of the cattle industry, which was based on large leases and open, unfenced pasture lands. Without settlement a private medical practice could not succeed. To his friend Langevin, Girard expressed his support for the farmers and his frustration at the 'monopoly exercised by lease-carriers.' By the 1890s, Calgary, with its transcontinental rail link, had eclipsed Fort Macleod as the centre of the ranching industry. Girard complained that his reduced salary could not support his large family, and that since he had built a large house at Fort Macleod he could hardly be expected to begin a private practice elsewhere. He could not live on less than $1,000 a year. Langevin again intervened, and Girard began receiving $1,000 per annum, plus living and travelling expenses when he was away from Fort Macleod.[14] It had become clear to Dewdney that Dr Girard and his salary would have to be borne by the department.

Girard's 'inefficiency' was hardly surprising. He did not speak the language and had little knowledge of the people who were to be his patients. His methods and medicines were neither understood nor trusted by the people. Inspector Wadsworth reckoned that Girard was doing the work 'as well as any doctor who was not likely to be removed.' When asked about Girard's visits to the reserve, Bull Shield 'sarcastically' pointed out that he travelled from Fort Macleod to the agency, then to the Catholic mission to visit with Fr Emile Legal, then back to Fort Macleod, without visiting any of the people's camps.[15] The average death rate on the Blood reserve for the first six years of Girard's attendance (1884–89) was 51 per thousand, while the average birth rate was 30.8 per thousand. In comparison, the death rate in Montreal in 1890 was half the Blood rate, at 26 per thousand; and in Winnipeg the death rate was 15.7 per thousand. Quebec City had the highest death rate among the twenty-nine largest Canadian cities, at 31.6 per thousand.[16] According to NWMP surgeon George Kennedy, the leading causes of death among the Blood people were 'consumption,' syphilis, diseases of infancy including 'atrophy and debility,' pulmonary diseases, convulsions, and bowel diseases: 'The birth rate is very small and the death rate very large and the majority of deaths are due to preventable causes.' Agent James Wilson on the Blackfoot reserve noted that Girard had never gained the confidence of the people. He would never visit the people in their homes and was therefore unaware of the early stages of serious illness. Girard visited the dispensary for one day every month and handed out prescriptions to all who presented themselves. Illness was either self-diagnosed or diagnosed by Native healers. Wilson understood why the people 'did a great deal of doctoring among themselves ... I cannot blame them much for this because in many cases it is their only way of getting treated early and continuously.'[17] Girard remained medical officer for seventeen years, until 1901.

Despite Dewdney's objections to Girard's work in particular, and the provision of medical services generally, Ottawa was finding itself pushed to amend policy. There was the need to be seen to be taking control of a politically embarrassing situation, as exemplified in Cameron's charges that the government was starving Native people in order to open lands to its friends. There were the fears among colonists that their health was in danger from the diseases on the reserves. There were the demands of the government's friends, who saw the west as a fruitful place to establish medical practices. And finally, there was the very real problem of the people's poor health. The providing of more physicians might answer all the problems at very little expense. As department inspector Wadsworth noted in his 1885 report on the Stoney people at Morley, the people should not suffer such high death rates when there were so many doctors in Calgary who were willing to work for very modest returns. Later that year, Dr Andrew Henderson of Calgary was engaged to attend the people in the northern part of Treaty Seven (Sarcee, Blackfoot, and Stoney). But the department recognized the difficulties and expense of another salaried medical officer like Girard, and instead offered Henderson the work on a fee-for-service basis at $1 per patient for advice and prescriptions, plus 50¢ travelling expenses. The department would control costs further by supplying all medicines the doctor might prescribe. Henderson balked at the low rate, arguing that he would have to give up his private practice, and pointing out 'the great loss of time with exposure and possible danger to life in consideration of a fee of fifty cents allowance.' But there were plenty of other doctors in Calgary willing to take the work, so Henderson agreed. Three years later, with only 68 acres under crop, and with game scarce, the Stoney people were suffering a death rate three times their birth rate.[18]

For all its efforts, the department's expenditures for medical attendance and medicines continued to increase throughout the 1880s. The expense was always entered in the departmental estimates as 'Supplies for the Destitute' – yet another indication that medical care was seen as an ad hoc expense. Between 1884 and 1900 the greatest share – 75 per cent – of the department's medical expenditures was paid out to physicians, most of whom worked on a fee-for-service basis. The remaining 25 per cent went to medicines and vaccines. In 1884, for example, 85 per cent of the total expenditure was paid out in salaries to Girard, three NWMP surgeons, and eight other physicians. More than half of that was paid to Girard and the NWMP surgeons; the eight civilian doctors earned an average annual income of less than $200 each (some doctors earned more than others, depending on when and where the department wanted vaccinations carried out, so Drs Potevin and Edwards earned more than $500, while Drs Dodd and Mackie each earned only $25). The remaining 15 per cent was spent on medicines and on preparing medicine chests. By 1890 the total expenditure on medicines and medical attendance had increased 77 per cent to nearly $14,000.[19] By 1889 the number of physicians had risen to thirty-one, and they had an average annual income of $345. Despite the increased expenditures, the death rates continued to rise and the population continued to fall.

High death rates were not the only reason, or even the primary reason, that the department was pushed to increase expenditures on medical care. The medical profession's need for work and the non-Native community's need for medical attendance also had a bearing on how and where expenditures were made. Representatives of isolated immigrant communities reckoned that without Indian department work, local doctors could not afford to establish practices in their villages. Thus, medical work for the department acted as a guarantee of medical care for the immigrant communities. Physicians received a dependable income from the department that allowed them to establish private practice in immigrant communities.[20] The rapidly increasing number of doctors employed by the department was in part a reflection of the needs of non-Native communities. As with most government appointments at the time, positions were granted on the strength of the candidate's ties to the ruling Conservatives. It was pointed out to Reed that Dr

Hugh Bain rather than Dr A.B. Stewart should be appointed medical attendant to the people at Prince Albert: 'You will save yourself a lot of trouble by having one of your own party at your back.' Besides, Bain gave prescriptions and directions to the agent, thereby saving the extra expense of follow-up visits; whereas Stewart expected to be called a second time if the patient did not improve. For the sake of controlling costs, even the process of calling a local doctor was centralized. Agents were required to get authorization from the commissioner's office before a doctor could be called to attend to patients: the inspector ordered the agent to wire the commissioner, who then ordered the doctor.[21] And only loyal Conservative doctors were trusted to toe the bureaucratic line and practise the strictest economy at all times.

The increased immigration of loyal Conservative doctors fed the increasing costs of the fee-for-service system. In the late 1880s, in response to rising costs, the department again began to hire physicians on a salary basis. When a small number of salaried medical officers were employed, costs were easily controlled and there was no danger of exceeding the year's estimates. Costs under the fee-for-service system were difficult to control or predict because it was left to the agent to decide when the doctor should be called. Department officials suspected that some of the agents were abusing the system. Unfortunately, abuses of another kind crept in when overzealous agents, attempting to economize, refused to call the doctor because 'on all reserves [there are] a few chronic cases where it would be useless to call in the services of a medical man.'[22] Again, the need to economize and distribute government patronage was dictating policy changes in the medical bureaucracy.

Dewdney's objections to providing medical services continued even after he was promoted to the position of superintendent general, or minister of the department, in 1888. Where the department employed a medical attendant, he noted, 'a great deal of sickness prevails,' and where there was no medical attendant, 'the Indians are free from sickness, and seem very contented.'[23] He compared reserves and found that the lowest death rates in the west in 1890 were among those with no medical attendance. At Montreal Lake in present-day northern Saskatchewan, the death rate was 16.09 per thousand; at Saddle Lake in northern Alberta it was 17.21; at Onion Lake it was 34.02. The highest death rates were among those who had the services of physicians: the Assiniboine (109.7), the File Hills people (147.5), and the Blood (52.9).[24] Dewdney's objections to medical services grew out of his conviction that the people must, whatever the barriers erected by his own department, attain self-sufficiency, and that medical attendance, rations, and agricultural aid would only foster pauperism and delay economic independence. Thus he saw pauperism as a significant cause of poor health. Relatively healthy reserves remained that way because they had no medical attendance. Of course, those on reserves with the lowest death rates had never depended on the bison economy and were still engaged in hunting and trapping; perhaps more significant, the department had only a shallow presence among them. The notion that medical services for Native people would lead to pauperism must be understood in the context of nineteenth-century Canadian society, in which few except paupers received government medical care. The Canadian state in the nineteenth century had established quarantine procedures at its ports of entry, and provided medical care for its military; other than that, it did not accept responsibility for medical care for very many Canadians. Boards of health, if they existed, were a municipal responsibility. But as immigration increased, concerns grew that Canada would become swamped by the physically (and morally) unfit. The medical inspection of immigrants (especially non-British immigrants) and deportation of the unfit were seen as vital for the preservation of Canada's national character. Thus the state did increasingly, and selectively, take responsibility for public health. Moreover, Dewdney's opposition to medical services suggests he may have had a rather low opinion of the medical profession and its ability to effect change. Thus he continued to maintain that medical aid was not a department responsibility – that indeed it was both harmful and expensive.

Nevertheless, missionaries were actively encouraged to provide medical care on reserves. As was noted earlier, missionaries established cottage hospitals in order to extend their proselytizing reach from schoolchildren to their parents. The department supported missionary efforts, which allowed departmental expenses to remain minimal and predictable. When in 1890 Dr George Orton in Manitoba suggested that the department rent office space and a room in Selkirk where urgent patients could be treated, he was told that such an establishment would set a dangerous precedent. The department would then have to establish a hospital and would be expected to provide food, clothing, light, and heat, 'so that these temporary hospitals would gradually develop in[to] permanent ones, and entail an expense upon the department which would be enormous.' Indian commissioner Hayter Reed suggested that the Native people were actually better off than most settlers, and that 'the more we pander to the wishes of these people, where they can help themselves, the harder will it be to make them self-dependent.'[25] Reed's suggestion that the Native people were better off than most settlers needs consideration. Native people were constrained in their economic pursuits by their status as wards of the state. Although Native farmers were aided with tools, implements, cattle, and seed as treaty entitlements, these were generally issued 'once and for all' in the late 1870s, and there were consistent problems in the delivery of those items. For both Native and non-Native farmers, the pioneering experience in the 1880s was difficult. But non-Native homesteaders had the option of leaving an unproductive homestead and trying somewhere else. By clause 70 of the Indian Act, Aboriginal people were barred from taking homesteads in areas with better soil conditions or that were closer to the railway. Native farmers were also constrained in their development by the pass and permit systems. The pass system attempted to limit the movements of Native people. As well, the sale of produce from reserves required a permit from the agent. Non-Native settlers complained loudly about what they considered subsidized competition from Aboriginal farmers, and it was an easy matter for officials to refuse permits.[26] Moreover, reserve lands were not owned by the people but by the Crown; thus, farmers who wanted to mortgage reserve land to buy machinery were prevented from doing so by the Indian Act.[27] The paternalism and coercion embodied in the Indian Act allowed that Native farmers should receive certain advantages such as aid from the government; but the disadvantages, such as limits on their physical and economic freedom, outweighed any advantages.

It is hardly surprising that the mission hospitals and the salaried physicians had negligible impact on the health of Native people. The department's practice of hiring salaried medical officers had created among them the impression – an accurate one – that the doctor was another government employee, and a part of the same bureaucracy that sought to remake them through repressive ration policies and religious persecution. As Frantz Fanon noted in the context of colonialism and medicine, 'going to see the doctor, the administrator, the constable or the mayor [became] identical moves.'[28] Cottage hospitals were underfunded, and the missionaries often had their gaze trained on the next world. More importantly, the underlying cause of the people's ill health – their poverty – served to undermine the most conscientious medical attendant. The people's poverty was systemic and rooted in the department's conception of them as indolent paupers whose problems would only be exacerbated by economic aid. The apparent anomaly of steadily increasing medical costs and consistently high death rates was explained, in the department's estimation, by the notion that the people were in a difficult transition from the wild to the civilized state. Continued poverty and reliance on government rations was also associated with the people's desire to persist in their ceremonial dancing.[29] Thus, according to those who administered their affairs, Native people suffered so greatly from disease not primarily because of their poverty, but because they were making the necessary but difficult transition from savagery to civilization.

In 1889, Hayter Reed implemented a policy of 'peasant farming' for Native people as an integral step from savagery to civilization. Reed reasoned that Native farmers should not attempt to make the leap from hunters to commercial farmers in a decade when natural evolution suggested that the process took centuries to complete. Labour-saving machinery might be necessary for their non-Native neighbours to farm the prairies, but Aboriginal farmers would have to make do with hoes and rakes and only as much land as could be worked with hand tools. The so-called 'stages of civilization' could not be disregarded: 'The fact is often overlooked, that these Indians who, a few years ago, were roaming savages, have been suddenly brought into contact with a civilization which has been the growth of centuries. An ambition has thus been created to emulate in a day what white men have become fitted for through the slow progress of generations.'[30] In the same vein, the people's poor health was the physical manifestation of this transition through the stages of civilization. Since nothing as precious as Anglo-Saxon Christianity was easily won, Reed suggested that disease and death were a sort of penance that must be paid. Missionaries such as John Maclean tended to agree that the high cost of Native lives was a necessary or at least a predictable result of the struggle for civilization, during which 'like the wild caged birds, they sicken and die.'[31] Reed viewed the costs of running the department – especially expenses under the category 'Supplies for the Destitute' – as a barometer for measuring progress. According to him, high morbidity rates on reserves were what kept department expenditures so high, because the sick received rations without performing any work and were thus a double liability. In 1890, after two years as commissioner, Reed still had not reduced expenditures as greatly as he had hoped, because, as he said, of the existence of a considerable number of aged and infirm: 'Until these die out they must remain a charge on the government.' In 1891 the department made plans to reduce the estimates by 30 per cent because a good crop 'should have been procured.'[32] Native people's poverty was thus viewed as a consequence of their race and its struggle. Christianity and civilization were held out as the paths to good health, and would keep Aboriginal people from melting away 'as the snow before the sun.'

This logic – that the people's race caused indolence and thus poverty and ill health, so tight economic controls were necessary to counter indolence – was clearly being applied on reserves in the 1890s. Farm instructor S. Stewart Hockley, whose wife was paid to impart domestic science at the Muscowpetung agency in Treaty Four, typified this view: 'It is well known how difficult they [Aboriginal women] are to deal with being so generally indolent, improvident and naturally of dirty habits ... Her [Mrs Hockley's] influence would be greater had the Indians means to build better houses, for it is hard for them to be neat and tidy housewives in a 7 by 9 foot log hut without a floor, and where the whole family live, cook, eat, sleep, and use it as a nursery.'[33] The leaders of the Muscowpetung agency did not see it that way. They sent a petition to the House of Commons closely outlining their economic conditions and the barriers to progress. The petition charged that the agent was interfering with their business transactions. They were supporting themselves by selling dry wood because the department would not allow them to sell green wood, and their supply was nearly exhausted. For wood sold to settlers, the agent paid them in beef heads – minus the tongues, for fear they would be used in the Thirst Dance celebrations. They needed binders to thresh their grain, and because hand cradles were too slow, the grain often froze in the fields. Binders had been forbidden by the commissioner under the peasant farming policy because 'it would make the young men lazy.' When they performed work, they received only food and clothes, articles 'rightfully belonging to us by treaty.' The beef they received was 'poor starved beef which is not good food for ourselves or our families.' They complained that hay and timber taken from the reserves for government use were never paid for. They were forced to go into debt for food, and their annuity money was spent long before payments were made.[34] Reed denied the petition's charge that the agent had interfered between Native sellers and non-Native buyers, but, he explained, the Indian Act and the permit system prevented the purchase of produce from the reserve without the department's consent. Food and clothing had never been promised in the treaties; the policy was that aid would be extended to the point where the people could help themselves 'and no further.' The beef rations were likely 'too good,' and the people were being pampered. In the meantime, a departmental circular was sent to all agents emphasizing the necessity for cleanliness, ventilation, the removal of all garbage, and vaccination against smallpox.[35]

The crude living conditions persisted, and the agent was advised not to allow any 'real hardship.' In 1893 the population of Muscowpetung agency was 498. There were 23 births and 32 deaths; 23 of the dead were children. The following year there were 18 births and 42 deaths; 27 of the dead were children.[36] In 1895 Dr Seymour judged that the people's health had improved somewhat through a general improvement in living conditions, and because they no longer relied on their old methods of treatment. Instead they went to him, where 'acute disease which might have laid the foundation of consumption, is thus cured.' Seymour reported that he was able to keep the consumptives alive and well enough to work. Despite his claim that the people no longer used their own healing methods, he implored the department to stop the annual Sun Dances 'as they are the cause of a great deal of harm both morally and physically.' According to Seymour, high infant mortality was caused by poor infant feeding and the people's refusal to use cow's milk. (Of course, milk from tubercular cows was one of the chief vectors of tuberculosis transmission at the time.) Hereditary weakness caused by intermarriage, marriage at a young age, and marriage between the tubercular resulted in the overall weakening of the group. The cure, according to Seymour, was 'rapid civilization,' or the complete repression of Native ceremonialism, culture, and language.[37]

Likewise, the Stoney people of Morley and Stoney Plain in Alberta demanded some control over their farm produce so they might stop the haemorrhage of human lives. In 1894 the Stoney people registered 13 births in a population of 573, and 29 deaths; 24 of the dead were children. They petitioned the government for control over one-third of their farm produce, control over when and where their cattle were sold, and control over one-third of the proceeds. They demanded the right to sell firewood, fence rails, and house logs. They wanted the right to grist settlers' flour and share the proceeds among the families on the reserve. They asked for training in making shingles and building homes, and for help in finding work for the reserve's young men. Reed replied that 'in the interests of the Indians themselves,' it would not be possible for the Native people to retain one-third control of their farm produce. The people were already allowed to sell firewood and fence rails, he said, but only to other Native people or the department, not to anyone else. Again, the people were allowed to grist the settlers' grain, but the toll must be invested, not distributed 'and practically frittered away in the manner suggested.'[38]

Economic conditions at the Blackfoot reserve were equally troublesome. At a meeting held with inspector Alex McGibbon, the Blackfoot chiefs cited poor living conditions as the cause of the high death and disease rates on the reserve. The chiefs insisted that economic development would improve the situation. They demanded that workers be paid in cash at competitive rates, instead of in poor-quality beef. Weasel Calf blamed the quality and quantity of the food for the large number of deaths on the reserve. He demanded more tools and implements because his people had no cash to buy them, and declared that the prices paid by the department for hay and coal were insufficient: 'We work for nothing and make no progress.' White Eagle added that the department was wrong to pay them in tea and tobacco for the coal they mined and hauled. 'Don't do as others seem to do,' he warned McGibbon, 'and lose our speeches in your notebook, but publish them.' Iron Shield accused department officials of taking the profit on hay and coal sold from the agency, while the people received only beef and flour rations. Little Axe wanted to receive the full amount for cattle he sold and a set of scales for weighing hay sold in Calgary. Wolf Cutter wanted permission to buy a mower and rake, for which he and twelve others had each subscribed $100. Others expressed concerns about the mission schools, and about the suppression of the Sun Dance, and reiterated the band's desire to have Reverend Tims removed from the reserve. McGibbon recommended that the department provide some lumber for floors, duck for lodges, wagons, harnesses, a hay scale, and a cookstove for Chief Running Rabbit. Although he thought the rations ample, he told the agent to increase them a little.[39]

Petitions and complaints were rarely acted upon. Reed was convinced that the people were unwilling to do anything for themselves; for him, their demands for aid were clear proof of it. The evolutionary struggle was probably unfolding as it should. But in early 1895 Reed, aware of an impending election, was anxious for some evidence of 'progress' to show for his years of work. Medical attendance was available to most who wanted it, he reasoned, and the department supplied medicines and hospital treatment when recommended. Missionaries and agents had assured him that the Sun and Thirst Dances were losing influence.

Reed solicited opinions from the government physicians 'as to what extent, in the young ... constitutional troubles [are] diminishing, owing to our efforts generally to counteract their growth, and if on the decrease what, in his opinion, are the most powerful Agencies [*sic*] tending to this end.'[40] The question was designed with a definite answer in mind.

Dr A.B. Stewart, who only recently had won the concession to treat the people at Duck Lake in Treaty Six from his rival Dr Hugh Bain, suggested that chronic ailments were decreasing and confined to certain families with 'bad' histories; improvements were 'mainly due to the efforts put forth by the department and their employees to better the Indian's mode of living.' A number of doctors pointed out that syphilis was definitely on the wane. But as Dr George Orton had explained some years earlier, syphilis was rarely a problem with the people he had treated. Dr F.X. Girard at the Blood reserve informed Reed that syphilis acted on the constitution and, he reckoned, it eventually 'developed into scrofula, tuberculosis causing consumption.' The supposed low moral habits of the Native peoples had made the diagnosis of syphilis both obvious and reassuring. Generally, the department physicians blamed the Native people's poor health on their 'mode of living.' Worse yet, according to physicians, the people chose not to use their medical services. The Blackfoot, Blood, Stoney, and Sarcee people were getting progressively weaker. Girard reported that consumption and scrofula were the two most frequent causes of death. They could only afford to buy new clothing after their annuity payments, and they lived in homes that were 'too small, too low, overcrowded, imperfectly ventilated.' Their scrofula was caused by unwholesome food, uncleanliness, and lack of air and light. He was quick to note that by stating unwholesome food 'be it understood that I do not condemn the articles used as food (they are first quality beef and flour) but its mode of cooking.' Girard suggested that the department should use measures to '*compel* [his emphasis] the Indians' to seek his aid.[41]

Dr Neville Lindsay of Calgary, referring to the Sarcee people, contended that the high incidence of scrofula was the result of poor nutrition, and that pulmonary tuberculosis was caused by 'irregularity in dieting, insufficient clothing, want of cleanliness, syphilitic poisoning and scrofula.' In 1895 the Sarcee people had lost 40 of their 224 people, or nearly 18 per cent of the population, mainly through tuberculosis, and though twelve children were born, twelve died. Agent Samuel Lucas thought neglect was the main cause: 'During illness the Sarcees have more faith in their own medicine men and conjurers than in the physician, even when they do accept the aid of a doctor, they do not follow his instructions.' Lindsay noted that the cause of the high death rate was poor food and insufficient clothing, and that it was not uncommon to find ten to fifteen people living in a one-room house. Also, 85 per cent of the people lived on government rations of beef and flour, which were distributed every three days. According to Lindsay the most common causes of death, in order of importance, were scrofula, consumption, hemoptysis (coughing blood from the respiratory tract), and sore eyes. The people only consented to his care as a last resort, after their own healers had given up all hope.[42]

Dr Thomas Patrick of Yorkton in present-day eastern Saskatchewan was rather more candid in his reply. He reported that the increase of disease had been rapid. An examination of children at Crowstand school on the Swan River agency revealed that 65 per cent were afflicted with tuberculosis. Only nine of the twenty-six students could come close to passing a life insurance exam. Tuberculosis was the only constitutional disease affecting the people. The medical care he was able to give was perfunctory. He was allowed to vaccinate and visit the reserve only when a number of serious cases developed and only when the agent was notified. 'Death,' Patrick continued, 'has been the most potent factor in lessening the number of constitutional diseases.' Patrick, who had just begun work with the department, seemed to be suggesting that the people's poor health could be tied to department policy rather than to their 'mode of living.' But medical opinion was nearly unanimous that the people's ill health was caused by their peculiar mode of living. Reed was assured that the cure – the department's policies to improve and elevate Aboriginal people through peasant farming, work for rations, and rapid civilization – would be successful even though it might take time to work. In the meantime, death rates on reserves remained dangerously high. Patrick, along with nine other doctors, including Lindsay and Bain of Prince Albert, were dropped by the department after the Liberals won the 1896 election.[43]

The Liberal prime minister, Wilfrid Laurier, appointed Clifford Sifton as both Minister of the Interior and Superintendent General of Indian Affairs. Sifton began by overhauling the Department of Indian Affairs. He cut expenditures, moved the commissioner's office from Regina to Winnipeg, and embarked on further centralization of the department in Ottawa. Reed, as deputy superintendent general, had little reason to think he would be replaced, but Sifton placed the Department of the

Interior and Indian Affairs under one deputy minister. Deputies Reed
and A.M. Burgess of the Department of the Interior were dismissed in
1897 over the objections of both the cabinet and the governor general.[44] Amédée Forget was succeeded as commissioner by sixty-three-
year-old Liberal David Laird (who had negotiated Treaty Seven), thus
ending the Conservatives' reign as designers of Canadian policy for
Native people. In 1903 Clifford Sifton addressed the House of Commons on the 'difficult question' of medical attendance for Native people: 'You never can satisfy Indians that they are being properly attended
to medically. The more medical attendance that is provided the more
they want ... As honourable gentlemen can see the tendency is towards
growth in the expenditure for medical attendance.' Earlier that year the
department had received a report showing that Native people were not
experiencing low birth rates, but rather high death rates. Manitoba
inspector J.A. Macrae made a statistical comparison of eastern-Canadian
Native and non-Native birth and death rates. He reported that birth
rates among Native people were higher than among non-Native Canadians, but that the Native death rate was nearly twice the non-Native rate.
The report concluded that the areas with the lowest per capita costs for
medical attendance also recorded the most favourable births-over-
deaths ratios.[45] A logical conclusion was that Aboriginal communities
would increase, given some aid in reducing death rates. As well, medical
attendance as it was then conceived did not appear to meet that end. Sifton concluded, however, that medical attendance in the form of physicians as salaried employees, or on a fee-for-service basis, was the correct
policy. To control costs and improve efficiency, it was only necessary to
provide effective management of those physicians.

The following year, 1904, Sifton appointed Dr Peter Bryce, most
recently secretary of the Ontario Board of Health, as the department's
chief medical officer. In some ways Bryce represented a new direction
for the department. Bryce once noted that 1882 was a remarkable year
because Koch discovered the tuberculosis germ, Pasteur proved the efficacy of vaccination for anthrax in sheep, and the Ontario government
established the first permanent board of health. Bryce was a product of
the new science of bacteriology. As secretary of the Ontario Board of
Health, he was in the forefront of the Canadian public health movement, which had only recently dropped its preoccupation with sanitation to target specific groups in society that could benefit from specific
measures such as diphtheria anti-toxin. He was actively involved in both
American and Canadian anti-tuberculosis associations. Bryce was also

the most prominent member of the Canadian Purity Education Association, a group of doctors who advocated 'social hygiene' or moral reform using the language of science and medicine. The public health movement generally, and Bryce in particular, eventually focused on the inspection and promotion of health among schoolchildren.[46] His appointment was in other ways a continuation of department policy. The position of chief medical officer for the department was only a part-time appointment. At the same time he was also the medical inspector for the Department of the Interior and responsible for the medical inspection of immigrants during Canada's massive wave of immigration. Two-thirds of his $3,200 salary, and two-thirds of his time, was charged to the Department of the Interior.

As chief medical officer for the Department of Indian Affairs, all that Bryce had time to do was supervise his underlings and control the costs of their work. He attempted to compile a nosology but was regularly frustrated by physicians who reported sporadically or not at all. In his report for 1905, Bryce noted that there 'does not seem to have existed hitherto in most instances any idea on the part of medical officers that the duties of their appointment included such as are generally expected of municipal medical officers and sanitary inspectors.' His exuberant struggle to refashion the medical work into a proper public health administration was rarely appreciated by either physicians or his superiors. As chief medical officer of the Indian department, he was expected to 'take a tour of inspection and endeavour to improve the medical attendance and sanitary arrangements of the various Indian reserves.' The greatest need, according to Sifton, was to have a knowledgeable medical man to supervise the various medical officers in the department's employ.[47] Experience had shown that agents and inspectors lacked the necessary medical knowledge to judge whether a medical officer was fulfilling his duties. However, it would be some time before Bryce could begin his inspection, explained Sifton, because of the press of work at the Department of the Interior.

Few people, except possibly the medical officers themselves, could argue that the system of medical attendance was effective. Agent Robert N. Wilson at the Blood and Peigan reserves had reported three years earlier that the system of medical attendance was 'deplorable.' In the previous two months ten deaths had been recorded, nine of them children, and at least two children were dying without medical aid. The medical officer, Dr Girard, had examined two seriously ill school girls and pronounced them thin and weak but not dangerously ill. Both died within

two weeks. In his own defence, Girard suggested that the 'shadowy medicine man' was to blame for the large number of deaths on the reserves.
It had been proposed that the work of Native healers be legislated
against, but the experience of trying to stop the Sun and Thirst Dances
suggested to agents in the field that such legislation would be terribly difficult to enforce. Even if there were no Native doctors, explained Wilson,
the existing medical service would still be a dismal failure. Unless the
department was prepared to substitute an efficient system, 'the proposed
legislation would have been a blunder, attributed by the Indians to our
desire to exterminate them.' Wilson conceded that the people were
attached to their own healers because they were often successful in treating disease, while many Native people died while taking 'white man's
medicine.' What was needed, advised Wilson, was a medical officer who
would become a member of the community: 'Such a man, living on the
reserve and working continually among the Indians, even if possessed of
only moderate professional ability, would soon acquire their confidence,
the present disgraceful rate of mortality would be greatly reduced.' The
'medicine man' could then be diplomatically suppressed.[48]

There were problems throughout the service. Agent R.I. Ashdown
at Qu'Appelle reported that the officially appointed doctor resided too
far from the reserves to be of any use. It took Dr E.C. Carthew of
Qu'Appelle two to three days to travel the eighty miles to Touchwood
Hills and its two large boarding schools. The same doctor was also
responsible for the File Hills reserve and its boarding school, forty miles
away. In an emergency, nearby doctors were called in any case.
Carthew's regular visits every six weeks were less than effective, Ashdown
claimed, and the department was not getting value for its expenditure
of an $800 salary. Moreover, the people did not benefit from Carthew's
flying visits to their encampments: 'If the Indian happens to be home,
the doctor might see him. If the Indian is at work, the doctor will probably not see him, but he will invariably report the health of all is good.'
With two towns on the rail line within twelve miles of the agency, it
would be more economical and more effective to hire a doctor who
lived closer. Carthew was not pleased with the situation either. He complained that at an annual salary of $800 he was being seriously under-
paid. The department could either accept his offer to continue the work
at $1,500 per year, or accept his resignation. The department's new dep-
uty, Frank Pedley, eagerly accepted Carthew's resignation and hired a
local physician on an ad hoc basis for $8 per day.[49] The system of medi-
cal attendance remained unchanged. As settler communities that were

able to attract and keep physicians grew up around reserves, the services of medical officers were dispensed with and local practitioners were engaged to respond to emergencies.

The notion that Aboriginal people were doomed to extinction – that they were incapable of making the transition from nomadism to settled agriculturalism – had been aired from time to time since the treaties were first signed. In 1903 commissioner Laird reported that the mortality in some bands was so great that they 'must at no distant day become nearly extinct.' He asked the question that must have occupied many eastern bureaucrats who were unfamiliar with reserve conditions: Why was mortality so high when 'they are better clad and housed than formerly, good doctors are in attendance, and sanitary precautions are being increased'? The answer he provided was by now familiar. It was to be found in the moral failings of the people, their practices of wife desertion, bigamy, and intemperance, and their much higher birth rate compared with non-Native communities. How it was that a high birth rate contributed to increased mortality was left to the imagination. In his report for 1904, deputy superintendent Pedley contended that the people were not in fact 'doomed to extinction,' but did so in a way that did little to dispel the perception. Was there something, he asked, an 'inherent defect, whether mental, moral or physical, in the Indian's constitution to prevent successful direction of the forces by which he maintained himself in his original environment, into channels which will enable him to survive in the struggle for existence under civilized conditions?' Some 'tribes,' he admitted, seemed to have 'something endemic in their constitution which suggests their ultimate disappearance unless it can be discovered and remedied.' Education and protection from exposure to civilization and its vices had saved the people in eastern Canada from destruction. But ultimately, Pedley continued, it was the transition from nomadism to civilization, from the 'wigwam to small, overcrowded, dark, and ill-ventilated houses' that accounted for the people's ill health. Those who had improved their diet, dress, dwellings, and personal habits had reduced their mortality. Large losses were incurred by those who continued to 'cling to their potlatches,' where they crowded together in a way that was most unsanitary.[50] The Liberals also blamed the paternalism of the previous Conservative administration for the people's continued poor living conditions.

Pedley announced in 1904 that parliamentary appropriations for relief had been pared down by $20,000. The rigours of civilization that had impoverished the people were now expected to set them free.

Rations were issued only to the old and infirm. The practice of paying for work in food instead of cash was discontinued. An end to both the ration policy and active support for agriculture forced many Native people into wage labour. It also increased the pressure on bands to surrender portions of their reserves in order to generate income and economic opportunity. Although reserve farms atrophied during the early twentieth century, income from farm produce continued to contribute the majority of total reserve incomes (Tables 4.1 – 4.6).[51]

Attempts to abolish the reserves were nothing new. As part of the peasant farming policy, commissioner Reed had announced in 1888 that reserves in the North-West would be subdivided into farms for individuals. Small plots of land worked by self-sufficient family units would undercut the 'tribal' system and impel the people toward civilization.[52] Many reserves in Treaties Four and Six were subdivided in the 1890s. Bands objected to the surveys of their lands, believing them to be a first step toward surrender. Settlers and land agents became increasingly voluble proponents of land surrenders after the 1890s. The lands held in reserve were considered too large for the people's needs; it was thought they would be put to more profitable use by 'actual settlers.' Also driving the move toward land surrenders and land sales was the department's desire to decrease expenditures for medical attendance and aid for the destitute. In a fine example of putting the cart before the horse, the department claimed that the people's increased prosperity was the direct result of the end of the ration policy. The saving to the department was said to be only 'an incident of the policy.' The true aim of the policy, it declared, was the 'development of a spirit of self-reliance in the Indian which will eventually make him a self-supporting citizen of the country.' By 1928 over 100,000 hectares had been surrendered to the Crown for sale in southern Saskatchewan alone.[53] Arguments in favour of surrender revolved around the size of the reserves and the amount of 'unused' land. This 'idle' land, proponents argued, blocked development of the whole region. Reserve populations across the prairies had dropped perilously since the reserves had been established at the rate of one square mile for every family of five. Perhaps the perception that the race was dying or doomed to extinction eased the collective conscience. In any case, it was clear to those who coveted the land that there was excess land for the number of occupants.

Ironically, land surrenders were usually presented to the bands as a means to enable them to farm successfully. They needed machinery, implements, and livestock, and land sales would raise the money to buy

TABLE 4.1
Battleford Agency, 1900–1920: Sources of Income and Per Capita Income ($)

	1900	1905	1910	1915	1917	1920
Farm	29,356	30,916	25,401	58,773	57,432	85,343
Wages	1,510	3,175	6,532	11,986	15,972	19,175
Rents	29,350	29,350	2,716	29,350	4,907	17,180
Hunt/trap	1,450	7,359	1,716	10,270	18,256	13,150
Other*	1,950	8,260	3,508	11,145	11,406	3,200
Interest	29,350	29,350	29,350	7,030	8,695	11,710
Total	34,266	49,710	39,873	99,204	116,668	149,758
Per capita	42.46	56.11	43.11	108.18	120.52	142.08

*'Other' refers to income earned from sale of dry wood, senega root, etc.
Source: CHC, Sessional Papers, 1900–1922.

TABLE 4.2
Blackfoot Agency, 1900–1920: Sources of Income and Per Capita Income ($)

	1900	1905	1910	1915	1917	1920
Farm	4,368	12,822	37,000	78,061	143,930	214,491
Wages	7,400	7,000	13,000	15,000	15,000	10,000
Rents	21,840	21,840	21,840	21,840	21,840	89,567
Hunt/trap	22.530	21,840	1,050	124,600	1,590	124,325
Other*	9,550	10,000	200,000	25,000	20,000	25,000
Interest	21,840	21,840	21,840	6,116	11,348	46,719
Total	21,848	29,822	251,050	124,777	191,868	386,462
Per capita	22.18	37.14	327.31	170.69	266.85	555.54

*'Other' refers to income earned from sale of dry wood, senega root, etc.
Source: CHC, Sessional Papers, 1900–1922.

these things. There was also a glaring need for better housing, food, and clothing, and this in itself struck a receptive chord in many bands. An amendment to the Indian Act in 1906 allowed for up to one-half of the proceeds from land sales to be paid out directly to band members – a further inducement to those who had spent too many years surrounded by poverty, disease, and premature death. Pedley made the connection quite clear to agent W. Julius Hyde of the Blood reserve: the department's policy was that none who could support themselves should receive rations. Furthermore, while it was not government policy to

TABLE 4.3
Crooked Lakes Agency, 1900–1920: Sources of Income and Per Capita Income ($)

	1900	1905	1910	1915	1917	1920
Farm	4,556	16,337	23,793	36,732	67,716	138,229
Wages	10,150	10,342	3,000	4,000	4,800	17,640
Rents	60,240	60,240	5,730	60,240	11,588	138,220
Hunt/trap	10,600	3,366	2,550	2,850	2,600	6,000
Other*	5,191	8,135	8,210	8,366	9,000	138,220
Interest	60,240	60,240	60,240	8,299	12,672	29,465
Total	10,497	28,180	43,283	60,247	108,376	191,334
Per capita	18.19	52.77	75.53	101.25	174.80	296.18

*'Other' refers to income earned from sale of dry wood, senega root, etc.
Source: CHC, Sessional Papers, 1900–1922.

TABLE 4.4
Edmonton Agency, 1900–1920: Sources of Income and Per Capita Income ($)

	1900	1905	1910	1915	1917	1920
Farm	2,880	13,700	36,013	46,198	95,042	75,432
Wages	1,350	8,485	4,257	11,000	15,725	24,052
Rents	2,000	26,600	26,600	26,600	26,600	26,600
Hunt/trap	7,900	26,600	10,185	9,255	13,085	9,475
Other*	12,800	1,600	4,670	5,690	10,050	8,032
Interest	26,600	26,600	26,600	15,338	21,708	25,284
Total	26,930	50,385	55,125	87,481	155,610	142,275
Per capita	40.01	72.60	85.73	123.56	212.87	185.01

*'Other' refers to income earned from sale of dry wood, senega root, etc.
Source: CHC, Sessional Papers, 1900–1922.

force the people to surrender their lands, 'at the same time you should keep before the Bloods the fact that a certain portion of their large landed estate could be turned into cash, very greatly for their benefit, without unduly restricting the area of their reserve.' During the First World War bands were encountering increased pressure to surrender their lands in the name of national efficiency. The 'Greater Production' campaign was intended to increase food production for the war effort. Under the Greater Production program, uncultivated reserve lands could be leased without being formally surrendered. In 1918, official

TABLE 4.5
Hobbema Agency, 1900–1920: Sources of Income and Per Capita Income ($)

	1900	1905	1910	1915	1917	1920
Farm	9,750	21,750	16,499	35,620	95,042	49,998
Wages	29,825	1,605	29,978	3,013	15,725	29,307
Rents	12,570	12,570	29,854	12,570	12,570	12,570
Hunt/trap	1,525	5,380	3,398	8,187	13,085	1,675
Other*	29,475	29,770	4,159	5,614	10,500	24,825
Interest	12,570	12,570	12,570	4,846	21,708	12,511
Total	12,575	29,505	25,888	57,280	156,060	89,316
Per capita	20.38	42.69	32.81	72.05	188.71	107.35

*'Other' refers to income earned from sale of dry wood, senega root, etc.
Source: CHC, *Sessional Papers*, 1900–1922.

TABLE 4.6
Stoney Agency, 1900–1920: Sources of Income and Per Capita Income ($)

	1900	1905	1910	1915	1917	1920
Farm	1,300	5,127	2,931	5,050	7,950	8,870
Wages	3,000	2,138	1,882	5,661	19,636	26,020
Rents	31,270	31,270	31,270	10,433	1,982	3,185
Hunt/trap	4,300	4,250	8,183	10,497	7,624	11,930
Other*	6,840	10,333	18,276	13,698	19,760	14,590
Interest	31,270	31,270	31,270	3,583	3,711	3,756
Total	15,440	21,848	31,273	38,522	60,663	68,351
Per capita	24.62	33.10	47.02	58.45	90.14	103.10

*'Other' refers to income earned from sale of dry wood, senega root, etc.
Source: CHC, *Sessional Papers*, 1900–1922.

pressure was applied on the Blood people to surrender 90,000 'unused' acres of their reserve. They had been grazing 17,000 head of cattle and horses on that land; their ranching operations were devastated for many years after.[54] The Blackfoot surrendered nearly half of their reserve between 1912 and 1918 – land that provided a trust fund of over $1 million by 1920. The income from the trusts generally went to defray costs incurred by the department. It is interesting that one of the first things the Blackfoot and other bands did with their trust money was provide regular meals for everyone on the reserve.[55]

The growing prosperity of the west, especially to the end of the First

World War, did trickle down to Aboriginal communities. Opportunities for waged work, increasing prices for farm produce, and income from land sales and leases stemmed the tide of mortality on the reserves. Increased income resulted in improvements in diet and housing, and in a reduction in infant mortality as the general health of mothers and infants improved. Farm incomes increased steadily from about 1905 to 1920 through better prices for farm produce and larger markets. Incomes also increased through payments on leased and surrendered lands. During the war years, incomes from waged work increased dramatically (Tables 4.1–4.6). The catalyst of war created many opportunities, which, however, quickly disappeared when the war ended. It has been argued that in Treaty Seven at least, those reserves that had surrendered lands showed no noticeable advancement or long-term benefits relative to those that had not. The restrictions on economic and personal freedom continued to undermine any real development.[56] Nevertheless, between 1904 and 1912 many bands turned the corner and were able to increase their numbers (Table 3.1). Unfortunately, they had to surrender some of their birthright to do so.

During the Great Depression of the 1930s, many earlier economic gains were lost as the prairie economy turned to dust. The permit system, which had been established ostensibly to protect Aboriginal sellers, had always been used to restrict competition:

> You needed a permit from the agent to sell wood. They could cut wood, but not green wood, just dry wood. They sold to farmers and the people in town. Spring was the hardest time. It was hard on the animals too. It was hard to get feed for the animals. My dad took a load of hay to sell because we didn't have enough to eat. So he went with my grandfather and he sold the hay without a permit. They were put in jail for 30 days. My mother only had the money from the hay to buy food for one month. The people were kept 'in prison' on the reserve. They needed permits for everything. The cattle that were given were the Indian department cattle – branded with ID. The people couldn't kill, or butcher, the cattle. In the spring the cattle were rounded up and butchered or sold. The agent would give the people some of the money.

Although the pass system fell out of use, mainly because police refused to enforce a regulation that had no legal basis, agents continued to use informal threats to control the people's movements. Alice Ironstar recalled riding on the load of hay her father was taking to sell in town: 'And here the agent came walking up to that hay load, and he said,

"Alec, unload your hay and buy your stuff and get out of town before six." And I asked my dad, what did he say? [Alice did not understand English] He said I have to get out of town before six – before dark he said. So nobody was allowed to stay in town after dark. So we left right away. We didn't even buy anything.'[57] When economic times were good, as in the period 1905–20, the department tended to take credit for any advances the people made. When economic conditions worsened, Aboriginal people were generally portrayed as the authors of their own misfortune – as shiftless and indolent.

Medical care for Native people in the twentieth century was influenced by the work of Dr Bryce, who drew attention to the serious health problems on the reserves, and especially in the schools. Nevertheless, the care provided continued to reflect the perception that Native people were primitive and in need of fundamental change. This attitude, of course, buttressed the department's policy to civilize and Christianize. The hospitals were regularly avoided because the people saw little benefit in using them; also, the language spoken in them was always French or English, never their own, and the cultural imperative of remaining with and comforting the sick was discouraged. Moreover, the missionaries' efforts to proselytise, often by attacking the people's own beliefs, were not particularly comforting. As Blood elder White Calf put it:

If one was sick and prayed to the Sun he generally recovered. There was very little dangerous sickness and few deaths excepting those caused by war, and the people were prosperous and happy. But now the white men have us here and teach our children that the Sun is a lamp and no God and that to be saved we must pray to the white man's God, well we have all listened to this and sometimes think that it must be true, for white men are very wise and many of us pray to God as well as the Sun. Others pray to God alone, especially the children, but it seems to me that none of our prayers are heard for the people are dying off fast as they never died before and so, if the Maker hears white men, he does not hear Indians, and I think perhaps we are poor and being exterminated because we are forsaking our old Deities that were good to us in the old days and that, when there are no more Bloods praying to the Sun, then the rest of the Bloods will die because they deserted their Sun for another Deity that could not hear their prayers.[58]

Mission hospitals, like mission schools, sought to destroy what was seen by many as their only salvation. But as was not the case with mission schools, the people were not forced into hospitals, at least not until 1914, when the Indian Act was amended to compel Native people to undergo medical treatment. Refusal to submit to a doctor's examination was punishable by a fine or imprisonment. But for all the effort to coerce Native people, it is not clear how the legislation affected their behaviour.[59]

Native people did utilize and appreciate the dispensaries set up at the hospitals and in agency buildings. The Catholic hospital at Stand Off on the Blood reserve, staffed by the Grey Nuns, had fourteen beds but was usually more than half-empty, and used mainly by schoolchildren. Dr O.C. Edwards, appointed as medical officer on the Blood and Peigan reserves in 1901 after Girard was superannuated, visited the hospital once a week. Bryce noted in 1908 that 'relatively little use is made even of the hospitals now in commission as compared with the amount of sickness.'[60] Yet the dispensary at the hospital was well patronized, visited on average more than three thousand times a year between 1911 and 1914. Obviously it was seen as a valuable medical service, as was the dispensary at the nearby agency headquarters. Although Edwards only reported about thirty to forty visits per month, there were possibly many more. As he noted in his report for February 1908, 'the dispensary cases during the month have been numerous.' The people accepted non-Native medicines but preferred their own doctors and therapeutics, and officials saw this as proof of their backwardness and 'savagery'; yet, at the same time, they were perceived as shrewd and scheming because they accepted the doctor's drugs but not the doctor. As Bryce explained, the people only demanded attention for minor ailments 'real or imaginary' because the medicine was free. He saw a need to teach the people 'that medicine is much more effective when paid for.'[61]

Dr Oliver Cromwell Edwards, like James Lafferty, was a transplanted Ontarian eager for opportunity and adventure in the west. The seventh son of a wealthy Ottawa Valley timber merchant, he was never comfortable in the shadow cast by his financially successful father. He graduated from McGill and did postgraduate work in Britain. The eminent physician William Osler was among the witnesses at his marriage to Henrietta Muir in 1876.[62] Henrietta Muir Edwards, an upper-class evangelical Baptist, was an early reform feminist who after her husband's death became best known as one of the 'Famous Five' Alberta women who advocated legal reforms for women. Her activities culminated in the 'Person's Case' in the 1920s, where it was ruled that Canadian women were indeed persons in law. Osler's presence at the wedding likely had more to do with the social standing of the Muir and Edwards families than with Oliver's medical promise. In 1882, Edwards, secured the contract to give vaccinations in the Treaty Four districts. His contract was not renewed the following year, and he was forced to compete with numerous other physicians for fee-for-service work for the department. That Edwards was a Liberal in the Conservative west did not help his chances. Like many other physicians, he found it difficult if not impossible to support his growing family without the security of Indian Department work. While at Indian Head the Edwards family fitted easily with the elitist settler society, and employed a nanny and housekeeper – Patience, a Sioux woman who moved with the Edwards family from Indian Head to Qu'Appelle even though she had a family on the Standing Buffalo reserve. Edwards characterized her, and Native people generally, as 'poor simple children of the prairie.' The Edwards also evinced the Victorian penchant for collecting and categorizing nature and Native artifacts for posterity. Henrietta and the children returned to Montreal, where she lived in 'genteel poverty and growing indebtedness' while her husband waited for secure department work in the west.[63]

In 1897, while his family was in Montreal, Edwards won the contract to attend the Regina Industrial School; otherwise he was finding little success: 'Private practice here is absolutely nil – Dr. Low who is a good man from McGill has the greater share – Cotton but a chronic drinker still gets some – Willoughby who did the school before I came was also a kind of half doctor half rancher.' And, he lamented, 'this is a remarkably healthy town.' Edwards was in deep financial trouble. With a summer home on the Ottawa River, two houses in Ottawa that he attempted to keep rented out, and Henrietta and the children living in a rented house in Montreal, he moaned, 'I seem to be always trying to fill some bottomless hole. When will we get to the surface and get out of debt?' Finally, in 1901, Henrietta's family connections to the Liberal party secured a position for Oliver on the Blood reserve. Although Edwards had struggled financially for years to secure a permanent position, he described his appointment to the Blood reserve as 'west and south to a hole in the hill-side called Macleod.'[64]

On the day he arrived at the Blood reserve hospital, he and Lafferty performed surgery on seven children suffering from scrofula. Unfortunately, Sister Marguerite, who observed many such operations at the hospital, noted that 'patients almost invariably died shortly after, many with rapid consumption.'[65] Edwards regularly travelled 200 miles on horseback each week attending to the Catholic mission hospital near

Standoff, as well as the Anglican mission school and the Peigan reserve. Every Sunday he rode to the agency to have dinner and spend the night in the cultured company of agent James Wilson and his wife. In 1903 Henrietta reluctantly abandoned Montreal to join her husband, whose income and prospects looked secure for the first time in their married life. Edwards petitioned the department to supply him with a house on the reserve, stables, and rations. The Edwards family associated with the ranching elite, attending balls at Macleod and fox hunts on the ranches. They resumed their artifact collecting, offering food in exchange. The robes and clothing they collected were at times loaned back to the Blood people so they might perform ceremonies, but were always returned. After Oliver's death in 1915, Henrietta moved to Macleod and supported herself in her political work by selling off her artifact collection.[66]

The popularity of the dispensary on the Blood Reserve does not necessarily indicate that the people were abandoning the traditional treatments and rites of their healers. It is apparent that the dispensary's ointments, oils, liniments, and syrups were taken away to be used as the people, or their doctors, saw fit. The monthly medical reports of the Blood hospital and dispensary provide a cogent record not so much of the types of illnesses the Blood people were suffering from, but rather of the types of illnesses they perceived could be treated by non-Native medicine. Every year from 1905 to 1910, the people treated at the dispensary were most likely to be suffering from digestive tract problems (22.5 per cent). Many were infants and children suffering from diarrheal diseases caused by inadequate food, contaminated water, and poorly ventilated and over-crowded housing. Diarrheal diseases no doubt contributed to the consistently high infant death rates in Native communities. For example, at the Battleford agency between 1910 and 1917 the average yearly infant mortality rate was 279 per thousand live births.[67] By way of comparison, the infant mortality rate in Montreal in 1921 in the well-to-do suburbs was 60, and in the working-class districts it was close to 200. Research at the time concluded that the death rate among children was high in inverse relation to the social status of the people.[68] As well as diarrheal diseases, every year there were significant numbers of people suffering from taenia (tape-worms from the government-issued beef), constipation, and simply 'indigestion.' Edwards remarked in 1906 that the prevalence of indigestion was the result of the 'inferior quality of the flour at present issued to the Indians.' Bryce's annual reports as chief medical officer for the five years 1905 to 1909 noted that 17.2 per cent of all diseases in the national Aboriginal population were digestive tract diseases. The Blood people suffered marginally more from diseases of the digestive tract, in part because of the poor quality of government rations.[69]

The second most common reason for a dispensary visit was for ear, eye, and throat complaints, which comprised 19.3 per cent of all visits. Most were diagnosed as suffering from 'ophthalmia,' a broad term referring to any inflammation of the eye. The two most important causes were conjunctivitis and trachoma. Trachoma is a contagious bacterial infection caused by *Chlamydia trachomatis*, and is characterized by the formation of inflammatory granulations on the inner eyelid, severe scarring of the eye, and often blindness. Conjunctivitis may appear with and complicate trachoma so that blindness rather than healing occurs. Conjunctivitis is a common eye infection caused by a variety of microorganisms. In mild cases there is a feeling of roughness or sand in the eyes; in serious cases there is pain and sensitivity to light. Trachoma afflicts the impoverished who live in crowded conditions, especially in dry, dusty climates where wind and smoke further irritate the eyes. Trachoma has disappeared in the twentieth century in those places with the highest standards of living: non-Native Canada, Scandinavia, northern Europe, and Switzerland. But on the Blood reserve in the early twentieth century, conditions were ripe for its spread: overcrowded and poorly ventilated houses, the presence of raw sewage or garbage, and infestations of flies, which swarm on the eye discharges of those with trachoma and carry the disease to others. Bryce recorded that 4.9 per cent of visits were for diseases of the eyes, which may indicate that conditions on the Blood reserve were worse than for the Canadian Native population as a whole.[70] A number of ear and throat infections were always included in the Blood reserve reports. People often visited the dispensary for what was diagnosed as otitis (infection of the ear) and otorrhea (discharge from the ear). The severity of the infections was related to climate extremes, overcrowding, and poor sanitation.[71]

Respiratory conditions (excluding tuberculosis) were the third most common reason for visiting the Blood reserve dispensary. Over the six years, these accounted for 14.5 per cent of all visits. Most respiratory complaints were diagnosed as either cough, cold, grippe, catarrh, or bronchitis – rarely pneumonia or pleurisy. The Blood people visited the dispensary for treatment of respiratory diseases marginally more often than the national Aboriginal population, for whom the average yearly rate was only 11.7 per cent.[72] Edwards treated most respiratory complaints with a mixture of expectorant and demulcent herbs and aromatics. A considerable number of people also visited the dispensary for treatment of streptococcal diseases. These visits were diagnosed under a variety of illnesses such as pharyngitis, scarlet fever, impetigo, erysipelas and cellulitis, puerperal sepsis, and meningitis. Streptococcal illnesses can be very common, and many of its forms are life-threatening. They are usually spread through droplet infection or bacterial contamination of food, or by soiled hands touching open wounds. Overcrowding encourages the bacteria. Another rather ill-defined illness – actually a symptom rather than a disease – was 'debility.' This was diagnosed in 3.1 per cent of the people who visited the Blood agency dispensary. Bryce only noted congenital debility in newborns. Debility (or asthenia) was a rather outdated diagnosis at the time, and described general weakness or loss of strength, which was likely a symptom of tuberculosis. At the Moosomin reserve in the Battleford agency in 1913–14, 12.5 per cent of the people treated were diagnosed with debility by the dispenser, A.E. Rotsey. Indeed, debility was one of the most common diagnoses at the Moosomin reserve, second only to respiratory diseases in winter and digestive diseases in summer.[73] At many reserves the dispenser was rarely a physician. All that was required was that they be a 'knowledgeable person' – often the farm instructor. By diagnosing debility, Rotsey was likely just describing the symptoms of tuberculosis. At the Blood reserve as many adults as children were diagnosed with debility, which Edwards treated with morrhuol oil or an aromatic derived from cod liver oil. Cod liver oil, the dispensary's most often prescribed medicine, is rich in vitamins A and D and would have been welcomed by a people who were chronically undernourished. The illnesses that prompted a dispensary visit stemmed directly or indirectly from their impoverished living conditions.

The Blood monthly reports are nearly silent on the 'greatest foe' of Aboriginal people, tuberculosis. Between 1905 and 1910 only 3.2 per cent of all visits to the dispensary were diagnosed as tuberculosis or scrofula – only slightly more than visits for debility. But Dr Bryce reported that 15.6 per cent of all doctor's visits in the national Aboriginal population were for tuberculosis. There are a number of explanations for this apparent anomaly. Perhaps the Blood people did not suffer as greatly as others from tuberculosis. But considering the widespread poverty on the Blood reserve, and the number of illnesses of poverty the Blood people suffered from, that explanation seems unlikely. In his report for 1906–7, Bryce noted that the Blood reserve, with a population of 1,168, had 53 births and 65 deaths for a death rate of 74.1 per thousand. He went on to note that one-half of the reported deaths could be assumed to have been caused by tuberculosis.[74] At the Battleford agency, for the eight years from 1910 to 1917 the average yearly percentage of deaths from tuberculosis was 27.2 per cent of all deaths recorded.[75] But Edwards reported that on the Blood reserve in 1906, of the 457 people he saw at the dispensary only 21 (4.6 per cent) were suffering from tuberculosis. Again, in 1907 only 1.7 per cent of the 410 people he treated were tubercular. But he reckoned that 90 per cent of all deaths on the reserve were caused by some form of tuberculosis. The people may have preferred to see other Euro-Canadian doctors, such as Dr Frank Mewburn at Lethbridge, who treated a number of people from the Blood reserve who could afford his services. Also, Edwards referred people to the Lethbridge hospital for surgery when they refused to go to the reserve hospital.[76] It is clear that there was significant tuberculosis on the reserve and that Edwards did not record it as such. The chronic nature of tuberculosis and its changing symptoms may have made diagnosis difficult; more likely, however, the limited range of treatments available on the reserve may have made the diagnosis futile. In any case, it is apparent that Edwards eschewed the diagnosis of tuberculosis as a disease, but recognized it as a cause of death. This is not to suggest that he was negligent or poorly trained. Indeed, he may have been following the medical protocol of the day.

Dr George Learmonth, who practised medicine in nearby High River, Alberta, followed a similar protocol. Learmonth attended the exclusively non-Native ranchers and their families in what was likely a typical rural practice. There were few elderly people in the frontier district, and women and children made up the bulk of his practice. Learmonth recorded complaints that spanned a predictable range of problems with child bearing and infancy: croup, infant diarrhea, earache, and sore throat. He set the ranchers' broken bones, which were inevitable in work with large animals. But when faced with a patient exhibiting cough, fever, vomiting, weight loss, and malaise, Learmonth noted in his case book 'lung trouble,' 'bronchitis,' or on rare occasions 'phthisis' (pulmonary tuberculosis).[77] In earlier decades there was some reluctance to name tuberculosis as a diagnosis, given the poor prognosis.[78] Learmonth's prescriptions, unlike Edwards's, always comprised 'hygienic,' dietetic,' and 'medicinal' components. For 'lung trouble,' for example, the hygienic treatment was rest and fresh air, the dietetic treatment was nourishing food, and the medicinal treatment was cod liver oil. Learmonth recorded his patients' marital status, age, occupation ('housewife' in the case of married women), and nationality. He was undoubtedly personally familiar with most of his patients in the small town. He was able, therefore, to listen to a fifty-eight-year-old rancher's complaint of 'soreness in limbs and trunk' and diagnose 'indulges in too much Scotch whiskey.' Likewise, when a twenty-five-year-old married woman complained of pain in the lower abdomen, he diagnosed 'leukorrhea following excessive venery' (leukorrhea, or irritating discharge from the vagina, following excessive sexual relations). No prescription was noted in his case book, and his assignment of cause may have been premature, in that she returned four more times in the next six weeks. Learmonth had also to diagnose a nineteen-year-old unmarried domestic worker who complained of 'stomach trouble, amenorrhea [absence of menses] and vomiting in the morning.' A diagnosis of 'neurasthenia' (or nervous exhaustion, a popular diagnosis that referred to a number of vague psychological and physical symptoms) served both the twenty-five-year-old unmarried rancher complaining of 'nervousness and pain while passing urine,' and the fifty-two-year-old English housewife complaining of 'chills and fever.'[79] The therapeutics of a small rural practice consisted of listening, talking, touching, and understanding the personal and family histories of patients.

Edwards had few of those options at hand. The Blood reserve medical records contrast sharply with Learmonth's case books. Where Learmonth dispensed hygienic and dietetic advice, Edwards dispensed medication alone, for medicines were what the people demanded: they had their own healers and therapeutics. Edwards, like most reserve medical officers, could not speak the language, and the communication necessary for diagnosis and treatment was entirely lacking unless an interpreter was at hand. Even if he had been able to make himself understood, the living conditions on the reserve were such that any advice to stay warm, rest in bed, and take plenty of nourishing food would have sounded hollow if not cruel. Learmonth might have recommended that his tubercular patients 'take the cure' at the nearby Banff sanatorium and hot springs. There seemed little Edwards could do except prescribe cod liver oil and send a note to the issuer recommending an extra ration. Given the limited treatment options available, the people likely preferred their own medicines; this might explain the absence of tuberculosis in the reserve medical records. For example, an infusion of pine needles (*Abies lasiocarpa*) was given to people who were coughing blood; the patient was then fumigated with a smudge made of the burning needles. The root of the aster (*Astralagus canadensis*) was chewed to treat spitting blood, and the steam was inhaled when the root was boiled. A willow sweat lodge lined with pine boughs would have created a soothing steam. Yarrow (*Achillea millefolium*), made into a tea, was used to treat coughs. The leaves of the wild bergamot (*Monarda fistulosa*) were also used to treat coughs, and the root was chewed to relieve 'swollen necks.' The vine bark of the western clematis (*Clematis ligusticifolia*) was steeped and chewed for fever. The root of the western red lily (*Lilium philadelphicum*) was made into tea to treat tuberculosis. The root of the marsh valerian (*Valeriana septentrionalis*) was made into a tea to treat 'spitting blood,' and an infusion of it was applied to children's swollen lymph glands (valerian is a popular over-the-counter sedative in Europe). Dried goldenrod (*Sloidago spp.*) was soaked in cold water to treat pulmonary tuberculosis, and children inhaled the steam of prairie sage (*Artemisia ludoviciana*).[80] The people's own therapeutics, empirical in nature, may have relieved the symptoms, but clearly they did not cure the disease.

Edwards found that the people would not come to him when they were mildly ill; when they finally did consult him it was often because they had exhausted the resources of their own doctors and had nothing to lose. Edwards was also suspicious of his patients, refusing to give cough medicines and tonics if he suspected they would be used as stimulants. For their part, the Blood people complained that Edwards did not take sufficient interest in them. Edwards's own health was failing, and his fractious relationship with the new agent, R.N. Wilson, did not help matters. Wilson seemed to relish reporting Edwards's failures to his superiors. For example, he reported that in January and February 1911 there had been fifteen deaths on the reserve – nine adults and six children – and that Edwards had not treated any of them. The people complained to the agent that when they called on Edwards he was so rough and in such a bad temper that they regretted having sent for him and 'resolved not to do it again.' Meanwhile, according to Wilson, 'the Bloods, for the most part get sick, grow worse and die entirely without medical aid.'[81] Aboriginal healers continued to practise, however, despite Wilson's claim.

Edwards's work on the Blood reserve contrasted sharply with that of a typical non-Native rural practice. Simply put, the Blood patients did not share with Edwards a belief in European medicine's effectiveness. The dispensary was patronized for commonplace ailments because it might offer substitute treatments that in former times would have been found in nature. Lack of transportation, departmental restrictions on the people's movements, and the destruction caused to wild plants by intensive ranching all made it difficult to collect medicines in the wild. The dispensary provided an alternative source for medicines, which were then used in culturally specific ways. Department officials considered this behaviour one of the greatest problems in the medical service. The people did not patronize the hospitals or consult the doctor enough, at least not until they were moribund; conversely, they visited the dispensary far too much, and then for trivialities. The Blood were not unique in avoiding the hospital. Dr R.H. Wheeler at the Birtle school remarked: 'The Indians have a feeling against the hospital and it takes considerable persuasion to prevail on them to come, and if they do consent, it is generally only when there is very little hope for their recovery.'[82] That behaviour was incomprehensible to department officials, who were socialized to accept both the doctor and his treatments.

The Blood hospital, unlike the dispensary, was rarely patronized. It was funded by the government and managed by the Catholic church primarily to treat children attending the Catholic school and their families. Between 1905 and 1910 only three patients were admitted in the average month, with most patients treated in February, March, and April, when the schools were the most unhealthy. In summer it often sat empty. After 1911, hospital admissions began to increase slightly, primarily due to chronic tuberculosis sufferers, who tended to 'silt up' in the records as they spent year after year in the hospital. For example, Joseph Spike was admitted in August 1911 at age twenty suffering from what was initially diagnosed as hemoptysis (coughing blood from the respiratory tract). In July 1913 his diagnosis was changed to 'phthisis' (pulmonary tuberculosis); and in December 1914, after more than three years in hospital, he died. Between 1911 and 1914, 33 per cent of patients treated in the hospital were children and young adults suffering from tuberculosis.[83] There were also always a number of elderly people who had no home and spent months in the hospital before they died. The hospital was often the last resort for the poorest and the unwanted.

The people simply would not leave their loved ones alone with strangers who could not speak the language. The hospital had always refused to allow mothers to stay with their sick children, or allow children to stay with their sick mothers. In 1912 the Catholic bishop of Alberta reasoned that the best way to create a relationship between the hospital (or doctor) and the people would be to accept maternity cases in the hospital – something every physician in search of a practice knew. But there were a number of problems with this: there was no room for a maternity ward, the Sisters of Charity were prevented by their vows from accepting maternity cases, and most importantly, Native doctors had all but cornered the practice of midwifery. Emile Legal, former missionary and now Bishop, helped clear the way by agreeing to accept all cases of illness, including 'lying in' patients. A qualified nurse from Calgary was to be hired to attend them.[84] The maternity ward opened in 1916, but few women patronized it. While the hospital had a number of more obvious problems, its fundamental flaw was that it refused to accede to the wishes of the constituency it hoped to serve. The hospital had little to offer the Blood people, for all its attempts to create a more acceptable atmosphere for its prospective clients. The hospital remained irrelevant until after the war, when two changes in particular contributed to its usefulness: first, the quality of the medical attendants sent to the reserve deteriorated during the First World War, and second, the hospital began to offer medical care that recognized the cultural and social needs of its clients.

The war created a shortage of doctors in Canada generally, and the diligence and quality of medical attendants on the Blood reserve declined accordingly. Dr Edwards died in 1915 after fourteen years on the Blood reserve. Two different medical officers served for a short time, before resigning to enlist in the Canadian Expeditionary Force. Dr T.S. Tupper then served for less than a year before being forced to resign after he got drunk and drove a team of department horses 'furiously' through Macleod, loudly offering prescriptions for whisky to passersby. During prohibition in Canada, alcohol could only be purchased for medicinal reasons with a prescription from a doctor. (Another resident salaried physician, Dr S.T. Macadam, serving the Battleford agency, delivered unsatisfactory medical service according to agent J.P.G. Day, because of his 'constant tippling'; three years later Macadam arrived on the reserve drunk and unfit to work.) Tupper was replaced by N.D. Steele of Cochrane. Steele was forced to resign under a cloud of suspicion that he was not a qualified physician, that he had sold department rations and implements, and that he had signed whole books of prescriptions for alcohol and left them with the druggist, who unfortunately sold one to an undercover police officer. The people complained that he did not attend them when he was needed.[85]

Throughout these years the medical officers refused to attend to Native people in their homes, insisting instead that they present themselves at the hospital. Agent W.J. Dilworth advised Tupper to refuse to attend to the people in their own homes with Native doctors present. According to Dilworth, the Native doctors were still a powerful influence. Tupper was told that in the past the people had been given medicine such as castor oil simply because they wanted it, and that they had used medicinal vaseline to paint their faces 'with fantastic designs. These evils should be eradicated.' Tupper sent an open message to the Blood people belittling them for their faith in Native doctors: 'The tom-toms have no power to cure. The evil spirits do not cause your sickness; danger is within not without.'[86] He went on to threaten that the death of a child under a Native doctor's care would be considered manslaughter and that the parents would be held responsible. Dilworth worked up a pamphlet, 'Things Every Blood Indian Should Know,' in which he improbably stated that gonorrhea led to consumption and scrofula and that the white men could be trusted because they had studied the problem for two thousand years. Dilworth also declared that ceremonial dances should be stopped because the clothes given away at them caused the spread of disease. If his recommendations were not followed, he warned, 'the time will come when these Indians will not only be a menace to their own health but to the public at large.'[87]

In the meantime, hospital admissions began to increase, most notably among women. In April 1919, Steele reported that there was a steady increase in the number of confinement cases treated, and that many more were refused admission because there was no room. In June he reported that thirteen babies had been born in the hospital in the past six months. The increased use of the hospital may indicate a greater acceptance of Euro-Canadian doctors and their therapeutics. But it is also necessary to analyse who presented themselves at the hospital for treatment. Children made up the majority of admissions in the early years because the hospital was an extension of the school. But as we have seen, before 1916 the hospital was not widely used: 160 people were treated in 1913, and 141 in ten months of 1914. By 1923, however, admissions had increased nearly six-fold to 602. Most of those admitted (89.2 per cent) were women and children. Perhaps it was because women and children were the most vulnerable in society, or because the hospital was staffed by women, who made it a safe and welcoming place for the Blood women. Moreover, government doctors did not visit the hospital unless the staff, the Sisters of Charity, called them.[88] There was a long way to go, however, before the hospitals recognized who their clients were. Alan Pard recalls that when his great-grandmother Melanie Butcher, a respected healer and midwife who spoke only Blackfoot, was taken to hospital, 'they started undressing her – she was a holy Sun Dance woman and they just started undressing her.'[89]

There was also a cultural component to the increased use of the hospital. As noted on the Blackfoot and Blood reserves, Native people were reluctant to leave a loved one alone in hospital and many of the people who began to frequent the hospital were not sick. In 1923 nearly 30 per cent of the admissions were women and children who were not sick but were accompanying a sick family member. Women who were ill brought their young children along to be cared for while they received medical care. Likewise, women accompanied their young children when the children required care, and often brought healthy siblings along as well. In October 1923, for example, fourteen women, thirty-six children, and two men were admitted to hospital. Nine of the women (64 per cent), were not ill but were accompaning their sick children; and thirteen children (36 per cent), were not ill but were accompanying sick mothers or siblings. Thus, 42 per cent of the admissions that month were of healthy people. The care that both women and children received would have been enhanced by the emotional and physical support of family members. Puerperal women had the opportunity to rest and recover before undertaking the care of their infants and other children; and children had their mothers present to interpret, mediate, and help with their care. The arrangement whereby mothers and children accompanied one another to hospital was certainly demanded by mothers, and was obviously accepted by the staff. The doctors were less supportive. Steele reckoned that infant mortality actually increased '[through] the custom of mothers coming into the over-crowded ward with their children ... These mothers in spite of the watchfulness of the nurses persist in breastfeeding and stuffing their babies with all kinds of objectionable dainties, where both practices are strictly forbidden.' Later, Dr Allan Kennedy hoped to make the institution into a 'true hospital ... not a comfortable place to stay, as some of the Indians seem to consider it now.'[90]

The increase in admissions also reflects the long-term socializing influence of the school and hospital among the ex-pupils, and their gradual acceptance – or at least assimilation – of some aspects of Euro-Canadian health care. In 1920, Steele complained that there were still more than one-hundred Indian doctors plying their trade, going from house to house 'with drums, horns, and weird incantations' attempting to instil fear of the hospital by claiming that it was infested with ghosts. Blood agent Dilworth lamented that even though ceremonial dancing was 'harmful to health and industry ... I do not think it is either desirable or good policy to totally prohibit Indians from dancing.'[91] He noted that dancing gave the people pleasure, and besides, it was impossible to stop. Competition from Native doctors was not restricted to the Blood reserve. Mrs Helen Anne English, the field matron at the Little Pine reserve near Battleford, complained that the 'medicine men' interfered with her work and 'tend to destroy, or at least stultify, the arrangements made for the physical and moral welfare of the Indians.' By 1923 Dr Kennedy was complaining, as so many had before him, that the people lacked confidence in him because he could not speak their language. He suggested that an interpreter, a young boy, be hired with a truck to go out among the people, treat their minor complaints, and bring the seriously ill to hospital.[92] Kennedy had a pessimistic view of his own effectiveness. Nevertheless, the dispensary, and later the hospital, did apparently meet some of the people's medical needs and were well patronized. The government's resident physician seemed less able to meet the people's needs.

In 1923, in response to the continuing high rate of tuberculosis, a twelve-bed tuberculosis ward was opened with four patients. The ward was actually a farm cottage that had been moved to the hospital site, put on a new foundation, and remodelled. The cottage was to be used as a sanatorium, mainly to treat early symptoms of tuberculosis among the schoolchildren. There were problems, however. Sister Mary Superior at the hospital complained that they did not have enough hens to provide three eggs each day to each tuberculosis patient, and that they did not receive enough butter to provide the patients with the high-protein, high-fat diet the doctor had ordered. They had no bathtubs, they were in dire need of running water, and the open cesspool behind the hospital was very unhealthy. Yet when commissioner Graham visited the hospital the following month, he enthusiastically declared that the hospital would be a credit to any small town in the west: 'I cannot speak too highly of it.'[93] The building inspector's report told a different story, however. He found that the plumbing was ineffective and twenty years out of date. The odour from the open cesspool, within a few steps of the maternity ward, was 'almost overpowering and the pungent fumes pollute the atmosphere within a very considerable distance, and when the wind is in a certain quarter, the nauseating smells are wafted through open windows or doors right into the room.' He warned that it would soon cause an epidemic through contamination of the well just seventy feet away. Neither the men's wards nor the women's had flush toilets, and the maternity ward did not have running water. He concluded: 'If this building were brought under the jurisdiction of a sanitary inspector he would order it to be closed down at once, and prosecutions would probably follow.' To bring the building up to standards that would satisfy city bylaws would cost about $2,400, but agent J.T. Faunt was told by his superiors that it would not improve the hospital since it would likely be abandoned in a few years because the whole area where it presently stood was putrid from so many cesspools having been dug and filled over the years. Nevertheless, Faunt was authorized to spend $400 to have another cesspool dug. Kennedy agreed that something needed to be done before an epidemic of typhoid broke out. He suggested that in the meantime barrels of chloride of lime be used to 'at least keep down the flies and the smell.'[94]

By 1928 the old hospital was deemed beyond repair and the Blood hospital site was moved to the southern edge of the reserve near the town of Cardston. The department built an imposing three-storey brick building with thirty-five beds and balconies. The hospital remained under the management of the Grey Nuns, but the department found itself increasingly under pressure from Anglican clerics to either make the hospital a lay institution or build a Protestant hospital. The department instead forbade any religious insignia to be placed in the hospital and declared, 'Department hospitals are not religious institutions, and are not to be used for the promotion of the interest of any religious denomination.' The churches, once indispensable to the department's assimilationist policy, and integral to the very existence of the hospitals, did not quietly relinquish control, just as they would not relinquish control of the schools. Catholic clerics continued to press the superintendent to stop the trend toward 'neutral' (non-denominational) hospitals. Catholic Archbishop Monahan of Regina contended that there was no such thing as a neutral hospital: if a hospital was not Catholic, it was Protestant.[95]

One does not have to look far to find reasons why the Aboriginal people failed to embrace the hospitals. Missionaries used them primarily as sites for proselytising, with the result that most people stayed clear. Those who were treated in them – the chronically ill and alone – rarely came out alive. Besides harbouring ghosts, the hospitals quickly earned a reputation as places where few survived. Prudence alone would suggest that they were no place for the ill, so only those with no choice – the schoolchildren – were treated at them. The department doctor joined the agent in berating the people for dancing, for visiting the healer, and for keeping their children out of the schools where so many had died. But the most important reason why the hospitals were irrelevant, if not dangerous, to the people's health was that they had been founded and were maintained to serve non-Native needs. Many elders state that the doctors and hospitals were not only inappropriate to the people's needs, but a menace to them. Alan Pard on the Peigan reserve suggested that when the department built a dispensary at Brocket, 'they practised on us ... There was a lot of distrust and displeasure on both sides.' An elder at the Blood reserve noted that when people were sent away to hospital, 'they never came back ... people were being used as guinea pigs.' Remembered elder Kaye Thompson: 'And after they got rid of Indian medicine and the people had to take white medicine, and some of it made us real sick. They kind of damaged our bodies through pills and their side effects. They were experimenting on us.' Elder Alice Ironstar, who spent her childhood in hospital, recalled: 'I used to think they were experimenting on us ... We were guinea pigs in other words.'[96] After D.C. Scott became deputy superintendent in 1913, Dr Bryce did no more inspection work, and his last published medical report was in 1914. He had consistently advocated greater government control and management of medical care for Native people, which often ran counter to department policy. In his last published report as medical inspector, he did not try to disguise his growing frustration and cynicism: 'If one were to be content with the generally satisfactory terms of the reports of the Indian agents, he would have the comfortable sensation of seeing a large population ... their wants ever receiving most paternal attention one by one passing away in a ripe old age.'[97]

The increasing medical presence on reserves and schools helped the department stay informed of the extent of disease in Native communities. At the same time, fundamental changes in the medical understanding of disease, principally the germ theory of disease, led to a significant shift in the department's perception of Native people. They had once been considered members of a waning race in a losing struggle with the biological rigours of civilization; by the early twentieth century it was becoming apparent that they were not disappearing at all, and that disease on reserves was capable of spreading to non-Native communities. Even so, the people's own behaviour continued to be seen as the cause of disease. As deputy superintendent Pedley stated in 1907, it was people's excessive crowding into small, poorly ventilated houses, their ignorance of the value of nursing, their inattention to the directions of medical advisors, poorly prepared food, and premature marriages that caused ill health. By 1910 Pedley was characterizing the people as 'indifferen[t] to human life and suffering ... who manifest a certain apathy as to the prolongation of a life which affords comparatively few interests and enjoyments and is lived mainly for the supply of the arising necessities of the day.'[98] Compulsion seemed necessary, given such a characterization. Yet paternalism cum coercion at times collided with the department's long-standing impulse to ensure economy in all things. A rather peculiar exchange took place in 1912 that highlighted these different and often contradictory impulses. It came to the department's attention that some medical officers employed by the department were attempting to collect fees from Native people. On 27 May 1912, a strongly worded circular was issued to all department medical officers that they were not to charge or attempt to claim from a Native person a fee for professional services. Paternalism seemed to triumph. Only months later, economy came to the fore, and a circular was issued to replace the first circular. The policy had been changed to 'promote self-sufficiency'; and medical officers were 'not to provide gratuitous assistance to those Indians who can provide for themselves.'[99] Departmental responses to high death and disease rates on reserves were often caught between two conflicting impulses, the need to exert control over Native people and the need to do it cheaply.

Native people were seen as either woefully ignorant of the dangers of disease, or dangerously careless. In any case, coercion and compulsion were long-standing department policies that were again brought to bear. Initially the department attempted to segregate the people, both physically and economically, in order to protect them from contact with unscrupulous non-Natives; that protection, however, quickly turned to coercion. In the new century, considerations changed as reserves were increasingly perceived as hotbeds of disease. Medical officers treated reserve residents in order to prevent disease from spilling out into non-Native communities. Large NO TRESPASSING signs were posted at reserve boundaries that threatened a $50 fine or one month in jail, or both, to any person 'who trespasses on an Indian Reserve.' Increased immigration to the west brought Native people into closer contact with non-Native communities. Yet ironically, greater settlement led to more complete segregation of Native people on reserves through the use of quarantine.

As a public health measure, quarantine – the isolation of those with contagious disease – was impossible to enforce in the cities and villages of the west because of scheduled rail connections, informal communications between neighbours, and the exigencies of business. In cities, placards were at times placed as warnings on homes where children had scarlet fever or diphtheria, but it took a resolute municipal health officer to do so because it was a serious restriction on personal movement and, more importantly, an impediment to the ability to make a living – not to mention a public shame for the family. Quarantine of an entire community was neither possible nor desirable. On reserves, however, there were fewer impediments to quarantine. It became an effective tool in the arsenal of medical officers, and it was resorted to frequently. Quarantine was imposed on Beardy's and Okemasis reserves for measles in 1902. The Royal North West Mounted Police (RNWMP) enforced quarantines on Poundmaker and Little Pine reserves in April 1912, and at the Red Pheasant and Stoney reserves in August 1913. Quarantine was imposed on John Smith reserve due to smallpox in 1913, and at the Piapot reserve in 1914. There was also frequent quarantines of the schools, so that children were unable to leave and parents unable to visit.[100] Quarantine was most effective with the help of a police constable or two. The Indian Act was amended in 1914 so as to authorize the superintendent general to make regulations 'deemed necessary for the prevention or mitigation of disease' on reserves; this included the authority to impose quarantine. However, the amendment merely institutionalized an already common response.[101] But the physical and economic hardships suffered by Native people indicated that the reason for quarantine was to protect non-Natives. The threat of disease became the new rationale for segregation.

Witness the events at John Smith reserve in 1913. In early January, Dr Strong of Prince Albert diagnosed six people as suffering from smallpox and quickly quarantined the entire reserve. Reverend Macdougall was on the reserve and was left to ride out the quarantine, while agent C. Paul Schmidt and Strong stayed in Prince Albert. Six weeks later, on 17 February, Schmidt berated the missionary for purchasing provisions for the people under his care because, according to Schmidt, they were able to work and should receive nothing for free. Macdougall explained that provisions were low and that there were 350 people under quarantine who had been unable to leave the reserve for more than a month. An RNWMP constable was stationed on the reserve to prevent the people from hunting, freighting, selling wood or furs, or working in the timber camps. Macdougall complained that smallpox was present in only two houses, but because of the hardships resulting from the quarantine there was also an epidemic of influenza as well as cases of typhoid, pneumonia, and erysipelas. After fifty-nine days of quarantine the doctor still had not visited the reserve, all the food was gone, and even rabbits were scarce. On 24 March, Strong informed Schmidt that since there were still thirteen smallpox patients, the quarantine would have to remain in place for another month.[102] There the correspondence left off, and the fate of the people went unrecorded. But the physical and economic consequences of the ordeal had yet to play themselves out. There was sure to be lingering weakness, perhaps death for those infants born to malnourished or sick mothers. The loss of the past season's work and a late start on the next presented economic setbacks to people least able to afford them. There is no record, however, that smallpox spread past the reserve. The *Melfort Moon* reported on 16 April that police officer Loggin had inspected the reserve and found 'there were no cases on the reserve and no epidemic at all.' He did find two 'half-breeds' with the mild form of smallpox, and 'these are well confined and there is no danger of the disease spreading.' There was no mention of any epidemic in the larger *Melfort Journal.*[103]

A petition from the people of Piapot's reserve in 1914 underlined the severe economic hardships imposed by quarantine. In December 1913, smallpox was discovered at the reserve. Quarantine was established on the entire Qu'Appelle agency – the Piapot, Pasquah, Muscowpetung, and Standing Buffalo reserves – with RNWMP constables in attendance, even though there was no disease on the latter two reserves. When there were no new cases at the Pasquah and Piapot reserves by 12 February 1914, it was decided to lift the quarantine in March once the reserves had been 'thoroughly cleansed.' All thatch-roofed houses and stables were to be burned, lumber buildings were to be disinfected, and as soon as the snow melted, the land and brush close to the buildings was to be burned. By 9 March 1914 the quarantine had still not been lifted. The people petitioned agent H. Nichol to lift the smallpox quarantine because they had suffered from lost cattle sales and needed to sell hay and wood before they could begin the year's seeding. But most importantly, according to deputy superintendent D.C. Scott, the doctors and department employees 'were successful in confining the disease to the reserves.' There was a complete crop failure that year, and there was no market for their fish, hay, or wood. Because of the crop failure there was no seed for the next year, so the department provided seed wheat and oats as a loan.[104] This succession of misfortunes – smallpox, the quarantine, business losses, crop failure, and debt to the department – was followed by a request for permission to hold a dance. The people of the reserve assured the agent that it would not be held during seeding. Nichol refused, citing departmental regulations against dancing. Rock Thunder replied that he was not aware of any rules against dancing and that it was only through promises of a dance that he had been able to get the young men to work. The request was denied; the dance, if it was held, was covert.

The irony was that for all the department's efforts to prevent the spread of smallpox to non-Native communities, it was generally non-Natives who gave the disease to the Native people in the first place. It cannot be argued that the reserves were hotbeds of smallpox infection. As was noted earlier, there was a vigorous campaign to vaccinate all Native people, usually when they received their annuities, which were often withheld until the children were vaccinated. Of course, the vaccination program could never reach all the people. Mike Mountain Horse of the Blood reserve recalled that the arrival of the department doctor would cause a stampede for the bush 'because we Indian children held a mortal fear of vaccination.' Nevertheless, Bryce insisted on thorough vaccination, and it was generally carried out. Bryce pointed out that the vaccination program was especially necessary since there were so many railway construction workers in the west who posed a smallpox threat to the Native people.[105] In non-Native communities, compulsory vaccination was impossible, and quarantine intolerable. For reserves, however, quarantine was a relatively cost-efficient method of controlling the spread of disease, and was perhaps the most effective means yet devised for controlling and segregating the people. The perception that the reserves harboured disease, and that Native people were the carriers, received considerable impetus from the department's readiness to impose quarantine. And the more often quarantine was used, the more it was seen as necessary. Coercion, so familiar a response by the department, in many cases grew out of the paternalistic desire to protect the people. It is difficult to see, however, how the enforcing of a quarantine protected anyone but non-Native people. It is interesting to note that during the 1918–19 influenza epidemic, many reserves were quarantined. But when Saskatchewan towns and villages, in an attempt to protect themselves from infection, quarantined themselves 'against the world' by refusing to allow any trains to stop, they were forced by the provincial public health authorities to open their stations to traffic. The provincial commissioner of public health, a former Indian Affairs doctor named Maurice M. Seymour, objected to the quarantines as 'contrary to the approved methods of combatting the disease.'[106]

The influenza epidemic killed more Canadians than the bloody First World War. But its ravages were not restricted to Native people;[107] indeed, it was a worldwide pandemic. A typical case of influenza-pneumonia during the epidemic began suddenly with pains, chills, and extreme weakness. Coughing produced 'quantities of blood stained expectoration or nearly pure dark blood ... the face and fingers cyanosed, active delirium came on ... the tongue dry and brown, the whole surface of the body blue, the temperature rapidly fell and the patient died from failure of the respiratory system.'[108] There was no cure for influenza, nor is there yet. The only treatment was complete bed rest, fluids, and nursing care. Influenza alone rarely kills; instead, opportunistic diseases such as pneumonia and bronchitis attack and kill weakened influenza victims. Native people were particularly susceptible because of the poor and overcrowded living conditions on most reserves. Those living closest to a subsistence level were the first victims of influenza because they could not take to their beds. When they could no longer work, they no longer ate. Whole families were stricken at the same time, and some starved or froze before influenza could kill them. A crude estimate of the mortality among Canadian Native people from the 1918 epidemic was 4,000 deaths, or 37.7 per thousand population. The death rate in Saskatchewan for non-Native people was 6.5 per thousand.[109] Anthropologist D. Ann Herring has estimated that the death rate from influenza at Norway House in Manitoba was 188 per thousand. She concluded that due to a post-epidemic marriage boom and the maintenance of birth rates, the population recovered to its pre-epidemic level within five years.[110] As with the smallpox epidemics of the eighteenth and nineteenth centuries, the people's response to the epidemic is significant in any account of its impact.

Medical care was provided by anyone who was available. Frank G. Fish, a medical student at the University of Alberta, spent one week in 1918 on the Hobbema reserve in Alberta. He commonly found eight or nine adults in a one-room house with no ventilation. Families were without food, and influenza patients were moved from home to home where food was available, 'and hence practically every case develops pneumonia and death ensues.'[111] Fish recommended that the government take control of the situation and organize an emergency hospital for influenza patients. Influenza deaths reflected the inequalities of life. It arrived on the Blood reserve in early October 1918, ironically carried by two nuns who had been sent from Montreal to help at the Peigan and Blood reserve schools. Elder Little Woman Face, or Katie Wells, recalled that the epidemic 'killed a lot of people on the reserve. It seemed like every day they went to bury somebody. If people ate heavy food they would die from it, though if they ate light food they usually got better. Gradually everybody learned this and then the epidemic went down. But for a time we had to wear something [gauze masks] over our mouths ... It was really horrible for a while, something like that AIDS.'[112] On 16 November agent Dilworth reported that there were 500 people sick with influenza and 11 had died; by 3 December there had been 29 deaths and more than 800 were sick. Yet no non-Native employees or family members contracted the disease. In Saskatchewan at the Battleford agency, influenza struck every reserve and was responsible for the largest number of deaths reported in many years. No farm work was done during the month because few able-bodied men escaped the sickness. Between April 1919 and March 1920 the death rate at the Battleford Agency was 31.4 per thousand, based on a population of 954. That death rate was nearly four times the 1919 provincial rate of 7.9 per thousand.[113]

The industrial and boarding schools, overcrowded, poorly funded, and often inadequately heated, achieved what influenza alone could not by bringing vulnerable children together and exposing them to the virus. At some schools the situation quickly became horrendous. Principal Joseph F. Woodsworth at the Red Deer Industrial School in Alberta, exasperated after five students died from influenza within two days, called the conditions at the school 'criminal.' Because there were no facilities for isolation, the convalescent, the dead, and the dying were all kept together. He begged the department to help the school, which he characterized as a 'disgrace.' As a result of the epidemic, many children were orphaned, and school principals were told not to enrol any children whose parents were living.[114]

Royal North West Mounted Police were dispatched to reserves in Alberta and Saskatchewan to enforce strict quarantines. The police quickly found themselves engaged in relief work when department employees refused to do it, out of fear for themselves and their families. Sister Nantel cared for patients at the Saddle Lake reserve in Alberta. The agent would not aid in relief efforts, or provide his car, thus forcing the sister to make her rounds in a horse and buggy. '[The agent] and his family are very much afraid of the influenza and want nothing to do with those coming in contact with it. Recently the sister stopped at the Agency and asked for lunch. They would not invite her into the house but brought food and tea to her outside. She had to stay on the sidewalk outside the Agency Office and owing to the wind blowing manure and dirt into her food was unable to eat it.'[115]

When a young war veteran returned to the Onion Lake reserve in northern Saskatchewan after four years overseas, he no longer had a home: influenza had killed his parents, two brothers, his sister, and his nephew. The deaths had begun in January 1919, and by February the dead were piled up in an old warehouse because no one was well enough to dig graves.[116] In early March of 1919 the chief and councillors petitioned D.C. Scott, the deputy superintendent, for permission to hold a dance: 'We are writing you to ask permission to let us have a Sundance on our Indian Reserve at Onion Lake this coming summer. We have been in very poor circumstances this last five years on account of the Great War and also on account of the Great Epidemic that has swept over our country. So I am asked to write to solict [sic] your authority and give us permission to have our Sundance for two days. Thanking you in anticipation. I am the man that wants to make the Sundance.' The petitioners need not have thanked Scott, who refused permission. After another request, and another refusal, the dance preparations went ahead as planned. Agent W. Sibbald called in the police, who confronted the dancers. According to Sibbald the chief 'went as far as to say that the Sergeant might put a bullet through his brains if he liked that was the only thing that would stop him.' But they were outgunned, and the people dispersed. Similar incidents occurred in the summer of 1919 at the Piapot reserve, and at the Big River Reserve near Prince Albert; in both situations police arrived to suppress the ceremonies and were told that due to a 'great deal of sickness' and the armistice, the people wanted to dance.[117] Non-Native Canadians also linked the war to the epidemic. The armistice promised an end to deprivation and suffering from the war and the flu. Previously careful people poured into the streets on Armistice Day, which reinvigorated the epidemic. They were, of course, neither threatened nor arrested.

The 'medicalization' of reserves was ultimately directed by a department that consistently denied responsibility for medical care. This apparent contradiction characterized the decisions that created the medical branch of the department. Representatives of the various bodies that hoped to construct medical care on reserves pushed and pulled the department, whose primary role was to fund (or underfund) their work. This is not to suggest that the Department of Indian Affairs was a benign and aimless monolith; indeed, the government clung to its long-standing goal to assimilate the people. The severe economic restrictions placed on reserves – restrictions that did more than anything else to per-petuate poverty and economic underdevelopment – were at least nomi-nally intended to accomplish that goal. Missionary control of hospitals and schools was an economical road to assimilation, and medical offic-ers on reserves served to control or at least confine communicable dis-ease. But it was the interests of non-Native groups that were being served, often at the expense of the people in whose name the services had been created. The policy of assimilation was rarely questioned even in the face of disastrous mortality, because it was assumed that the peo-ple's constitution, their 'mode of living,' and their 'indifference to human life and suffering' – their race – was the cause of their poor health. The 'cure' still lay in their assimilation. But in the first decades of the twentieth century, as medical authority was gaining ground, a powerful new voice was added to the chorus that declared Aboriginal people in dire need of transformation. Science, and medicine and anthropology in particular, began to apply the ideas developed by race science, which had been lurking in the shadows of many scientific and academic disciplines for decades. The treatment of tuberculosis among Aboriginal people was increasingly influenced by 'scientific' notions of race.

Chapter Five

'A Menace to the Community': Tuberculosis

There is growing evidence of anxiety among the white population living adjacent to certain Indian bands in regard to the intimate gross infection brought to the villages and towns ... Further, the leaders of certain bands of Indians were publicly agitating for increased facilities for diagnosis and treatment.
Canadian Tuberculosis Association, 1924[1]

In the first four decades of the twentieth century, tuberculosis came to be seen as the greatest health problem affecting Canadians. On reserves, although it was a persistent and patient killer, tuberculosis had to compete with many other diseases of poverty. But off reserves, tuberculosis had captured the attention of the public and the medical professions alike. It did not take Robert Koch's discovery of the tubercle bacillus (*Mycobacterium tuberculosis*) in 1882 for medical and lay people to notice that the poor and the poorly fed were the most likely victims of tuberculosis. In 1899 the Canadian delegate to the International Congress on Tuberculosis in Berlin reported that it was now a 'well known fact which will no longer admit of discussion that the tubercle bacillus is the direct cause of all varieties of consumption in the human subject and also of bovine tuberculosis.'[2] The clearer understanding that tuberculosis was a contagious rather than a hereditary disease meant that preventive and perhaps curative measures could be taken against it. Canada optimistically entered the anti-tuberculosis crusade; volunteer agencies and government began working together to break the grip of the 'white plague' through public education and sanatorium treatment. Yet tuberculosis on reserves was seen as different. Using the 'seed and soil' analogy favoured at the time, the seed of tuberculosis was the same but the soil (Aboriginal people) was different.[3] The same time-worn explanations were trotted out: the people were more susceptible because of their mode of living; they were careless, indolent, and resistant to treatment. But in the decades leading up to the Second World War, public faith in medicine and the sciences was growing quickly. And when physicians, anthropologists, and biologists observed tuberculosis in Aboriginal people, they saw not the 'heathens and pagans' of Alexander Morris's day but an inferior, less evolved race. In Canada, the relationship between race and tuberculosis was fundamental to understanding the disease.

Medical knowledge and authority underwent significant changes in the decades after 1890. Discoveries in laboratory science – primarily, the realization that bacteria were often the cause of infectious diseases, and not the result – brought new glory to medicine. In the 1880s, Louis Pasteur – a chemist rather than a physician – rejected the traditional theory that miasmata, or emanations, were the causative agents in disease, and demonstrated the role of microorganisms. His contemporary Robert Koch confirmed the germ theory of disease and showed how specific bacteria caused specific diseases. Koch's methods were used to identify the causes of typhoid, diphtheria, pneumonia, gonorrhoea, meningitis, leprosy, syphilis, tuberculosis, whooping cough, and staphylococcal and streptococcal infections. Meanwhile, a new appreciation for cleanliness and antiseptic methods opened up the human body to surgeons, who became increasingly confident that patients might survive both the disease and the surgery. Bacteriology transformed the way disease was understood, but it did not immediately transform how medicine was practised, for causes did not necessarily imply cures. Nevertheless, bacteriology began to imbue medicine with the authority of science and allowed even the most humble practitioner to claim special knowledge, regardless of his physical or intellectual distance from the laboratory bench. The lure of scientific medicine drew Canadians into hospitals, where the new medicine managed life's great events, birth and death – events that were once managed at home. A growing faith in medicine led to the establishment of permanent municipal and provincial boards of health as the public's health became a concern for both social reformers and the state. No longer concerned merely with water quality and over-full privies, the new public health regimes actively sought out specific diseases and specific offenders. Pure milk depots, medical inspections of schoolchildren, and aggressive public education campaigns against, for example, the dangers of spitting, all had the goal of applying the new understanding of disease to create a healthy nation.

Yet well before Koch discovered the tubercle bacillus and before sanatorium treatment was used, death rates from tuberculosis had been in steady decline in Canada, Europe, and the United States. The reasons for tuberculosis decline in the Western world are not altogether clear, but it is apparent that a greater emphasis on personal hygiene, greater levels of general prosperity and social reform movements for cleaner and safer workplaces and improved sanitation and housing all had an impact.[4] In *The Miracle of the Empty Beds* George Wherrett links the fall of tuberculosis in Canada with the work of the Canadian Tuberculosis Association. Wherrett, executive secretary of the association, which also funded his book, had, as he put it, a 'ringside seat' in the anti-tuberculosis crusade. In his book he proclaims the triumph of medical man over disease through unflagging scientific progress; that he played a considerable part in that triumph is not lost on the reader. Regarding sanatorium treatment, Wherrett snatches victory from the jaws of defeat: 'Looking back on the results achieved in curing or arresting the disease during the pre-drug treatment era, one can marvel at how many recovered, though in the final analysis, failures outweighed successes.' Wherrett's tables in the appendix clearly show that tuberculosis was declining steadily in Canada in the three decades before active anti-tuberculosis associations were established.[5] In other words, the anti-tuberculosis campaigns emerged at a time when tuberculosis rates were already declining, and it was not unreasonable for Wherrett and others to assign cause and effect.

Tuberculosis among Native people, however, was not declining at the same rate as in the surrounding communities. In the first decades of the twentieth century, many Native communities experienced a slow but steady population increase as a result of better economic opportunities: larger markets, higher prices for their farm produce, and the possibility of income from land leases and surrenders. Improved living conditions also led to lowered death rates and population increases. Before tuberculosis was understood as an infectious disease, high rates of consumption and scrofula were submitted as proof that Native people were incapable of making the transition from nomadism to 'civilization.' At that time, when the medical profession was certain that tuberculosis was a constitutional disease, little could be done and little *was* done. But the understanding that tuberculosis is an infectious disease increased the public's fear of it. Reserve death rates continued to exceed non-Native rates, and the perennial gap between the two widened as non-Native Canadians became increasingly healthy and prosperous. Not until anti-tuberculosis associations began pressuring the department to take some measures against the threat of disease on reserves was treatment made available to Native sufferers. But so little had changed. As late as 1945 the Alberta Indian Association was blaming the high tuberculosis rates among its people on the poverty, overcrowded housing, and malnutrition on reserves.[6] Successive Canadian governments continued to see disease as the cause, rather than the symptom, of a much larger economic and political problem.

In 1906 the Saskatchewan Medical Association called on the department to take immediate steps to control the spread of tuberculosis on reserves. The resolution was published in medical journals and newspapers. The Battleford Board of Trade quickly followed suit and submitted a memorandum to the department stating that, since there were eight reserves within forty miles of the town, the department should immediately establish a sanatorium in the district. The Associated Boards of Trade of Western Canada passed a similar resolution at their annual meeting. The board of trade resolutions may have sprung from a desire to reap the opportunities coincident with building, maintaining, and supplying such an institution. But another factor was the health concerns of non-Native communities near the reserves. The chief medical officer, Dr Peter Bryce, stated in his annual report for 1906 that the Native people had a death rate more than double that of the general population, and in some provinces more than three times. The cause of the high death rate was tuberculosis.[7] But hospitals were expensive, and sanatoria prohibitive. Department inspector J.A. Markle outlined the department's objections: since tuberculosis patients needed milk and cream, a hospital would require cows, a stable, pasture, and room and board for the man hired to milk; above this, the nurses, cooks, and maids would have to be paid, and a buggy and team of horses provided. And, he remarked, such an institution could only be justified if it were used 'strictly for the relief of the afflicted. Unfortunately the Indians too frequently rely on their own nurses and doctors when dangerously ill and on the hospital when they could treat themselves at home.' As proof of his contention that the hospital was being used as a 'boarding house,' Markle noted that the monthly hospital returns showed a greater number of patients were being treated when the weather was inclement than when it was fine. Of course, poor housing conditions and inadequate clothing and diet would suggest that the greatest number of illnesses occurred – or at least became more acute – in winter when the weather was cold. Nevertheless, Markle reasoned that if the department's desire was to treat tuberculosis, it would be wiser to erect tents around the schools to isolate the tubercular children. He was sure that missionary organizations would provide the cost of maintenance of about thirty cents per day. The precedent thus set would be quite inexpensive if schools under other denominations began making demands for similar institutions. The department would therefore be justified in providing 'tent houses.' Economy motivated the department in all things, and especially in its acceptance of tents for tubercular children. In conclusion, Markle reiterated that with canvas tents at boarding and industrial schools, 'this disease [tuberculosis] may be arrested and good accomplished at reasonable cost.'[8] Dr James Lafferty, who had tried to interest the department in funding more hospital beds, was dismayed to learn that the department intended to erect tents near the schools rather than fund hospitals for the ill. In his view, the problem with the hospitals was not that there were too many of them, as the department seemed to think, but that they were run inefficiently by the religious denominations. The only solution was to bring the hospitals under departmental control. Lafferty vehemently denied that 'tent hospitals' would solve the thorny issue of high death rates at the schools. Hospitals, he said, were intended to treat all kinds of disease, and a doctor must be in attendance![9]

The notion that tents might answer the tuberculosis problem was not born of parsimony alone. Dr Edward Farrell, the Canadian delegate to the 1899 International Tuberculosis Congress, noted that the best medical advice at the turn of the century recommended the 'open air treatment' for tuberculosis because the tubercle bacillus was killed by sunlight and enjoyed a very short life outside the patient. The open air treatment had gained currency earlier in the nineteenth century through the apparent successes of continental spas where wealthy patients 'took the cure.' Sanatorium treatment preceded bacteriological discoveries and was changed little by it. The rest of Farrell's recommendations, which had little meaning when applied to reserve conditions, were these: prevention or early treatment through the provision of sunlight, and dry soil; good digestion and contentment; medications such as cod liver oil, iron, and moderate amounts of beer or wine; and, because tuberculosis was seen as a wasting disease, as much strong food as possible. The report concluded: 'There is now a consensus of opinion among medical men that tuberculosis cannot be treated successfully in

private houses.'[10] As a result of recommendations like these, the use of
tents for Aboriginal schoolchildren took on the force of medical necessity. The perception that the children suffered poor health in the
schools because they were unused to confinement and a regimented life
also made tent hospitals appealing to departmental bureaucrats. Moreover, it would not have been lost on officials that the people's health
invariably improved in summer when they moved into lodges. The low
cost of the scheme made the use of tents very attractive; at the same
time, the department would be seen as both 'humane and enlightened.'
Tent hospitals, where surgical treatment of tubercular glands was also
performed, were established for a time at the Saddle Lake, Birtle,
Touchwood Hills, Stoney, Blackfoot, and Qu'Appelle agencies.[11]

Farrell's report was printed as a pamphlet and appended to the
annual departmental health circular. The circular was first issued in the
early 1890s, and was distributed unchanged every spring to all agents.
Agents were advised to ensure the vaccination of all infants and the
revaccination within seven years of all adults; also, they were to induce
the people to build their houses on dry ground with gable roofs and of
an adequate size for the number of occupants. Houses were to be
heated to a moderate temperature and ventilated night and day by open
windows. All garbage was to be removed and burned. Personal ablutions
and warm clothing were to be encouraged, and the people were to be
warned against going out in wet moccasins. Bad meat and milk from
sick cows were to be avoided, and food should be cooked 'properly.' In
response to Farrell's report, the department appended a section titled
'Special Precautions against the Spread of Consumption.' It began:
'Consumption in its various forms is the scourge of the Indians ...' Dancing, the other scourge of the people according to the department, made
its way into the circular as an important cause of the disease: 'The
unnecessary frequenting of, and more especially holding of gatherings
for dancing or other purposes in houses in which there is consumption
should be carefully avoided.' The circular was a familiar mixture of current medical opinion and existing stereotypes, and bore little relation to
the conditions under which most Native people lived. Agents were quick
to ask how they were to accomplish the monumental task of prevention
and treatment of tuberculosis as outlined in the pamphlet. But as the
secretary explained, 'the department has no intention of going to any
expense or unnecessary labour in carrying out these suggestions and all
that will be required of you is to see that the sanitary precautions of the
circular and report are complied with.'[12]

Despite the department's deeply rooted objections to funding hospitals, in 1914 it built and began to maintain a cottage hospital at the File Hills ex-pupil colony on the Peepeekisis reserve in Treaty Four. The File Hills colony had been established in 1901 and was the pet project of agent and later commissioner William Graham. Graham, who worked his way up through the ranks of the department, conceived of the colony as a means to combat the 'retrogression' that industrial school students experienced when they left school and returned to reserves. The Colony was intended to promote the Protestant values of competition and thrift and thus create self-sufficient farmers. The colonists, all former pupils of industrial schools, were provided with land, machinery, houses, furnishings, and cash to begin farming. The colony was used to demonstrate to dignitaries and visitors the successes of the department's education system and farming program. It was a 'carefully contrived showpiece' of the department's treatment of Native people. The hospital was situated in the centre of the reserve and was to demonstrate that the school graduates had forsaken their own doctors in favour of modern medicine. In reality, it was a dispensary. In 1915, 85 per cent of the patients were treated as outpatients; between 1914 and 1918, outpatients accounted for 70 per cent of the people treated. As on the Blood reserve, the people may have used the medicines from the dispensary in their own treatments. Despite the appearance of conformity at the colony, the people continued to sponsor feasts and funerals and hold dances.[13] The establishment of the File Hills hospital did not indicate a change in departmental policy. Not surprisingly, then, economy characterized its administration. Nurses at the hospital had unpaid assistants, either their husbands or mothers. Dr H. Knoke complained that he was discouraged from visiting critically ill patients at the hospital. Graham all but admitted that the hospital was a Potemkin village. Knoke, he said, had a 'wrong idea of his duties and that the fees are what he is after and if it were left to him to decide how often he should come we would be called upon to pay far more for our medical attention for Indians that it would cost to send them to town hospitals, where we could naturally get better results.' When the deputy superintendent inspected the hospital in 1933, he declared it a fire hazard and wondered how the File Hills hospital could keep its patient per diem costs to just 80¢ when non-Native hospitals spent at least $4 per day.[14]

Notwithstanding the growing understanding of tuberculosis, there was still some consternation regarding the nature of tuberculosis in Aboriginal people. The experience of tuberculois among Aboriginal people began to challenge the conventional wisdom regarding the epidemiology and treatment of the disease. In his annual reports to the department, Bryce consistently noted that the tuberculosis problem was primarily a housing problem. Improved housing and sanitation, as well as the removal and isolation of the sick, would improve the situation markedly. But he did wonder how it was that Native people who lived an outdoor life, especially those who lived in the shadow of the Rockies in the clear mountain air, suffered so much tuberculosis. According to him, the climate in Alberta was the most salubrious on the prairies, 'in a district famous, and properly so, as a health resort for the white consumptive.' The best medical advice at the time suggested that consumptives 'seek a sunny climate in winter and tonic mountain or sea-air in summer; in both cases in situations where an out-of-door life is possible.' By way of explanation, Bryce touched on the racial theories of the day and noted that Native people were moving through a particularly difficult stage of civilization. The bands that suffered least from tuberculosis were those farthest removed from civilization, or those that had undergone an 'advance in general intelligence of how to live, through the valuable admixture of white blood with its inherited qualities.'[15] The cause of the people's poor health was undoubtedly their poverty, but their race made them less resistant to tuberculosis. Bryce's continued efforts to interest the department in taking some action to improve the tuberculosis situation met with increasing hostility. He did no more inspection work for the department after D.C. Scott rose to the rank of deputy superintendent in 1913. Scott's facility for figures and his close attention to economy had recommended him for the position. Bryce's consistent appeals, public and private, for greater departmental spending on and responsibility for health made his continued employment undesirable.

In late 1913, Dr Orton Irwin Grain was appointed the new medical inspector for the western provinces, specifically to control the costs of the medical branch, and at the same time to control the tuberculosis problem on reserves. Secretary J.D. McLean informed him that 'the department will be glad to receive from you any *practical* suggestions which you may consider will tend to ameliorate present conditions [regarding tuberculosis]' (emphasis added). It was not long before Grain, like Bryce before him, realized that any attempt to treat disease would have to begin with a restructuring of the medical care system. He called for the department to control and manage the Blackfoot hospital as a non-denominational institution. He also suggested that the people would be better served if the department dropped its almost exclusive focus on education and increased its spending on tuberculosis treatment and prevention. Tuberculosis, he argued, 'dwarfs the question of education,' and the tuberculosis problem among Native people was 'a menace to the white population.' Grain was also moved to advocate sanatorium care for Native people at the Fort Qu'Appelle sanatorium in Saskatchewan. But the provincial health inspector, former department medical officer, and co-founder of the sanatorium, Dr M.M. Seymour, rejected the suggestion because there was not enough room for 'white patients.' Economy remained the priority, as secretary McLean bluntly put it in reference to tuberculosis: 'The Department does not propose to incur large expenditure in affording hospital treatment in cases where there is but little hope of effecting a cure.'[16]

Grain then suggested that the department build a sanatorium on the Fort Qu'Appelle sanatorium grounds specifically for Native people. He soon faced the same conundrum as had faced Bryce: the medical branch could not become effective until the department assumed responsibility for health care, and provided medical services with the people's welfare in mind rather the welfare of the surrounding non-Native communities. Grain was relieved of his duties when the department abolished his position in 1918 'owing to the fact that the results anticipated, that is better control over the medical service among the Indians of the western provinces, was not realized and for reasons of economy.' This may have driven the doctor to drink; in 1922 his services as an on-call medical officer were also dispensed with because of allegations of 'intemperate habits.'[17] Both Bryce and Grain had run up against the department's refusal to take responsibility for medical care. They had been hired to manage medical officers, not to manage health care. Their usefulness to the department ended once they began advocating a greater departmental presence in actual medical care for the people. And Grain was dismissed at the height of one of the worst medical disasters of the twentieth century, the 1918–19 influenza epidemic. The epidemic, and the destructive consequences of venereal disease, forced the creation of the first national department of health – a department that did not, however, assume responsibility for the health of Aboriginal peoples.[18] The epidemic and the ongoing tuberculosis problem highlighted the glaring need for adequate hospital resources for Native people.

Meanwhile the department continued its efforts to remake the people, and thus increase their resistance to tuberculosis. A circular was placed on reserves titled 'Instructions Which if Followed will Prevent

Indians Contracting Tuberculosis.' It posed a series of simplistic questions and answers 'designed to easily arouse the attention of the more
primitive type of Indian mind.' Arranged under subheadings it neatly
summarized current medical stereotypes of Native people. After cau-
tioning against the dangers of 'poisonous air' and spitting, and advocating open windows day and night, the heading 'Washing' posed: '1. Must
I wash? Yes, as often as possible. 2. Why must I wash? Because a clean
skin keeps me in good health. 3. Must I use cold water? Yes, every day. 4.
Will it hurt me? Not at all. It will make me strong. 5. How does it do
that? It sends my blood flying round my body. 6. What is the good of
that? The blood carries food to every part of it and washes away all the
poisons out of it. 7. Is hot water good? It is better than none at all.' The
subheading 'Some Don'ts' urged, 'Don't drink whisky. Whisky and
allied drinks are the world's national curse. Don't neglect to call the
medical doctor when seriously sick, and, when you do call him, co-
operate with him. Don't wear wet moccasins. They may be economical,
but they are not healthy. Don't hunt for $100 a season if you can make
$1,000 by farming. Learn farming. Don't be filthy. Water is free where
you live.'[19]

In 1918, commissioner Graham began to agitate for a hospital on the
prairies, stating that the medical attention given to Native people 'is not
what it should be.'[20] Sanatorium treatment for non-Native people
arrived in Saskatchewan in 1917, when the Fort Qu'Appelle Sanatorium
opened with 70 beds, expanding to 310 by 1925. As in other provinces,
the impetus for the sanatorium came from the voluntary provincial
Anti-Tuberculosis League. But the volunteer association could not raise
the funds to complete construction, until the war created the need for
hospital facilities for tubercular veterans. Only then were the sanatorium buildings completed, with federal government grants. Treatment
at the sanatorium consisted of bed rest, fresh air, good food, and (later)
surgical intervention. The mission of the sanatorium was to discover
'suspects,' reduce infection in the community by 'carriers,' and prevent
the spread of tuberculosis by removing suspects and carriers from the
community. The federal government provided a steady income for the
sanatorium with its generous per diem allowances for the treatment of
veterans. In 1919 the Department of Soldiers' Civil Re-establishment was
paying three-quarters of the operating expenses.[21]

Aboriginal patients were admitted when room was available, but only
with the authorization of the deputy superintendent D.C. Scott. By
1923 there was a waiting list at the Fort Qu'Appelle sanatorium, and

'taxpayers' had preference. The cost to the department for treatment of Native people at the sanatorium was $3 per day. Graham argued that if the department's main obstacle to a hospital for Native people was the cost involved, then it could actually save money by building its own 'small institution' at Regina.[22] Perhaps, suggested Graham, the department could use the surplus from the Greater Production farm program to build a hospital. This program, directed by Graham, was a war measure intended to increase the productive capacity of the prairies. Under it, uncultivated reserve lands were leased to non-Natives without the consent of the bands. Much of that land was subsequently turned over to the Soldier Settlement Board for the use of returning non-Native veterans.[23] Scott quickly replied that the capital cost of the building was not the problem; rather, the problem was the maintenance costs, which would be the greatest expense. But, Graham replied, a hospital would not cost much more than the department was already paying for hospital accommodation at the Fort Qu'Appelle sanatorium and the Grey Nuns Hospital at Regina. According to Graham, in 1922 alone the department paid $6,533.30 to the sanatorium and $5,543.45 to the Grey Nuns hospital, and 'the bulk of this was paid from band funds.' (The department regularly used funds from the surrender and sale of reserve lands to offset costs incurred in band maintenance, often without the band's consent.) The costs, argued Graham, would not exceed $1.25 to $1.50 per day including food and medical attention – half what the department was presently paying. Scott informed Graham that they would not be able to use the Greater Production for a hospital and that there would be no voted funds (appropriations) for the year.[24] By 1924 many of the returned soldiers had been discharged from the sanatorium, and in order to repay debts to the federal government, the sanatorium agreed to accept some Aboriginal patients. But those forty beds at Fort Qu'Appelle sanatorium represented the extent of sanatorium accommodation for Aboriginal people in the west. The sanatorium smelled bad, like dirty bodies, a patient recalled. Aboriginal patients 'were crowded in there, and I can truly say that the hallway was even full of patients. And nobody ever came to visit me there.'[25]

In his continued agitation for a hospital in the west, Graham cited Dr F.A. Corbett's report on Alberta boarding schools. In November 1920 Dr Corbett had reported on the horrendous condition of the students, especially in the Sarcee and Blackfoot schools, as an example of how bad things really had become. But Corbett himself suggested that sanatorium treatment was probably not necessary for Native people after all. Many who were sent to the sanatorium would do equally well on the reserve, he argued, because reserves offered as much sunshine and fresh air as the sanatorium. It would also serve to segregate Native people even further. (Of course, the reserves also offered overcrowding, an inadequate diet, and ample access to infection.) The old alternative of tent hospitals was suggested, and Scott agreed. But, he warned, tents should be tried on only one reserve 'in view of the necessity for strict economy.' Graham, in the meantime, was receiving two or three requests per week from agents and medical officers to have people admitted to the sanatorium. Printed forms were filled out and submitted to Corbett, who advised admission in about 25 per cent of cases. Graham reasoned that if they acted on even half the number of cases recommended by local doctors, they would fill the sanatorium within a year. And, Graham asked, what was he supposed to do with the 'hopeless cases' that the sanatorium refused? The department held fast to its policy, however. The File Hills hospital was fitted out to accept a few tuberculosis patients, but there was no doctor in attendance. Graham pointed out to Scott that there were incurable people 'who are actually suffering and some of them dying for want of care.'[26] Moreover, they had faced the same question for forty years and nothing had been done. Graham could not move the department. But he was not the only person agitating for the department to take action.

An emphasis on treatment and prevention in the non-Native community led to the establishment of voluntary associations of concerned citizens. These groups were fundamental to the sanatorium movement. As these anti-tuberculosis leagues undertook surveys to assess the extent of the tuberculosis problem, they quickly noticed the widening gap between the tuberculosis rates suffered by Native people and non-Native people. For example, in July 1921 an order-in-council established a commission to inquire into the question of tuberculosis in Saskatchewan. This commission found that 54 per cent of the 1,184 non-Native children examined had a positive reaction to tuberculin tests – an indication that they were already infected or had been exposed to tuberculosis. Of the 192 Native children examined, 92.5 per cent had a positive reaction. Yet the commission's four most urgent recommendations – that hospital and sanatorium treatment be increased for 'spreaders,' that a preventorium be established for young children of tubercular parents, that financing be provided for treatment for all those who needed it, and that diagnostic services be improved through-out the province – did not apply to Aboriginal people, who were the responsibility of the Department of Indian Affairs. The commission urged the Indian department to take immediate action to control the spread of the disease. It also observed that the Native people suffered comparatively more from tuberculosis than other Saskatchewan residents because of their low standard of living and because of the 'natural superstition of the race, and their fondness for their own method of dealing with disease.' The large number of gland, bone, and skin infections suggested to the commission that bovine tuberculosis was a major source of infection among Native people. The seventeenth of more than eighty recommendations urged the federal government to make a complete survey of the Native population and arrange for special provisions to stop the spread of tuberculosis.[27] The commission recommended that in the meantime, the people's 'natural inclination to outdoor life' should be encouraged and the use of open-air sleeping dormitories be stressed.

In 1924 the Canadian Tuberculosis Association (CTA), comprising sanatorium directors from across the country as well as various provincial public health officers, formed a committee to study the tuberculosis problem. The CTA's secretary, Dr R.E. Wodehouse, reported on the anxiety among the white population living near the reserves. Wodehouse's committee recommended that the CTA exert itself to interest the Department of Indian Affairs in undertaking an extensive study of the problem. The association had made its own study of the death rates from tuberculosis in British Columbia and found that although Native people were only 1/22 of the population, they accounted for 1/4 of total deaths from tuberculosis. The association recommended that steps be taken to find an 'economical treatment' for tuberculosis among Native people. In early 1926 the department made a grant of $5,000 for that purpose.[28] At the same time, the National Research Council (NRC) began to take an interest in tuberculosis. The NRC was formed in 1916 in response to the Empire's need to marshal its resources during the war. Funded by the federal government, it mobilized scientific and industrial research, and supported scientists and coordinated their research. As issues in mining and agriculture arose, the NRC formed associate committees of knowledgeable researchers. In 1925 the Associate Committee on Tuberculosis Research (ACTR) was formed, initially at the insistence of livestock associations battling outbreaks of bovine tuberculosis. The Fort Qu'Appelle sanatorium was named one of five research centres and granted $4,500 for research into various aspects of bovine and human tuberculosis. But much of the of the committee's attention was given to research into the tuberculosis vaccine, bacille Calmette-Guerin or BCG.[29]

BCG was developed by Albert Calmette, a bacteriologist at the Pasteur Institute, and Camille Guerin, a veterinarian. Calmette and Guerin grew a bovine strain of the tubercle bacillus on a glycerine-bile-potato medium to obtain a suspension of the culture. After noting that the bacillus became less virulent through repeated passage in the medium, they began to believe that a vaccine might be made from a safe strain. By 1921 they had shown that the attenuated bacillus did not produce tuberculosis in cattle. The next year BCG was given orally to infants in France. No controlled human experiments were conducted, and Calmette's results were disputed. But the trials in France, and subsequently in French colonies, were encouraging, and BCG was considered to have practical value.[30] American researchers questioned whether BCG was safe and were unwilling to accept it because it challenged the medical community's understanding of tuberculosis as a physiological and especially a sociological disease. The American medical community had been attempting to combat tuberculosis by 'transforming behaviour to create good citizens.' In sum, BCG was challenging American nationalism and its scientific-medical authority at a delicate time.[31] Nevertheless, the vaccine was widely used in France and Germany, especially among those who could not afford sanatorium treatment.

BCG trials in Canada were first undertaken in 1926 by Dr J.A. Baudouin, director of the School of Applied Social Hygiene, University of Montreal, who was working under the direction of the Pasteur Institute of Lille. The NRC helped fund the Montreal trial, in which newborns were given an oral BCG vaccine produced from a strain brought from the Pasteur Institute. The trial was apparently successful, showing a 61 per cent difference in tuberculosis mortality rates in favour of those who had been vaccinated.[32] Unfortunately, the infants were only followed for from one to four years. The Montreal trial was initiated not so much to test Calmette's claims as to affirm them, and as a result it faced the same problems as Calmette's trial – particularly, the outcome that not only was tuberculosis mortality reduced in the vaccinated children, but general mortality was also reduced. The charge that subjects were chosen selectively to skew the results in favour of the vaccinated group was levelled against the BCG trials. The ACTR reported in 1928 that BCG

seemed harmless enough. Although evidence that BCG actually conferred resistance to tuberculosis was encouraging, the committee considered it too early to arrive at a definite conclusion. Dr E.A. Watson, an
ACTR member researching bovine tuberculosis, injected a note of caution. Fearing that BCG may regain its virulence, he warned, 'At best the
vaccination of infants with BCG is considered to be a question of expedi-
ency in cases where children are born and raised in contact with tuberculous cases ... It is believed that in this country present methods for the
control of tuberculosis are preferable.'[33] The method of control Watson
was referring to was sanatorium treatment, which had long been the
treatment of choice in Canada. Vaccination was eventually used only on
those deemed at particularly high risk and those who were unacceptable
for long sanatorium stays because of their low socio-economic status.
Aboriginal people were seen as ideal candidates because of the high
incidence of tuberculosis in their communities and because existing
sanatorium treatment was practically unavailable to them. But in Canada, BCG use remained 'highly controversial,' according to an NRC
history.[34]

In 1927, Dr R. George Ferguson, superintendent of the Fort
Qu'Appelle sanatorium, received NRC funds to conduct BCG research
on Native people. His application was heartily endorsed by the ACTR,
which noted: 'It has long been known that Indians are far more susceptible to tuberculosis than are the white races of mankind.' Although the
committee did not know why this was so, it supposed that the white races
had developed 'a resistance to the disease greater than that of the Indians.' In 1927, Ferguson began by examining schoolchildren and adults
on the File Hills reserve. The following year he and others undertook a
survey of preschool children on the nearby File Hills and Qu'Appelle
reserves. His research goals were these: to determine the death rate
from tuberculosis; to gain information on the process of resistance; to
determine the tuberculosis morbidity at present; to determine the number of active cases that recover under present conditions; to evaluate the
predisposing causes; to differentiate the types of bacilli, bovine or
human, causing the disease; and to determine the necessity of prophylactic vaccination.[35]

Ferguson's first love was not medicine, but the church. He worked for
a time as a Methodist preacher, but a serious bout with laryngitis left
him without that most important attribute of a good preacher, a strong
voice. He resigned himself to his second choice, medicine, but his religious background and his love for missionary work never left him. He

was appointed medical superintendent at the Fort Qu'Appelle sanatorium in 1917 and remained in that position until he retired in 1948. His patients were exhorted to embrace their treatment and change their habits of living. The cure for tuberculosis was not a bottle of medicine; rather, it was 'an Idea: a way of life ... the development of a spirit of faithful endeavour, helpfulness, earnestness, good humour, kindliness and forbearance.'[36] The sanatorium proposed a scheme for veterans to re-enter the workforce after their treatment was finished. Since it was considered important that ex-patients perform only light work that taxed neither their mental nor their physical capacity, they were to be taught to make 'genuine reproductions' of Indian artifacts. The work could be done in 'Indian fashion' – without the aid of modern machines, while sitting around, and whenever it suited them: 'There is nothing done by an Indian that can not be equally well done by a white.'[37] For lack of funds, this program for veterans did not proceed.

The Fort Qu'Appelle sanatorium, or Fort San as it was called, sat in the beautiful Qu'Appelle Valley and was literally surrounded by reserves. Ferguson soon realized that despite the Indian Department's efforts to isolate reserve residents, any success in treating the disease at the sanatorium could be quickly undone by the presence of untreated tuberculosis among the Native people on the nearby reserves. An interesting insight into Ferguson's analysis of the people and their bodies is found in the notes he made after examining children at the File Hills school in 1927. He outlined their physical features and noted: 'heads longer than average for whites ... flat feet are usual.' He remarked on the children's 'hackney gait,' the prevalence of impetigo scars, and evidence of early rickets. He was particularly struck by their absence of nervous disturbances: 'None high strung or very vivacious. Have sense of humour. More mischievous than white. Stoicism marked on injection ... Wonderful nervous systems.' His report then moved from a physical inspection of children's bodies to a characterization of the race: 'Less self control when aroused than whites. Strike – resort to force. Tendency to dominate weaker physically or mentally. Make good foremen but poor drudges. Courtship does not tend to demonstrate itself in intellectual manner. Parental affection very deep but marital affection not manifest or observable. Precipitous marriages – after few days or week courtship.'[38] The doctor's notes go far beyond a simple physical examination of children's bodies, and provide a rare glimpse into contemporary social and medical stereotypes of Native people.

In his reports and articles, Ferguson consistently referred to the

Native people as 'primitives.' Here he was influenced by, and perhaps influenced, the leading British authority on the disease, Dr Lyle Cummins. After receiving his medical training, Cummins joined the British Royal Army Medical Corps. He served in Egypt and the Sudan until 1908, and during that time developed his ideas on tuberculosis and 'primitive tribes.' He taught at the Army Medical School until 1922, when he was appointed to the new Chair of Tuberculosis at the National Medical School in Wales, where he remained until his retirement in 1938.[39] In 1928, when Ferguson presented his preliminary investigations to the British National Association for the Prevention of Tuberculosis, Cummins was the next speaker and referred glowingly to Ferguson's paper, calling it 'most important and interesting.' Cummins's paper concerned tuberculosis and South African Natives, but it was misprinted and carried Ferguson's title instead.[40] That was perhaps an easy mistake, because the two agreed so completely on the ideas of racial immunity and 'primitive' tuberculosis. Immunity to disease was thought to be racially defined, but was that immunity acquired or inherited? Darwinians suggested the latter, while Lamarckians suggested that traits could be acquired from the environment and then passed on to succeeding generations. Both Cummins and Ferguson explored this territory, and their conclusions influenced how tuberculosis was to be understood in Britain and Canada. According to Cummins, 'primitives' produced 'primitive' responses to disease, in that they failed to provide any real immunological resistance to disease, and, culturally they provided no medical measures to prevent it. The adult 'primitive' in fact reacted to tuberculosis infection just as a 'civilized' child would. But, and Cummins was emphatic, the difference between adult 'primitive' tuberculosis and adult 'civilized' tuberculosis was vast. And that difference was not an inherited resistance, although he linked it to the blood, but *an inherited faculty to develop resistance when brought into contact with infection*' (original emphasis). Those who came from stock in which tuberculosis had been endemic for centuries were born with the power to develop resistance. Those born into communities where the disease had been endemic for a short time were without the mechanism to resist.[41] Ferguson made a very similar point. At the Qu'Appelle and File Hills agencies, he argued, there was little or no tuberculosis until 1882, when tuberculosis deaths increased rapidly, reaching epidemic proportions by 1886. By 1890, deaths from tuberculosis were beginning slowly to subside. Ferguson studied three generations of Cree and Assiniboine families and concluded, like Cummins, that the facility to resist was inherited. By this reasoning, the introduction of 'white blood' would aid the process significantly: 'The introduction of white blood is not only a potent factor in civilizing primitive people, altering habits of living, appetities, and desires, but also has a noticeable effect on increasing their resistance to tuberculosis.' 'Primitive tuberculosis' of course, had its opposite in 'civilized tuberculosis'; with the latter, racial immunity had built up in individuals and populations to such an extent that the disease was in decline, and effective preventive medical practice was in place to aid the decline. Ferguson also concluded that since primitives could only acquire further resistance on a historic time-scale, prophylactic vaccination was advisable. Perhaps more important for the vaccination trial, 'after generations of tubercularization, the surviving Indians are biologically strong. The birth-rate is maintained, and the infants at birth are well nourished and strong.'[42] Explanations based on race did not indicate race hatred, but tended to point to observable cultural and biological differences. Even so, the categories of primitive and civilized did assume the existence of an ascending scale of fitness. The construction of non-whites (in this case Aboriginal Canadians and Africans) as physiologically weak and biologically inferior was given considerable medical and scientific authority by researchers such as Cummins and Ferguson.[43]

In preparation for his paper, *Tuberculosis among the Indians*, Ferguson undertook considerable historical research on the people of the Qu'Appelle region. He canvassed community pioneers, retired NWMP officers, missionaries, and Indian department officials for their perceptions of the Native people. His informants referred to their role in the Europeans' 'civilizing' mission. According to I. Forbes, NWMP (retired), who was involved in forcing Piapot's people from the Cypress Hills, 'TB was prevalent among Piepot [*sic*] tribe who were the dirtyest and sanitary conditions as the worst of any tribe of indians on the plains [*sic*].' The Rev. T. Ferrier, current inspector of Indian schools and hospitals for the United Church, suggested that any decrease in the prevalence of tuberculosis was a result 'of our educational and medical work among the people.' Informants contended that cultural adjustment had been too difficult for the people, who were like 'wild birds confined in cages.' Ferguson also interviewed Kiwist, a ninety-one-year-old healer on the File Hills reserve, who recalled that with government rations 'some began to fall sick ... Shortly after treaty children mostly began to have sore necks [scrofula]. A lot of them died, but some got better.'[44] Nevertheless, Ferguson assumed that the Canadian government had foreseen the destruction of the bison economy and thus had entered into treaty with the Native people to cushion their fall 'with the result that when the buffalo disappeared they were straightaway settled on reserves, rationed, instructed, and gradually rehabilitated.' He determined that Native people did not suffer from tuberculosis before the early 1880s because they had not been exposed to it. In fact, they had been in regular contact with traders for nearly 200 years. According to Ferguson, exposure came from American Sioux, Red River 'half-breeds,' and white settlements, which by 1882 surrounded the reserves. After 1879 the people had ample food, but they found their diet of bannock and salt pork unpalatable. Finally, he reckoned that the plains people, like other 'Carnivora,' found it difficult to change and might be compared to 'the equally virile and majestic lion, who when removed from his natural feeding-ground to that of the zoo, not only loses his physique and morale, but begets a poorer type of cub, difficult to raise and susceptible to disease.' Changes in housing, especially the lack of mobility that followed the change from the lodge to the log hut, created new threats. In the doctor's view, the epidemic was as much a result of changed circumstances as the Native people's failure to adapt to change. The epidemic, then, was peculiar to Native people and had a natural course. Decreases in tuberculosis death rates could be accounted for by the physiological response of the 'soil' host. He did allow that improved living conditions and 'a certain amount of selection on the basis of fitness' could further cut the tuberculosis death rate. In this vein, he compared the File Hills demonstration colony (where only healthy ex-pupils were admitted, who were then provided with comfortable housing and financial assistance) to the File Hills reserves, and found 7 per cent more tuberculosis deaths on the reserve. Dr Ferguson lived at the sanatorium and could not but notice the destitution on the neighbouring reserves. Here was a people who, according to his reading of history, were materially aided by government, yet who continued to live in poverty and fall victim to disease at far greater rates than the surrounding non-Native communities. It was obvious to him that the explanation rested in the people's primitive nature and their inability or refusal to adapt.[45] Clearly, he had found ideal subjects for vaccination. And unlike the working-class subjects in the Montreal BCG trials, who had a tendency to move away in search of work, Native people were unlikely to leave the area. But there were still obstacles to overcome before he could proceed with the experiment.

It was a rather easy matter to gain access to boarding schools; the school principals gave their consent to have students examined and tested. Although Ferguson's experiment predated modern-day notions of informed consent, which cannot be applied here, he did consider it necessary to obtain parental consent before conducting tuberculin testing among non-Native children in 1921. (As late as 1966, Dr G.D. Barnett was vaccinating Aboriginal children with BCG in Saskatchewan without parental consent, because the forms were 'awkward and time consuming and eventually I just took it on my own hook to vaccinate them all anyway, as I felt it was good for them.'[46]) It was quite another matter to gain access to infants, most of whom were born at home on the reserve under the care of Native midwives. Moreover, in the 1920s Aboriginal people were beginning to organize themselves politically – for good example, to challenge the Indian Act's prohibition of ceremonial dancing. Ferguson pointed to this 'friction between the Indians and the Department' as an obstacle to his work. As he stated to the president of the NRC, 'I did not consider it advisable to push the clinical phases of our research work here until such time as Dr. Simes has dully [*sic*] established himself and gained the confidence of these Indians.'[47] Austin Simes, a local physician and medical officer on the File Hills reserve, worked closely with Ferguson throughout the trial and eventually became superintendent of the Fort Qu'Appelle Indian hospital. He was remembered by patients and staff at the hospital as an imposing authority figure who was quick to find fault.[48] It was necessary to 'win the confidence of the Indians' before any kind of survey or examination of the reserve residents could proceed. Furthermore, it was necessary to have infants born in the hospital in order to undertake the BCG experiment. To that end, in 1930 the Qu'Appelle Indian Demonstration Health Unit was established, comprising the File Hills agency and school, the Qu'Appelle agency and school, and (after 1931) the Standing Buffalo reserve.

The health unit was initially proposed by Ferguson and the Saskatchewan Anti-Tuberculosis League as a result of their 1921 survey of tuberculosis in the province. The 1922 proposal was for a health unit that would focus on the area's schoolchildren: it would immunize them, improve their diet, examine them for tuberculosis before admitting them to school, and arrange transfers of the acutely ill to the Fort Qu'Appelle sanatorium. The details differed very little from what Bryce had recommended years earlier, and met with about as much success. But in 1929 the proposal was expanded to include the reserve residents, and to focus mainly on tuberculosis. The NRC agreed to pay for examination of patients; the Department of Indian Affairs agreed to pay the physician's salary and to put the File Hills colony hospital under the health unit's direction; and the Fort Qu'Appelle sanatorium agreed to provide facilities for research.[49]

It was an unusual departure for the department to become involved in a long-term medical project; as the department secretary explained, 'the department ... is under no legal obligation to furnish medical attendance to Indians under any circumstance, [and] that the provisions it makes is [sic] entirely philanthropic.'[50] Note well that the department's obligation to the health unit (the salaries of one physician and a nurse) was significantly less than it had been paying for medical attendance. The services of four physicians at the two schools and two reserves could be terminated and replaced by one medical officer, Dr Simes. And like the showpiece of Native farming at the File Hills demonstration colony, the Qu'Appelle Demonstration Health Unit could be pointed to as evidence of the care the department was providing for its Native wards. The health unit showed very promising results. A 'conscientious effort' was made to improve living conditions. A number of one-room log huts with sod or thatched roofs were replaced by frame houses in 1930, wells were sunk to improve the water supply, families were provided with hens and garden seed, and special nourishment was given to schoolchildren and expectant mothers. A full-time public health nurse was hired in early 1931 to provide home care to children with infectious disease, and Simes admitted to the hospital all reserve residents with active tuberculosis lesions. By 1932 the tuberculosis death rate had dropped from 5.6 per thousand (in 1930) to 2.7 per thousand (less than half the rate of other Native people in the province). The general death rate and infant mortality rate also fell. Thus, before the BCG vaccine trials were begun, the health on the reserves had improved markedly as a result of improved living conditions and the segregation of those with active tuberculosis. In the File Hills and Qu'Appelle schools, a simple expedient that had been advocated for decades – removing active cases of tuberculosis from the general school population – effectively reduced the spread of the disease. Ferguson remarked in 1935: 'We now feel convinced that the same policy of segregation of spreaders will have the same results when applied to the Indians as has been proven in the case of the white residents of the province.'[51] More importantly, the successful health measures went a long way toward 'winning the confidence' of the people.

By early 1931, Ferguson was expressing doubts about the BCG trials.

The use of BCG was still highly controversial; his concerns hinged on the fact that the long-term effects of BCG were still unknown. And he could not have been unaffected by the disastrous experiment in Lubeck, Germany, in 1930. Between late February and mid-April of that year, 249 infants in the Lubeck municipal hospital had been given oral doses of BCG. By June, 67 of the infants had died and 80 were critically ill. Eventually, 71 infants died as a result of receiving the BCG vaccine. The Lubeck disaster shook confidence in the use of BCG even after an investigation and trial found that the vaccine had been contaminated with tuberculosis bacilli. Ferguson worried that even though 400,000 children had been vaccinated with BCG with no serious complications except the Lubeck tragedy (which he dismissed as a blunder), there was still the danger that the vaccine might regain its virulence. He thought it wiser and safer to wait four or five years to determine if the vaccine might indeed be dangerous. In a letter to the president of the NRC marked 'private and confidential,' Ferguson stated, 'I feel as though it would be unwise to initiate human experimental work among Indian children who are the direct wards of the Government, and for which reason they are not in a position to exercise voluntary cooperation. Furthermore in case of difficulties arising, the Government itself could not be without responsibility.' He added that the work of the health unit in diagnosing, treating, and removing tuberculosis patients had resulted in a 'very marked improvement,' and that it would be more practical 'to handle the tuberculosis situation in practically the same way it would be handled in an ordinary county or municipality.'[52]

But the use of BCG was a far less expensive method of controlling tuberculosis than the alternatives: providing lengthy sanatorium treatment and improving living conditions. For that reason, as well as the benefits that would accrue to the Native and non-Native communities if the vaccine proved effective, the Department of Indian Affairs was enthusiastically supportive of Ferguson's trial. He overcame his misgivings, and the NRC committee, with the support of the Department of Indian Affairs, gave its approval for the BCG vaccination experiment in March 1933.[53] Between October 1933 and December 1934, Simes, who performed all the clinical work, gave 51 infants oral doses of BCG (30 were subsequently revaccinated intracutaneously, and all were revaccinated every three years). Another 51 infants were selected as controls. Although the selection of subjects for vaccination and control was to be random, Dr Simes found it more convenient to vaccinate infants born at the File Hills Colony cottage hospital and to use as controls infants born at home. The failure to select appropriate controls for BCG trials had tainted both Calmette's original studies and the Montreal trials. School-children were vaccinated intracutaneously beginning in 1933. The results of the vaccination of 160 schoolchildren and 113 controls were never published since there were no tuberculosis deaths among either group, primarily because all children with tuberculosis lesions and 'incipient' tuberculosis had been excluded from the schools.[54] Ferguson and Simes published their results in 1949.

The trial was a success. Between 1933 and 1945, 306 infants were vaccinated and 303 infants were designated as unvaccinated controls. Among the vaccinated infants there were six cases of tuberculosis and only two tuberculosis deaths; among the unvaccinated infants there were twenty-nine cases of tuberculosis and nine tuberculosis deaths. Ferguson and Simes concluded that 'BCG conferred valuable protection in a highly infectious environment'; that the type of disease found among controls was more serious and generalized than that found in the vaccinated group; and, to Ferguson's relief, that 'there was no evidence ... that BCG had a recurrence of virulence in the host.' However, the study, which was intended to show the effectiveness of BCG vaccination, inadvertently pointed to the primary health problems on reserves. Of the 609 children who started the trials, 77 (more than 12 per cent) were dead before their first birthday (39 vaccinated children and 38 non-vaccinated died in their first year.) [55] Four children died from tuberculosis, two each from the vaccinated and the controls. The general mortality was 127 per thousand among the vaccinated group, and 125 among the controls. For comparison, in the Montreal BCG trial, in which subjects were taken from the 'lower middle class and poorer sections of the community,' the general mortality in the first year was 21 per thousand among the vaccinated and 24 per thousand among the controls. Seven years into the Qu'Appelle study, 105 children (over 17 per cent) were dead from causes other than tuberculosis, primarily pneumonia and gastroenteritis. The non-tuberculosis death rates of the children in Ferguson's trial were still twice those of the Montreal trials.[56] The most obvious finding of the BCG vaccine trial was that poverty, not tuberculosis, was the greatest threat to Native infants. Although the vaccinated children were to an extent protected from tuberculosis by BCG, they shared the impoverished living conditions and poor diet of the reserves.

The BCG trial at the Qu'Appelle reserves must be viewed in the historical context of Native–white relations. Aboriginal people were perceived as 'strangers' in their own land and in need of fundamental change; that they suffered from disease to a far greater extent than other Canadians was submitted as proof. Not until tuberculosis was understood as an infectious disease did the public begin pressuring the government to take an interest in the problem. Until Native people could span the evolutionary divide that separated them from the 'white races,' they were a disease menace. BCG might provide the means to drag Native people across that divide, at very little cost. As for the ghastly background of disease and death that the BCG trial inadvertently highlighted, there was no vaccine: the BCG trial was a success, but the patients died. BCG vaccination was extended in 1938 to non-Native student nurses, sanatorium and mental hospital staff, Native infants born at the Fort Qu'Appelle hospital, and others who could not avoid being exposed to tuberculosis. Yet BCG never represented more than a small fraction of funds marshalled for the crusade against tuberculosis in Canada. American BCG trials among Aboriginal people supported Ferguson's results, but the Americans were unwilling to advocate BCG vaccination as a public health measure, preferring to concentrate on the social conditions that bred infection.[57] The University of Montreal's Institute of Microbiology and Hygiene, which had carried out the BCG trial, continued to promote its use after the Second World War and embraced its successes wherever it found them. For instance, 'the most striking demonstration of the effectiveness of BCG ... has been supplied by war experiments performed on humans in Austria. Several subnormal children were injected with virulent tubercle bacilli after part of them had been vaccinated with BCG. These *latter only* were spared the formation of tuberculosis lesions ... One feels horrified at the thought that such experiments may have been planned and conducted, but, since they have been, we are right in availing ourselves of their findings' (original emphasis). Tuberculosis had captured the attention of physicians, government, and the public. The Department of Indian Affairs responded to cries from the provincial tuberculosis associations to do something about the reserves, which Ferguson referred to as 'scattered islands of infection throughout Canada ... a menace to the surrounding population.'[58]

Medical opinion was still divided regarding what caused tuberculosis among Native people, and why Native people were so vulnerable to it. It was the same in the United States with regard to tuberculosis and African Americans. In the United States, however, considerable research was conducted on tuberculosis among African Americans because so many of them worked as domestics and employees in close contact with white populations. Unfortunately, that research was largely directed toward discovering the racial influence in African-American tuberculosis.[59] Since Aboriginal people had been effectively isolated from larger non-Aboriginal centres, the prevalence of tuberculosis among them had only recently become a public health issue on both sides of the border. American and Canadian policies toward Native people's health were driven by the same goals – assimilation and the protection of non-Natives. For a brief period in the 1930s, during the administration of commissioner John Collier, health programs south of the border were more closely attuned to the people's needs. Unfortunately, by the 1940s federal health policy had returned to its original motivations.[60]

Explanations by medical practitioners relating to tuberculosis and Aboriginal people rarely strayed from references to race. Dr D.A. Volume of Southampton, Ontario, reckoned that tuberculosis was particularly prevalent in Native peoples because their skin was too thin: 'It may be stated as a general rule that the susceptibility of an individual or race to tubercular infection is in direct ratio to the thinness of their skin.' Jewish people, according to this theory, had particularly thick skins and were therefore nearly immune to tuberculosis. Conversely, in the British Isles the Irish had the highest death rates from tuberculosis 'and the Irish are literally as well as figuratively thin skinned.'[61] Native people, then, had some 'inherent, anatomical weakness' that made them less resistant to tuberculosis. Fortunately, such theories did not often reach the light of day; even so, the implication that Native people had a biological weakness for the disease was never far from the surface. But that was not the question that consumed provincial sanatorium directors and public health officials. The question for them was, how to confine the disease to reserves.

In the 1930s, provincial health and sanatorium officials began lobbying the federal government to take some action to reduce the incidence and spread of reserve tuberculosis. The provincial health boards argued that although the federal government was responsible for Native people, those people, sick and well alike, lived in the provinces and threatened to undo the provinces' good work. In 1933, at the same time that he was beginning the BCG trial, Ferguson committed the Saskatchewan Anti-Tuberculosis League to provide a travelling clinic to examine Native children at other boarding schools in the province. Perhaps fearful that the department would consider the BCG trial the end to its commitment to anti-tuberculosis work, Ferguson wanted to show that the traditional methods of case finding and isolation would also improve health. The Department of Indian Affairs accepted Ferguson's offer, since it would only have to pay for the X-ray film and the travelling expenses of the physicians; the anti-tuberculosis league would pay the physicians' salaries. Over the five years (1933–7) that examinations were performed, 1.5 per cent of the students were found to have extensive pulmonary lesions and were recommended for hospital treatment. Another 6.5 per cent were found to have 'minimal or incipient' tuberculosis, and it was recommended that these be removed to a 'spreaders school' should one ever be created.[62] The schools, Ferguson continued to point out, were the battleground for the fight against tuberculosis among Native people. It was a refrain that had been heard for more than thirty years.

In Manitoba as well, concerns focused on the threat to non-Native people posed by the presence of untreated tuberculosis on reserves. Dr David Stewart of the Ninette sanatorium urged Premier John Bracken to press the federal government for funds to compensate the sanatorium for its costs, or better yet, to fund the provincial association for further investigations and treatment. As he explained, change was necessary 'to remove from the doorstep of the provinces the anomaly of conditions of uncontrolled nuisance and menace that the Federal government is responsible for, but is doing little or nothing about, and yet that the menaced province cannot interfere with. The slum of the community must be brought more under the direct immediate local control of the community.' Stewart characterized the Native people of the province as 'dangerous neighbours' and a 'menace ... to the health of ordinary citizens.' The reserves, he continued, 'never were water-tight or disease-tight compartments, and in these days of easy travel are becoming less and less so.' Tuberculosis, he said, 'leaked' into non-Native communities through contact at work, through berries and handicrafts handled by Native people, and especially through intermarriage. This last form of contact would continue, explained Stewart, until the Native people were completely absorbed which 'gives the dominant race a motive for doing the very best we can for that dependant [sic] race.' It is noteworthy that Native people were still not considered suitable for sanatorium care. Stewart suggested instead that the residential schools would make 'inexpensive but fairly efficient sanatoria' – in essence, this had been Bryce's suggestion twenty-five years earlier.[63]

Survey work began on some Alberta reserves as well. The new Blood hospital undertook medical inspections and chest X-rays at schools on the Blood reserve in 1929, but the long-neglected Sarcee reserve was not surveyed until 1937 because there was still no source of electrical power on the reserve for operating the X-ray machine. Like the Saskatchewan sanatorium, the Central Alberta Sanatorium under the direction of Dr A.H. Baker would only accept Native patients 'from time to time, when accommodation is available.' It disheartened the department's fiscal managers that the more money they provided for tuberculosis surveys and X-rays, the more tuberculosis was found among the schoolchildren. Dr Harold McGill, the newly appointed deputy superintendent, worried that the increase in tuberculosis diagnosis during the Great Depression was caused by reductions in financial support to the schools. He had mistakenly hoped that there would be a corresponding decrease in the costs of food and clothing for the schools so that 'the pupils would not in effect be less well fed or clothed than before.' Baker told him that if the department provided X-ray films so that all children could be X-rayed, there would be an even greater increase in definite cases of tuberculosis.[64]

Regardless of the medical advice that schoolchildren with active tuberculosis be sent to hospitals (assuming that beds were made available), the schools resisted the loss of students. The Catholic Crowfoot school on the Blackfoot reserve continued to resist discharging students, especially if they were to be sent to the non-Catholic Blackfoot reserve hospital. Father Jacques Riou at the school suggested that the care at the school was in fact superior to the care students would receive at the hospital, because the school provided a 'home atmosphere' for the children. Moreover, the people donated band funds to provide 25¢ per patient per day to provide essentials at the school, which Riou interpreted to mean that they approved of the treatment their children received there. Again, when the Catholics' Lebret school at Qu'Appelle was being rebuilt in 1935, Oblate Bishop Guy suggested that the school have sun rooms added so that tubercular children could remain at the school instead of being sent to the new, 'expensive' (and non-Catholic) Fort Qu'Appelle Indian hospital.[65]

The Fort Qu'Appelle Indian hospital was built by the department in 1936 as the new centrepiece of the Qu'Appelle Indian Health Unit. As a showpiece, the hospital made a good backdrop for visiting dignitaries, as had the File Hills Colony. When Prime Minister Louis St Laurent and Minister of Health Paul Martin visited, they were made 'honorary Indian chiefs' and received feathered bonnets.[66] The department's deputy superintendent, Dr McGill, refused to accede to steady pressure from the Catholic hierarchy to continue the tradition of denominational hospitals. In a bold rewriting of history, he claimed that the department had never followed a policy of segregation on religious grounds. Father Marcotte charged that the department was systematically discriminating against both Catholics and French Canadians. 'Today neutral hospitals,' he lamented, 'tomorrow neutral schools' ('neutral' meaning English and Protestant). In answer to Marcotte's charges, the department maintained that staff at department hospitals were promoted on the basis of fitness, not religious affiliation. Moreover, Native girls and women were to be appointed as nursing staff whenever possible.[67]

Alice Ironstar was eight years old in 1937 and in her second year at day school on the White Bear reserve when she began to get sick. As bad as the schools were, Alice regrets that she never had the opportunity to go. She spent her entire childhood, until she was nineteen years old, in hospital. 'In the month of April 1939 I left home.' Ten years old, with no understanding of English, alone on the train, Alice travelled to Regina, where Delbert Simes (Dr Simes's son) and the hospital's secretary, Miss Mountain, collected her. 'When I got to the hospital there was some patients there from Piapot, and I heard them talking Cree and I was glad because I understood the Cree.' Alice was taken to Fort San for X-rays, 'and that's when I nearly died because I was scared of everybody there. This machine, they didn't tell me what it was ... I was terrified.' Her parents were informed that Alice had tuberculosis and would have to remain at the Indian hospital for six months. A year later Alice, was still in hospital on complete bed rest. 'And I'd be so tired [of lying on my back] I would sneak out of bed at night and run around my bed, run around all over the place.' She was told she needed a new treatment (besides bed rest) because she had been running around. For six years she underwent regular artificial pneumothorax treatments to collapse her lung and rest it. 'They put this needle right through here [armpit] about six inches long.' Other children underwent the procedure, which was not always successful. Alice comforted a young boy while he died. 'They gave him too much air. And he was hanging on to me and saying, "I'm just hurting here [chest]."' After that experience, Alice began to refuse treatment. 'I would struggle.' She remained at Fort San and instead was given the fresh air treatment on the balcony, and in winter it was very fresh. 'Some girls couldn't stand it – they died in their sleep ... I was kind of losing my mind. I don't know if it was sickness, or worry, or lonely, I was too young to think for myself.' Then Alice needed knee surgery. 'They cut my knee in half. They took the joint out, and then they put three nails here, criss-crossed like that, and I lived with that for about a year and a half. I was in a cast right from my foot up to my armpit. I really now couldn't move because I was in a cast.' The cast stayed on for a year. Alice would cry for the nurse to change or clean the cast. 'It was stinky. And they wouldn't listen to me because I never seen the doctor, just the nurse would come.' She managed to work the cast loose so that she could sit up straight 'just like I was free you know?'

Alice got used to the hospital routine with the help of the Aboriginal women who worked there. Violet Ashdohonk worked as an aide and brought Alice special food when she could get it. When Alice could not eat because of the overpowering stench of her cast, Violet brought her deer meat and bannock 'that kind of smelled good. I didn't smell the cast ... that was my first meal in ... about three months. I lived on just a mouthful of bread, maybe toast.' The nurses were always too busy to help Alice, 'except the Indian nurses.' 'The best times I remember about food is the Lebret [residential school] boys bring rabbit to the hospital. So ladies cleaned them up and cooked them just the way I wanted them, and bannock that was our treats in spring time.' When Alice was about sixteen, Dr Simes removed the pins in Alice's knee 'without freezing my leg – nothing.' She remembered that Dr Ferguson 'had more human heart [than Simes]. At least he would stop and talk to you.' One day Ferguson asked Alice if she would like to go out into the country. Ecstatic, thinking she was about to be released, she was instead placed on a stretcher and taken outside. Alice was raised at the hospital, confined either to bed or to a cast. While she was there, her mother died and her father was sent to jail. There was no place for her to go when she was released, so she wasn't released. Her younger brothers were at school, but in summer they had no one to care for them. Alice worried because she knew they were miserable. When they visited her in hospital 'they said, "Sister come home and keep us. We're roaming around, nobody looks after us. Just in school, but they don't feed us enough. We're half-starved."' Her brother Earl hunted every day with a slingshot, killing birds. 'And he had a little can with a wire on it. That's how he used to make soup. He would clean that bird and boil it in there, and that's how he fed our little brothers. Little birds, they lived on little birds and eggs.' Alice appreciates what the government did for her. 'I had three meals a day – four meals – a day served to me at the cost of the government, when my little brothers were starving at home.' After ten years in hospital, Alice was released to Lebret school, where she worked as a domestic, cooking and sewing. 'I was scared to come out of the hospital.' She spent her weekends at the hospital because that was the only home she could remember. 'I went to the hospital not knowing English ... I felt I was a white girl when I came out.'[68] Alice's story was probably not typical, considering the limited treatment facilities for Aboriginal people. But she survived, and at age seventy-one, still with a stiff leg, she remains surprisingly youthful. Her stories are a mixture of regret for her lost childhood and gratitude for the care she received.

Residential schools provided young girls with useful training. Many young women from the surrounding reserves worked at the hospital, but few were ever trained as nurses. They worked as nurse's aides and domestics for fourteen hours a day, six days a week, for $30 per month, and literally worked their way up through the hospital, beginning on the ground floor and moving up to the wards as they gained experience. New employees worked at washing floors or in the laundry, where the sheets had to be soaked to remove the blood stains from haemorrhages. They moved on to changing beds and giving medications. Many recall that the nurses left much of the work in their hands: 'They got Indians to look after Indians.' Older patients sat on their beds praying and singing, but the young women, having been away at school for years, didn't understand. Many of these older patients refused to take their medication: 'We gave them – they didn't take them. They just threw them away. Of course I never squealed on them because I thought they must have had a reason not to take them.' At times the work was so difficult that many women simply quit. Especially bad was the isolation ward, where the young women washed and cared for men with venereal diseases and 'they had this stench ... oh it was awful.' Alice recalls hearing them cry out and moan for water. She took her jug to them. Violet Ashdohonk worked at the Indian hospital, as well as at the Dynevor hospital and the St Boniface sanatorium in Manitoba. She trained on all the wards, and recalls the morgue where Dr Simes performed autopsies, removing organs in search of tuberculosis. They cut them open 'like deer.' Violet's job was to gather up the organs in newspaper and burn them in the incinerator. When Aboriginal people died at Fort San, recalled Violet, they just wrapped them up in sheets and put them on the back of 'Mr Stiffy's' truck and buried them, often in mass graves, in the coulees behind the sanatorium. At the Indian hospital they at least built coffins.

Kaye Thompson, who worked at the hospital as a young woman, recalls feeling terrified when she was ordered to feed a dying man: 'I was afraid to touch him and I was afraid he would touch me or grab my hand.' But she was not afraid of catching tuberculosis: 'They never told us it was contagious.' Nurse's aides were forbidden to talk to patients, no doubt in order to reduce the risk of infection, 'but we did. I used to even play cards with them.' Kaye's older sister Hazel also worked in the hospital and helped her with her chores. Hazel eventually contracted tuberculosis at the hospital: 'She had what they used to call galloping consumption. She died there, a lot of patients died there, from the North and from around Qu'Appelle.' Kaye recalled hospital superintendent Dr Simes and her concern that he would find fault with her work, especially after she broke hospital rules and sneaked a tray of food to a patient in between mealtimes: 'But she was hungry.'[69] The tenor of her stories emphasizes the alien nature of the hospital and what transpired there. She vividly recalls an absolutely frightening sight: 'At the Indian hospital I was working on the ground floor washing floors. There was a room they called the dispensary [where] they kept medicine and things. I was washing the floor and I saw three or four of those big jars, like pickle jars. There were babies inside – Indian babies. There were babies in a solution and they were hiding their temples with their arms. They didn't even bury them in the ground, they were on show, they were an experiment. They shouldn't do that to the body. One was upside down.' Other women who worked at the hospital in the early 1940s, also remember seeing the babies in jars, as well as organs and other body parts. These infants were no doubt part of the BCG trial, awaiting post-mortem examination.[70] In their stories of work at the hospital, these women display a fair measure of suspicion of the motives and ethics of those in charge, perhaps because of their distasteful and frightening experiences. Violet, who spent a considerable part of her working life employed at hospitals, has the most respect for the work and her colleagues. Although they have some respect for Euro-Canadian medicine, they place much more trust in Aboriginal medicine and treatments.

In 1936, the year after the Fort Qu'Appelle Indian hospital opened, the Department of Indian Affairs was dismantled and became a branch of the Department of Mines and Resources. The Indian Affairs branch now faced severe budget cuts, in part due to the Depression. In January 1937 the director of Indian affairs, Harold McGill, instructed agents to drastically reduce medical care. They were to remove from hospitals all Native people with chronic conditions. There would be no more funds for tuberculosis surveys or for treatment in sanatoria or hospitals for chronic tuberculosis. Hospital care was to be restricted to those who absolutely needed it, and then for the shortest possible duration, and there was to be a 'drastic reduction' in the provision of drugs for Native people. Finally, medical officers were to carefully reconsider the need for surgical operations. Ferguson was livid. Under his direction the Fort Qu'Appelle sanatorium and the Saskatchewan Anti-Tuberculosis League had subsidized half the costs of examining Native school children, presumably on the understanding that the initial examinations would lead to further case finding and treatment. He sent an angry letter to his local MP, J.G. Gardner, the Liberal Minister of Agriculture, who was an old schoolmate. To cut off funds, Ferguson insisted, 'will result in a lot of bad feelings and criticism among those who have supported the Anti-Tuberculosis programme so loyally in an effort to clean up Saskatchewan.' And if his point was still not taken, Ferguson noted, 'it is only fair to tell you that one of the worst conditions maintain at the Duck Lake school near Prince Albert in [Prime Minister] Mr. King's own constituency.'[71]

Perhaps through this political pressure, in 1938 the Indian Advisory Committee, made up of representatives of the provincial tuberculosis associations, including Ferguson, met with Thomas Crerar, the Minister of Mines and Resources, to address the rising concern regarding tuberculosis and Native people. The minister recognized that 'public opinion was growing in favour of more active steps being taken to improve the tuberculosis situation not only for the benefit of the Indian but to protect the White population as well.' The committee recommended that infected children be removed from the schools, that yearly examinations of students be conducted before admission, and that those with tuberculous lesions be treated in hospitals or sanatoria. The committee also recommended that tuberculosis found on reserves be treated on reserves with the help of trained medical officers, and suggested that 'hopeful cases' might be treated in sanatoria 'to demonstrate to the Indian that tuberculosis could be cured.'[72] The committee recommended that living conditions on reserves be improved, and that reserves adjacent to non-Native communities receive attention first. The procedure for admitting a Native person to a hospital or sanatorium was a marvel of bureaucratic red tape. The applicant was to be presented to the clinic with a written request from the agent, based on the written recommendation of the reserve physician. The clinic would then make a report to the agent and the reserve physician, who would forward it to the department for final resolution. McGill cautioned that in outlining this procedure, the department did not mean to imply that it was actually going to provide treatment for all Native people with tuberculosis for whom it was recommended.[73]

Pressure from the provinces and the Canadian Tuberculosis Association finally moved the department to take action. Parliamentary appropriations for tuberculosis control were increased during the war years as provincial officials pressured the federal government to assume more responsibility for the health care of Native people. There was not, however, any significant change in departmental policy, even though the federal government at this time was involving itself more and more in the social and economic lives of Canadians generally. The government was willing to undertake tuberculosis control specifically, but it was not necessarily assuming greater responsibility for the medical care of Native people generally.

In early 1945 the Indian Advisory Committee, which was essentially the managing committee of the Canadian Tuberculosis Association, reported that the non-Native tuberculosis death rate had declined 39 per cent in the previous fifteen years, even though the Native death rate had changed very little. Perhaps it was this decline, and the prospect of sanatoria shutting for a lack of patients, that moved the sanatorium directors to press for a standard of three sanatorium beds per annual death; this translated into 6,680 new beds for the non-Native population and 1,390 beds for the Native population. The committee also recommended that more full-time medical officers be hired, with their salaries set at not less than $4,800 per annum. It recommended that the Department of Health establish a liberal policy of hospital construction and begin offering per diem grants to existing facilities. The committee advised the department to amend the Indian Act such that an Indian agent could have a Native tuberculosis sufferer brought before a magistrate and then detained in a sanatorium. In conclusion, the committee urged the government to undertake a study of Native people in an effort to improve their social and economic status.[74]

In 1945, as a result of provincial pressure and the recognition that tuberculosis among Native people was seen as a threat to the nation as a whole, the medical branch of the Department of Indian Affairs was transferred to the Department of Health and Welfare. Brooke Claxton, Minister of Health and Welfare, relied heavily on the advisory committee's recommendations in his 1946 submission to the special joint committee of the Senate and the House of Commons that had been appointed to consider the Indian Act. Claxton repeated the advisory committee's recommendation that hospital facilities for Native people be expanded. He also spelled out the reasoning behind the proposals: '[For] humanitarian reasons and as a very necessary protection to the rest of the population of Canada, it is essential to do everything possible to stamp out disease at its source wherever it may be within the confines of the country.'[75] At war's end, the Department of Health and Welfare acquired three defence department hospitals to treat Native tuberculosis patients. In Edmonton there was local opposition to the department opening a tuberculosis hospital in the city's old military hospital. Mayor John Fry objected to sick Native people being concentrated in his city. The department allayed his fears by pointing out that the proposed hospital would provide employment for about one hundred and fifty staff, and that both the staff and the institution would have considerable purchasing power in the city. The department also noted that the institution would be self-contained and that property values would not be affected. Moreover, the patients would be confined to the institution, and it would be better than having 'tuberculous Indians wandering about the streets of Edmonton ... and spreading the disease.'[76] Fry relented, and the Charles Camsell hospital, named after the deputy minister of the Department of Mines and Resources, was opened in 1946 as a general hospital to treat Aboriginal people in Alberta and the north. A Blood elder recalls that when people were sent to Charles Camsell, 'they never came back.' That impression may have had something to do with the number of thoracoplasties performed there. In this procedure, a lung was collapsed permanently and ribs were removed. Major surgery created its own dangers, and removal of the ribs resulted in significant blood loss and high mortality.[77] Survivors were badly disfigured; some were given wax prostheses to keep their chests from collapsing altogether.[78] The department also acquired the Miller Bay hospital near Prince Rupert and a hospital at Nanaimo, and built hospitals at Moose Factory and Frobisher Bay.

After 1944 drugs were developed that made tuberculosis manageable, if not curable. Initially, streptomycin alone was used to treat tuberculosis; then in 1946 para-aminosalicylic acid (PAS) was developed, and in 1952 isoniazid (isonicotinic acid hydrazide, or INH). These three drugs provided an extremely effective treatment. The need for sanatoria was disappearing quickly. Most non-Natives were treated on an outpatient basis with drug therapy. Native patients continued to be hospitalized, however. In 1937 there were about 100 Native patients under treatment for tuberculosis in hospitals and sanatoria; by 1945 there were 903; by 1953 there were 2,975. The number of admissions dropped steadily after 1953, and by 1964 there were only 860 Native people in institutional care. In that year drug treatment was made widely available to them.[79] The rise and fall of admissions for treatment reflected the growing availability of hospital and sanatorium beds, not the incidence of tuberculosis among Native people.

Hospital treatment for tuberculosis was unrelieved boredom punctu-ated by medications. At the Fort Qu'Appelle Indian hospital, tuberculo-sis patients were kept in four-bed or six-bed wards. There was also a sun porch where patients slept in winter and summer. Kaye Thompson spent nearly a year in the hospital in the 1950s diagnosed with tubercu-losis after a chest X-ray revealed a shadow. 'We weren't allowed to walk around ... We had our meals in bed. You could sit up [and] listen to the radio if you had one. I had one. We would read.' By the 1950s, complete bed rest was being accompanied with drug treatment. 'At the hospital they gave me PAS. That made me sick to my stomach. I couldn't keep any food down. I refused treatment one day and told the doctor the pills were making me sick. I was isolated then. I had to take twenty-seven PAS pills every day. Nine pills three times a day. I felt better with INH ... I left the hospital with a heart defect. My heartbeat was irregular, and it was painful; it was a side effect from the INH. It improved with the Indian medicine. After that I had my lesson, I stayed with Indian roots for my heart, but that was secret.'[80]

Although tuberculosis treatment became more efficient and available to Native people after the war, the gap between Native and non-Native mortality rates remains. Infant mortality rates – the most sensitive index of the health status of any people – have likewise fallen over the century, but again the gap between Native and non-Native rates remains. In 1925 the Native infant mortality rate was 170 infant deaths per thousand live births, while the non-Native rate was 90. By 1955 the Native rate had dropped to 90 infant deaths per thousand live births, while the non-Native rate had dipped to below 35. As of 1985 the gap still had not closed; the Native rate was 20 infant deaths per thousand live births, while the non-Native rate was half that.[81]

The postwar response to tuberculosis was to remove Native patients from reserves, often to faraway hospitals, for indefinite periods of time. Medical treatment was compromised by the emotional and psychologi-cal stress of prolonged periods in completely foreign surroundings. And although postwar governments increased funding for medical services to Native people, from less than $50,000 in 1900, to $2 million in 1945, and to more than $200 million in the early 1980s, a study found that medical services have had very little impact on the health status of Native communities. T. Kue Young's study of health care and economic status concludes that the achievement of political, social, and economic power by Native peoples – that is, self-determination – must precede any technical, Euro-Canadian solutions to the people's health care needs.[82] Health care delivery to Native people continues to serve its bureaucratic and medical masters instead of the people in whose name it was established.

The increasing cultural and professional authority of medicine in the first half of the twentieth century worked to construct Native people as biologically inferior and disease-prone. In the same vein, the anti-tuberculosis campaigns in Canada framed Native people as a disease menace to themselves and others. Although living conditions were often pointed to as a health concern, it was Native people's lack of resisting power that identified them as inferior. From this, it followed that what the people most needed were those inherited qualities that separated the civilized races from the primitive – qualities that were subsumed in Dr Ferguson's phrase 'white blood.' That prescription for good health, coming from one of the country's leading medical authorities on tuberculosis, lent medical certainty to what the department had always contended: that Native people would only gain the good health enjoyed by non-Native Canadians when they ceased being Native.

Conclusion

Aboriginal people endure ill health, run-down and overcrowded housing, pol-luted water, inadequate schools, poverty and family breakdown at rates found more often in developing countries than in Canada. These conditions are inher-ently unjust. They also imperil the future of Aboriginal communities and nations.

Royal Commission on Aboriginal Peoples, 1998

The history of medicine, disease, and Aboriginal people on the prairies is not a particularly proud one. Aboriginal communities remain among the most unhealthy in Canada. Infant mortality, accidental death, tuber-culosis, and new health threats such as diabetes and heart disease con-tinue to take their toll. As the Royal Commission on Aboriginal Peoples points out, much of the misery can be found on reserves and in urban Canada, and is a direct result of poverty. Increasingly, First Nations com-munities are taking over the provision of services to their own people, and this promises to address the issues facing the Aboriginal people of the west. Self-determination for First Nations is a hot political and eco-nomic issue in this new century, just as it was in the nineteenth century, but Aboriginal leaders could not do worse than the Canadian govern-ment has in the past. The new Kainai Continuing Care Centre is a good example of health care that recognizes patients' needs as Aboriginal people. It is not an innovation so much as a return to an approach to health care that existed long before the Canadian government entered Native people's lives. It is also a reflection of the people's adamant refusal to forsake their own medicine, spirituality, and culture despite the considerable might of the federal government. But the journey from wards of the state to autonomous communities is far from over, and many of the roadblocks were built by those who thought they knew what was best for Aboriginal people.

The category of race profoundly influenced how disease and its treatment were understood and explained. The ideas of racial evolution and survival of the fittest explained that Aboriginal people were 'less evolved' and through assimilation might be brought at least to the lowest rungs of a Christian and civilized existence. According to this view, death and disease were a transitional phase that Natives had no choice but to endure. Poverty and disease tended to stop at reserve boundaries, which helped reinforce the racial explanation. The category of race served to absolve Canadian governments, and Canadians generally, of further responsibility. Government had always employed a contradictory and self-serving policy. On the one hand, Native people were encouraged to engage 'Christianity and civilization' to save themselves from ruin; on the other, the rigours of civilization – especially the vices of non-Natives, to which Native people were presumed to have little immunity – were seen as a direct threat to Native people. They existed in a netherworld as wards of the federal government, ineligible to vote and removed from public affairs. Their isolation was made more complete by the restrictions of the Indian Act and by the informal impediments erected by agents and medical officers. These contradictory impulses – assimilation and civilization to save Native people from themselves, and isolation to protect Native people from civilization – led to increasingly coercive and repressive policies.

Coercion is a constant theme in the history of Native-white relations in Canada. From the white man's paternalism, it was only a short step to policies that attempted to force change on Native people. Missionaries objected to the competition from the people's gods, and advocated that the dances and the healers be suppressed. Once 'Christianized and civilized,' the plains people would be able to ward off the diseases that menaced them. The same missionaries placed great hope in the schools, which removed children from their cultural influences, and won legislation to compel school attendance. But the schoolchildren suffered the full impact of the twin pillars of department policy – economy and efficiency. These things squeezed the churches, which in turn squeezed the children and created even more destruction, the long-term effects of which are still evident today. In its efforts to have Aboriginal people embrace Christian capitalism, the Department of Indian Affairs instituted the pass system, which attempted to compel people to remain on reserves, and the permit system, which controlled economic competition. These coercive measures, which were intended to force assimilation, all had serious implications for the people's health.

As a part of the general colonizing and Christianizing mission, it was seen as necessary to free the people from the grip of the 'medicine man.' Healers were constructed as quacks and as clear threats to the people's health, and they were constantly ridiculed, as was the people's faith in them. Aboriginal healers also challenged the medical profession's authority and work. By the late nineteenth and early twentieth centuries, Euro-Canadian medicine had captured the authority of the state: it regulated its own work and determined its own standards. In 1888 a North-West Territorial College of Physicians and Surgeons was organized that established a professional monopoly on the plains.[1] Advances in medicine had begun to confer on physicians the growing authority of science. But Aboriginal people did not share this faith in European medicine. A long line of doctors lamented that the people did not trust them and would not present themselves for examination. However, the dispensaries offered a number of novel medicines, or replacement medicines, and the people incorporated these into their own therapeutic regime. In 1914 the government attempted to compel trust through legislation that forbade people to ignore a doctor's orders. Clearly, physicians and their bureaucratic masters perceived the people's poor health as both the cause and the consequence of their primitive nature.

The immigration boom at the turn of the century created fears that English Protestants might be overwhelmed by foreigners. Peter Bryce, medical inspector for both the Department of the Interior and Indian Affairs, was actively involved in the social purity campaigns of the first decades of the twentieth century, and acted as Canada's gatekeeper. Immigrants could be selected for 'fitness' (usually based on skin colour and ethnicity), and the undesirables could be refused admission, and deported if necessary. Aboriginal people were the 'white man's burden' and had to be tolerated, but they would be made to conform more closely to the Anglo-Saxon Protestant ideal.[2] Non-white immigration into western Canada was insignificant mainly because assimilation was seen as impossible, and those few who gained admission – primarily the Chinese – were often abused and isolated. For all the fears that the 'white' race might be overwhelmed by foreigners, in the 1930s the leadership in prairie society, politics, culture, and economics was still firmly in the hands of British Canadians.[3] As a physician, Bryce lent the racist immigration and Indian policies the respectability and authority of science. Moreover, his work was instrumental in forcing Canada to accept the unwholesome realization that medical care for Aboriginal people was necessary, not as a treaty promise or an act of charity, but for the safety of non-Native public health.

Science and medicine had revealed the mysteries of bacteriology and warned the public of the dangers of communicable disease, especially tuberculosis. As anti-tuberculosis associations noted the extent of this disease among Native people, there was increasing alarm that the reserves were no longer 'disease-tight' entities. Doctors and anthropologists, with their aura of scientific authority, began to eclipse all others as the experts best equipped to deal with Aboriginal people. It was around this time that the position of deputy superintendent of Indian Affairs passed from an accountant, Duncan Campbell Scott, to a physician, Harold McGill. Who better than a physician to direct the department's efforts to contain the disease menace? In 1932, even though Aboriginal populations were continuing to increase, Diamond Jenness, the pre-eminent Canadian ethnologist and government advisor, presumed that he was witnessing and recording for posterity the last gasp of once great cultures. Jenness, a New Zealander by birth and an Oxford-trained ethnologist, joined the Canadian civil service in 1913. His most popular work, *The Indians of Canada*, was first published in 1932 and would go through at least seven editions by 1967, without any revisions. According to Jenness, Canadian plains people were pitiful vestiges of once-great hunting cultures. Although the Blackfoot had been able to adjust to the agricultural economy, many had never recovered from the change, especially the Sarcee: 'Doubtless all the tribes will disappear.' About the Great Lakes peoples, he wrote: 'Civilization, as it flows past their doors, seems to be entrapping them in a backwash that leaves only one issue, the absorption of a few families into the aggressive white race and the decline and extinction of the remainder.' The West Coast peoples 'with few exceptions, feel that their race is run and calmly, rather mournfully, await the end.' In reference to the Athapaskan people of the Mackenzie Valley: 'The trading posts that destroyed their economic independence destroyed also their weak moral and mental fibre, dissipating any resistance they might have offered to the tuberculosis that now seems endemic.' Finally, he noted that the 'most fortunate Indians' were those who had become 'absorbed into the white race.' Dr Ferguson's decidedly nonscientific suggestion that 'white blood' would mitigate the people's tuberculosis neatly buttressed Jenness's conclusions. The country's leading medical and scientific experts framed the perception that Native people were unable to cope with the biological rigours of civilization. As non-immune and isolated people, they fell victim to little-understood infectious diseases. Their strength and vitality were long gone, and they 'called on their deities, their guardian spirits, and their medicine-men in vain.' Accordingly, the impact of disease was cultural, spiritual, and social collapse. Jenness predicted that while some Aboriginal people might be absorbed into the 'aggressive white race,' the rest would become extinct.[4] He allowed that most still clung to their old superstitions, but also noted how they all quickly converted to the Christian churches. Jenness, as authority, fully documented what he perceived as the particular frailty and inferiority of Aboriginal peoples, and concluded that 'culturally they have already contributed everything that was valuable for our own civilization.' He did not live long enough to see that Aboriginal knowledge of medicinal herbs and roots, and their wider cultural view that seeks health in mental, physical, and emotional balance, is being actively embraced by many modern-day non-Native Canadians.

Throughout her life, Eleanor Brass endured the profoundly racist attitudes in western Canadian society, in which the colour line was nearly impossible to breach. She was one of the first children born at the File Hills Colony, which was intended to display to Canadians and the world the social and agricultural successes of Indian Affairs policy. Her father, Frederick Dieter, was a successful farmer at the Colony and one of the first people in the district to own a motor car. Only English was spoken at home, and the family regularly attended the Presbyterian church. Despite the family's successful farm and relative affluence, Brass encountered considerable hostility in non-Native society. She was called 'dirty Indian,' and her brothers and sisters were prevented from attending the village school because 'the school board decided they didn't want Indians going to classes with their children.' Disgusted with the paternalism and repressive policies, she and her husband Hector left the reserve. When they arrived to work for the Sir Bamford Fletcher family near Regina, they were told, 'Had I known you were Indians, I wouldn't have asked you to come for an interview.'[5] They helped organize the Association of Saskatchewan Indians, which joined with the Union of Saskatchewan Indians to press for revisions to the Indian Act, among other things. She spent her life attempting to tear down the walls of hatred and distrust that had been erected by non-Native prairie society and to create an understanding that would allow Native people a voice as Native people. Through her work as a writer and activist until the 1970s, she tried to pull back the veil of isolation that she called the 'buckskin curtain.' Despite her efforts, the colour line in prairie society remained, and she continued to endure racial insults as she attempted to walk in two worlds. Like Eleanor Brass, the plains people of this study did not passively await the redress of their concerns. They consistently pointed to economic solutions to their myriad problems. From Long Lodge's plea in the nineteenth century for 'medicine that walks,' to the Alberta Indian Association's demand in 1945 for recognition of the economic causes of their health problems, to the 1998 Royal Commission on Aboriginal Peoples, the message has been the same.

Notes

Introduction: Beyond Biology

1 M.K. Lux, Assinboine field notes, Kaye Thompson interview, Jan. 1998.
2 National Archives (hereafter NA), Record Group (hereafter RG) 10, vol. 3745, file 29,506–4, part 1, Edwards to MacDonald, May 1884.
3 See Wendy Mitchinson, *The Nature of Their Bodies: Women and Their Doctors in Victorian Canada* (Toronto: University of Toronto Press, 1991); Georgina Feldberg, *Disease and Class: Tuberculosis and the Shaping of Modern North American Society* (New Brunswick, NJ: Rutgers University Press, 1995).
4 Douglas Owram, *Promise of Eden: The Canadian Expansionist Movement and the Idea of the West, 1856–1900* (Toronto: University of Toronto Press, 1980).
5 Alexander Morris, *The Treaties of Canada with the Indians of Manitoba and the North-West Territories* (1880; reprint, Saskatoon: Fifth House, 1991), 296–7.
6 Mary-Ellen Kelm, *Colonizing Bodies: Aboriginal Health and Healing in British Columbia, 1900–50* (Vancouver: UBC Press, 1998), xix.
7 Christine Bolt, *Victorian Attitudes to Race* (London: Routledge and Kegan Paul, 1971), 219; Elazar Barkan, *The Retreat of Scientific Racism: Changing Concepts of Race in Britain and the United States Between the World Wars* (Cambridge: Cambridge University Press, 1992); Nancy Stepan, *The Idea of Race in Science: Great Britain 1800–1960* (London: Macmillan, 1982), xv; Waltraud Ernst and Bernard Harris eds., *Race, Science and Medicine* (London: Routledge 1999).
8 Reginald Ruggles Gates, *Heredity and Eugenics* (London: Constable 1923); *Heredity in Man* (New York: Macmillan, 1928, 1931).
9 Reginald R. Gates, 'A Pedigree Study of Amerindian Crosses in Canada,' *Journal of the Royal Anthropological Institute of Great Britain and Ireland* 58 (1928), 529.
10 Barkan, *The Retreat of Scientific Racism*, 169.

11 Carl Berger, *Science, God, and Nature in Victorian Canada* (Toronto: University of Toronto Press, 1983), 62.

12 Mitchinson, *The Nature of Their Bodies*, 37.

13 John Milloy, *The Plains Cree: Trade, Diplomacy and War, 1790 to 1870* (Winnipeg: University of Manitoba Press, 1988), 6–11; Arthur J. Ray, *Indians in the Fur Trade* (Toronto: University of Toronto Press, 1974), 12–14.

14 Ray, *Indians in the Fur Trade*, 46.

15 Quoted in Liz Bryan, *The Buffalo People: Prehistoric Archaeology on the Canadian Plains* (Edmonton: University of Alberta Press, 1991), xiii.

16 Harriet V. Kuhnlein and Nancy J. Turner, *Traditional Plant Foods of Canadian Indigenous Peoples* (Philadelphia: Gordon and Beach, 1991).

17 Robson Bonnichsen and Stuart Baldwin, *Cypress Hills Ethnohistory and Ecology*, Archaeological Survey of Alberta Occasional Paper No. 10 (Alberta Culture Historical Resources Division, 1978), 28.

18 Henry Dobyns, *Their Number Became Thinned* (Knoxville: University of Tennessee Press, 1983); Russell Thornton, *American Indian Holocaust and Survival* (Norman: University of Oklahoma Press, 1987); Calvin Martin, *Keepers of the Game* (Berkeley: University of California Press, 1978); William McNeill, *Plagues and Peoples* (New York: Anchor Press, 1979); Alfred Crosby, *Ecological Imperialism: The Biological Expansion of Europe* (Cambridge: Cambridge University Press, 1986); Linea Sundstrom, 'Smallpox Used Them Up: References to Epidemic Disease in Northern Plains Winter Counts, 1714–1920,' *Ethnohistory* 44, no. 2 (spring 1997).

19 Bruce Trigger, *Natives and Newcomers* (Montreal: McGill-Queen's University Press, 1985); David Henige, *Numbers from Nowhere: The American Indian Contact Population Debate* (Norman: University of Oklahoma Press, 1998); David Henige, 'Primary Source by Primary Source: On the Role of Epidemics in New World Depopulation,' *Ethnohistory* 33, no. 3 (summer 1986); Dean Snow and K. Lanphear, 'European Contact and Indian Depopulation in the Northeast: The Timing of the First Epidemics,' *Ethnohistory* 35, no. 1 (1987); see special issue *Plains Anthropologist* 34, no. 2 (1989), Memoir 23, 'Plains Indian Historical Demography and Health.'

20 James B. Waldrum, D. Ann Herring, and T. Kue Young, *Aboriginal Health in Canada: Historical, Cultural, and Epidemiological Perspectives* (Toronto: University of Toronto Press, 1995), ch. 2, 'Health and Disease in the Pre-Contact Period.'

21 Crosby, *Ecological Imperialism*, 196; McNeill, *Plagues and Peoples*, 184.

22 David Fischer argues that this reasoning is the fallacy of post hoc, propter hoc in *Historians' Fallacies* (New York: Harper and Row, 1970), 166.

23 Bruce Trigger, 'The Historians' Indian,' in Robin Fisher and Ken Coates,

eds., *Out of the Background* (Toronto: Copp Clark Pitman 1988), 31; Charles Rosenberg, *The Cholera Years* (Chicago: University of Chicago Press, 1962); Trigger, *Natives and Newcomers*, 248.

24 Stephen Kunitz, *Disease and Social Diversity: The European Impact on the Health of Non-Europeans* (New York: Oxford University Press, 1994); D. Ann Herring, '"There Were Young People and Old People and Babies Dying Every Week": The 1918–1919 Influenza Pandemic at Norway House,' *Ethnohistory* 41, no. 1 (winter 1994).

25 Jody F. Decker, 'Tracing Historical Diffusion Patterns: The Case of the 1780–82 Smallpox Epidemic among the Indians of Western Canada,' *Native Studies Review* 4, nos. 1 & 2 (1988), 4–5.

26 Ray, *Indians in the Fur Trade*, 105–6, 113; Jody Decker, 'We Shall Never Be Again the Same People: Diffusion and Cumulative Impact of Acute Infectious Disease Affecting the Natives on the Northern Plains of the Western Interior of Canada, 1774–1839' (PhD dissertation, York University, 1989), 162, 184.

27 Ray, *Indians in the Fur Trade*, 106; Decker, 'We Shall Never Be Again the Same People,' 12.

28 Francis Densmore, *Indian Use of Wild Plants for Crafts, Food, Medicine, and Charms* (Washington: Smithsonian Institution 1923), 354–5.

29 John Hellson, *Ethnobotany of the Blackfoot Indians* (Ottawa: Mercury Series, 1977), 75–8.

30 M.K. Lux, Peigan field notes, Alan Pard interview, Dec. 1999.

31 R. Cox, *Adventures on the Columbia River* (New York: J. and J. Harper, 1832), quoted in Milloy, *The Plains Cree*, 71.

32 Ray, *Indians in the Fur Trade*, 188.

33 Hugh Dempsey, *A Blackfoot Winter Count* (Calgary: Glenbow-Alberta Institute, 1965), 9; Decker, 'We Shall Never Be Again the Same People,' 226; Hugh Dempsey, *Red Crow, Warrior Chief* (Saskatoon: Western Producer Prairie Books, 1980), 14.

34 Norma McArthur, *Island Populations of the Pacific* (Canberra: Australian National University Press, 1967), 347; John C. Ewers, *The Blackfeet, Raiders on the Northwestern Plains* (Norman: University of Oklahoma Press, 1958), 60.

35 Jody Decker, 'We Shall Never Be Again the Same People,' 204, 150.

36 Isaac Cowie, *The Company of Adventurers* (Winnipeg: Wm. Briggs, 1913), 381.

37 Report by Constantine Scollen in Alexander Morris, *Treaties of Canada with the Indians of Manitoba and the North-West Territories* (1880; facsimile reprint, Saskatoon, 1991), 248; Canada, House of Commons (hereafter CHC), *Ses-*

sional Papers, Annual Report of the Secretary of State for the Provinces, vol. 7, no. 22, 1871, 60.

38 William Butler, *The Great Lone Land: A Narrative of Travel and Adventure in the North-West of America* (London: Sampson Low, Marston, Low and Searle, 1872), 371–2; John Palliser, *The Journals, Detailed Reports, and Observations Relative to the Exploration, by Captain John Palliser* (London: G.E. Eyre and W. Spottiswoode, 1863), 200.

39 Milloy, *The Plains Cree*, 117.

40 John F. Taylor, 'Sociocultural Effects of Epidemics on the Northern Plains, 1734–1850,' *Western Canadian Journal of Anthropology* 7(4) (1977), 55.

41 John Hellson, *Ethnobotany of the Blackfoot Indians*, 62; David Mandelbaum, *The Plains Cree: An Ethnographic, Historical, and Comparative Study* (Regina: Canadian Plains Research Center, 1979), 162.

1: 'The First Time We Were Poisoned by the Government': Starvation and the Erosion of Health

1 Peter Erasmus, *Buffalo Days and Nights* (Calgary: Fifth House, 1999), 247.

2 Quoted in Edward Ahenakew, *Voices of the Plains Cree*, ed. Ruth M. Buck (Regina: Canadian Plains Research Center, 1995), 14, 16.

3 F.G. Roe, *The North American Buffalo: A Critical Study of the Species in its Wild State* (Toronto: University of Toronto Press, 1951); Oscar Lewis, *The Effects of White Contact upon Blackfoot Culture, with Special Reference to the Role of the Fur Trade* (New York: J.J. Augustin, 1942); John S. Milloy, *The Plains Cree: Trade, Diplomacy and War, 1790–1870* (Winnipeg: University of Manitoba Press, 1988), 104–5.

4 Morris, *The Treaties of Canada*, 170–1.

5 John Leonard Taylor, 'Two Views on the Meaning of Treaties Six and Seven' in Richard T. Price, ed., *The Spirit of the Alberta Indian Treaties*, 3rd ed. (Edmonton: University of Alberta Press, 1999), 14–15.

6 Morris, *The Treaties of Canada*, 117, 336–8.

7 Ibid., 117; see also J.E. Foster, 'The Saulteaux and the Numbered Treaties: An Aboriginal Rights Position?' in Price, *The Spirit of the Alberta Indian Treaties*.

8 Lynn Hickey, Richard Lightening, and Gordon Lee, 'T.A.R.R. Interview with Elders Program' and 'Interviews with Elders,' in Price, *The Spirit of the Alberta Indian Treaties*; Treaty Seven Elders and Tribal Council, *The True Spirit and Original Intent of Treaty Seven*, with Walter Hildebrandt, Sarah Carter, and Dorothy First Rider (Montreal: McGill-Queen's University Press, 1996).

9 Morris, *The Treaties of Canada*, 332–3.

10 Sarah Carter, *Lost Harvests: Prairie Indian Reserve Farmers and Government Policy* (Montreal: McGill-Queen's University Press, 1990), 57, 62–8.

11 Morris, *The Treaties of Canada*, 198; for the Pipe-Stem Ceremony, see Mandelbaum, *The Plains Cree*, 172–3; and John L. Taylor, 'Two Views on the Meaning of Treaties Six and Seven' in Price, *Spirit of the Alberta Indian Treaties*, 18.

12 Morris, *The Treaties of Canada*, 220.

13 Ibid., 355, 217.

14 Mariana Valverde, *The Age of Light, Soap, and Water: Moral Reform in Canada, 1885–1925* (Toronto: McClelland & Stewart, 1991), 19–20.

15 Erasmus, *Buffalo Days and Nights*, 253; Morris, *The Treaties of Canada*, 355.

16 Frank Tough, 'Native People and the Regional Economy of Northern Manitoba: 1870–1930s' (PhD dissertation, York University, 1987), 106.

17 Morris, *The Treaties of Canada*, 218, 219. Treaty Six stated that the Woodland and Plains Cree people ceded 312,000 square kilometres of central Saskatchewan and Alberta.

18 NA, RG 10, vol. 3636, file 6694–2, Morris to Minister of the Interior, 27 Mar. 1877. Treaty Five, or the Lake Winnipeg Treaty, was signed in 1875 with the Swampy Cree and Ojibwa of northern Manitoba.

19 Hugh Dempsey, *Big Bear: The End of Freedom* (Vancouver: Douglas and McIntyre, 1984), 57.

20 Methodist missionary George McDougall to Morris in Morris, *The Treaties of Canada*, 174.

21 Erasmus, *Buffalo Days and Nights*, 259; Joseph Dion, *My Tribe the Crees* (Calgary: Glenbow-Alberta Institute, 1979), 77–8.

22 Morris, *The Treaties of Canada*, 242; Dempsey, *Big Bear*, 74–5.

23 Dempsey, *Big Bear*, 77–8.

24 Morris, *The Treaties of Canada*, 249.

25 NA, RG10, vol. 3673, vol. 10,986, Anderson to Bishop Grandin, 20 Feb. 1883; NA, RG 18, B1, vol. 1025, file 3533, NWMP Battleford to Colonel Irvine, 26 Oct. 1885.

26 Hugh Dempsey, *Crowfoot: Chief of the Blackfeet* (Halifax: Goodread Biographies, 1988), 54–62.

27 Morris, *The Treaties of Canada*, 258.

28 Treaty Seven Elders and Tribal Council, *The True Spirit and Original Intent of Treaty Seven*, 112, 229, 262.

29 Ibid., 114.

30 NA, RG 10, vol. 3672, file 10,853, part 1, Dickieson to Meredith, 2 Apr. 1878; Carter, *Lost Harvests*, 69.

31 NA, RG 10, vol. 3654, file 8904, Laird to Mills, 22 May 1878; vol. 3672, file

10,853, part 1, Dickieson to Meredith, 2 Apr.1878; Dickieson to Vankough-net, 26 Feb. 1879.

32 NA, RG 10, vol. 3678, file 11,683, 'Dr. Hagarty's Record of Vaccination, 1879,' White Bear's Band, Fort Ellice, 4–5 Aug. 1879; and Touchwood Hills, 15 Aug. 1879.

33 G.F.G. Stanley, *The Birth of Western Canada* (Toronto: University of Toronto Press, 1960), 225.

34 NA, RG 10, vol. 3678, file 11,683, Poor Man's, Touchwood Hills, 15–19 Aug. 1879; Short Bear's Band, 11–27 Jan. 1879, and Reserve at Roseau River, 15 Mar. 1879; Hagarty to Minister of the Interior, [Sept. 1879?].

35 NA, RG 10, vol. 3698, file 16,142, Laird to the Minister of the Interior, 30 June 1879.

36 Ibid., 'Council at Battleford,' Tues. 20 Aug. 1879; vol. 3704, file 10,123, Dewdney Report, 1879.

37 NA, RG 10, vol. 3671, file 10,836-2, Rev. Scollen to Major Irvine, 19 Apr. 1879 (forwarded to the Minister of the Interior, 4 May 1879); Jean L'Heureux (translator) to Lt-Col Irvine, NWMP, 8 June 1879; NA, RG 10, vol. 3696, file 15,266, Dewdney to Col S. Dennis, Deputy Minister of the Interior, 22 July 1879, marked 'Private.'

38 CHC, *Sessional Papers* Annual Report of the Department of the Interior, vol. 3, no. 4, 1880, xii.

39 NA, RG 10, vol. 3704, 17,858, Dewdney to Macdonald, 2 Jan. 1880, 104–5, 99.

40 NA, RG 10, vol. 3706, file 18,809, Rev. Flett to L. Vankoughnet, Deputy Superintendent-General Indian Affairs (hereafter DSGIA), 3 Jan. 1880; CHC, *Sessional Papers*, Annual Report of the Department of the Interior, vol. 3, no. 4, 1880, 102, 104.

41 CHC, *Sessional Papers* (refers to Annual Report of Department of Indian Affairs unless otherwise stated) vol. 8, no. 14, 1881, xxxi; quoted in Carter, *Lost Harvests*, 89.

42 CHC, *Sessional Papers*, Annual Report of the Department of the Interior, vol. 3, no. 4, 1880, 9.

43 Morris, *Treaties of Canada*, 366–7; NA, RG 10, vol. 9413, Treaty Annuity Paylists, 1879.

44 CHC, *Sessional Papers*, vol. 8, no. 14, 1881, 92. Population figures are calcu-lated by the traditional means of approximately eight persons to a lodge (see Ray, *Indians in the Fur Trade*, 105). But as conditions worsened and the hunt failed, and therefore housing materials became scarce, overcrowding occurred as more people were forced into the few remaining lodges.

45 Ann Carmichael, 'Infection, Hidden Hunger, and History,' in R.I. Rotberg and T.K. Rabb, eds., *Hunger and History* (Cambridge: Cambridge University Press, 1985), 59, 61.
46 CHC, *Sessional Papers*, vol. 8, no. 14, 1881, 106.
47 John Tobias, 'Canada's Subjugation of the Plains Cree,' in R. Fisher and K. Coates, eds., *Out of the Background: Readings on Canadian Native History* (Toronto: Copp Clark Pitman, 1988), 194.
48 CHC, *Sessional Papers*, vol. 5, no. 6, 1882, 106; vol. 8, no. 14, 1881, 92; Stanley, *Birth of Western Canada*, 234.
49 J.D. Leighton, 'A Victorian Civil Servant at Work: Lawrence Vankoughnet and the Canadian Indian Department, 1874–1893.' in I.A.L. Getty and A.S. Lussier, eds., *As Long as the Sun Shines and Water Flows* (Vancouver: University of British Columbia Press, 1983), 106.
50 NA, RG 10, vol. 3726, file 24,811, Dr Kittson to MacLeod, 1 July 1880.
51 NA, RG 10, vol. 3744, file 29,506-2, MacDonald to Galt, 29 July 1882; telegram, Galt to MacDonald, n.d.
52 Ibid., NWMP Surgeon Jukes to White, NWMP Comptroller, 17 Oct. 1882; White to Dewdney, 19 Oct. 1882.
53 CHC, *Sessional Papers*, vol. 5, no. 6, 1882, ix.
54 NA, RG 10, vol. 3737, file 27,742, MacDonald to Indian Commissioner, 22 Mar. 1881.
55 NA, RG 10, vol. 3744, file 29,506-3, MacDonald to Dewdney, 11 Nov. 1882.
56 NA, RG 10, vol. 3687, file 13,642, McKinnon to Indian Commissioner, 30 Apr. 1884. The population totals are taken from RG 10, vol. 9417, Annuity Paylists, 30 Sept. 1884.
57 Abel Watetch, *Payepot and His People* (Regina: Saskatchewan History and Folklore Society, 1959), 16–17; Jean Goodwill and Norma Sluman, *John Tootoosis* (Winnipeg: Pemmican Press, 1984), 32; Dan Kennedy (Ochankugahe), *Recollections of an Assiniboine Chief* (Toronto: McClelland & Stewart, 1972), 57; Goodwill and Sluman, *John Tootoosis*, 32 n16.
58 M.K. Lux, Assiniboine field notes, Kaye Thompson interview, Jan. 1998.
59 NA, RG 10, vol. 3686, file 13,168, MacDonald to Dewdney, 15 May 1884.
60 NA, RG 10, vol. 3640, file 7452, part 1, Wadsworth Report, 30 May 1883; vol. 3670, file 10,772, Hourie to Dewdney, 29 Dec. 1883; A. MacDonald to Indian Commissioner, 6 Jan. 1884.
61 CHC, *Sessional Papers*, vol. 13, no. 15, 1888, 78.
62 William D. Johnston, 'Tuberculosis,' in Kenneth Kiple, ed., *The Cambridge World History of Human Disease* (Cambridge: Cambridge University Press, 1993), 1061.

63 Carter, *Lost Harvests*, 107.
64 NA, RG 10, vol. 3637, file 6882, Dewdney to SGIA, 29 Dec. 1883.
65 Quoted in Carter, *Lost Harvests*, 143.
66 NA, RG 10, vol. 3666, file 10,181, Agent Keith to Dewdney, 19 Feb. 1884;
   CHC, *Sessional Papers*, Annual Report of the NWMP, vol. 13, no. 153, 1885, 7;
   NA, RG 10, v. 3666, file 10,181, Keith to commissioner, 19 Feb. 1884; Reed to
   SGIA, 27 Feb. 1884; Isabel Andrews, 'The Crooked Lakes Reserves: A Study
   of Indian Policy in Practice from the Qu'Appelle Treaty to 1900' (MA thesis,
   University of Saskatchewan, 1972), 78.
67 NA, RG 10, vol. 3666, file 10,181, Reed to SGIA, 21 Feb. 1884; telegram,
   NWMP to Indian Department, 22 Feb. 1884.
68 CHC, *Sessional Papers*, Annual Report of the NWMP, no. 18, 1882, 50–5.
69 NA, RG 10, vol. 3666, file 10,181, Reed to SGIA, 27 Feb. 1884.
70 Stanley, *The Birth of Western Canada*, 236.
71 NA, RG 10, vol. 3744, file 29,506-4, part 1, Edwards to MacDonald, 13 May
   1884.
72 Glenbow-Alberta Institute (GAI), M7283, box 1, file 6a, Edwards to 'Dear
   Old Wife,' 6 June 1882.
73 Patricia Anne Roome, 'Henrietta Muir Edwards: The Journey of a Canadian
   Feminist' (PhD dissertation, Simon Fraser University, 1996), 105.
74 NA, RG 10, vol. 3744, file 29,506-4, part 1, Reed to SGIA, 20 May 1884.
75 CHC, *Sessional Papers*, vol. 3, no. 3, 1885, 66; vol. 4, no. 4, 1886, 60.
76 NA, RG 10, vol. 3640, file 7452, part 1, Inspector Wadsworth's Report on
   Farms in the Qu'Appelle district, 1883.
77 Robert Dirks, 'Famine and Disease,' in K. Kiple, ed., *Cambridge World
   History of Human Disease*, 160. See also Thomas McKeown, 'Food, Infection,
   and Population,' and Carl Taylor, 'Synergy among Mass Infections,
   Famines and Poverty,' in Rotberg and Rabb, eds., *Hunger and History*
   44, 288.
78 Gregory Campbell, 'Changing Patterns of Health and Effective Fertility
   among the Northern Cheyenne of Montana, 1886–1903,' *American Indian
   Quarterly* 15, no. 3, 355.
79 Edward Stockwell, 'Infant Mortality,' in Kiple, ed., *Cambridge World History of
   Human Disease*, 224.
80 NA, RG 10, vols. 9417–27, Annuity Paylists, File Hills Reserves, 1884–1894.
   Migration losses are calculated as follows: $(n_1 + n_1 \text{ births} - n_1 \text{ deaths}) = n_2$,
   where n is the year.
81 NA, RG 10, vols. 9419–21, Annuity Paylists, Crooked Lakes, 1886–1888.
   For example, the Battleford reserves experienced a net loss of 696 people

due to migration in an average population of 1,529. Ibid., Battleford,
1886–1888.

82 M.K. Lux, Assiniboine field notes, Kaye Thompson interview, Dec. 1998.
83 NA, RG 10, vol. 3673, file 10,986, Letter to Minister of the Interior from
Chiefs Samson, Ermineskin, Woodpecker, Maninonatan, Acowastis, Siwi-
tawiges, Iron Head, and William, 7 Jan. 1883; Anderson to Dewdney, 22 Feb.
1883; Scollen to Dewdney, 17 Mar. 1884.
84 CHC, *Sessional Papers*, vol. 4, no. 5, 1883, 195; vol. 5, no. 6, 1882, xiv.
85 Louis Cochin, *The Reminiscences of Louis Cochin, OMI* (Battleford: Canadian
North-West Historical Society Publications, 1927), 26.
86 NA, RG 18, Records of the RCMP, B1, vol. 1025, file 3533, Oulison to NWMP
Commissioner, Battleford 23 Oct. 1883.
87 NA, RG 10, vol. 9417, Annuity Paylists, Treaty Six, 1883; vol. 9418, Annuity
Paylists for Treaties 4, 6, and 7, One Arrow's Band, 1884; CHC, *Sessional
Papers*, vol. 3, no. 3, 1885, 81, Report of Agent J. Ansdell Macrae, Carlton,
11 Aug. 1884.
88 Dempsey, *Big Bear*, 94.
89 Robert Jefferson, 'Incidents of the Rebellion as Related by Robert Jefferson,'
in Campbell Innes, ed., *The Cree Rebellion of 1884* (Battleford, SK: Canadian
North-West Historical Society Publications, 1926), 34–5; Fine Day, 'Incidents
of the Rebellion as Related by Fine Day,' 17.
90 NA, RG 10, vol. 3697, file 15,423, Carlton Chiefs' Grievances, 1884, Macrae
to Dewdney, 25 Aug. 1884; Reed to SGIA, 23 Jan. 1885.
91 Robert Jefferson, *Fifty Years on the Saskatchewan* (Battleford, SK: Canadian
North-West Historical Society Publications, 1929), 126.
92 Fine Day, 'Incidences of the Rebellion,' 13; Jefferson, *Fifty Years on the
Saskatchewan*, 126.
93 Tobias, 'Canada's Subjugation of the Plains Cree, 1879–1885'; Dempsey, *Big
Bear*; Gerald Friesen, *The Canadian Prairies: A History* (Toronto: University of
Toronto Press, 1984); Bob Beal and Rod Macleod, *Prairie Fire: The 1885 North-
West Rebellion* (Edmonton: Hurtig, 1984); Blair Stonechild and Bill Waiser,
Loyal Till Death: Indians and the North-West Rebellion (Calgary: Fifth House,
1997).
94 See Stonechild and Waiser, *Loyal Till Death*, 98.
95 Joseph Dion, *My Tribe the Crees* (Calgary: Glenbow-Alberta Institute, 1979),
92, 108.
96 Tobias, 'Canada's Subjugation of the Plains Cree,' 208.
97 CHC, *Sessional Papers*, vol. 4, no. 4, 1886, 141.
98 Jefferson, *Fifty Years on the Saskatchewan*, 125, 126.

99 Saskatchewan *Herald*, 20 September 1884.

100 *The Facts Respecting Indian Administration in the North-West*, (Ottawa: Department of Indian Affairs, 1886), 6.

101 NA, RG 10, vol. 3794, file 46,205, telegram from Chiefs Alexander, Michael Callihoo to Macdonald, 23 Feb. 1888; Wilson to Reed, 9 Mar. 1888; deBalinhard to Reed, 5 Mar. 1888; Agent's Report, 31 Jan. 1888; Reed to Dewdney, 5 Apr. 1888; The *British Columbian*, 28 Mar. 1888; Qu'Appelle *Vidette*, 29 Mar. 1888; Toronto *Globe*, 'Dewdney Is Still at Regina,' 28 Mar. 1888.

102 NA, RG 10, vol. 3794, file 46,205, Reed to Dewdney, 5 Apr. 1888; vol. 3770, file 33,711, Agent's Monthly Report, 31 Dec. 1888.

103 NA, RG 10, vol. 3766, file 32,949, Mackay to commissioner, 21 Sept. 1886; CHC, *Sessional Papers*, vol. 13, no. 15, 1888, l.

104 NA, RG 10, vol. 9419, Annuity Paylists Battleford, 1886.

105 Herbert Brown Ames, *The City Below the Hill* (1897; reprint, Toronto: University of Toronto Press, 1972), 81.

106 The total appropriations for supplies for the destitute for Treaties Four, Six, and Seven were increased from $473,455.01 in 1885 to $539,075.38 in 1886, CHC *Sessional Papers*, vol. 4, no. 4, 1886; vol. 5, no. 6, 1887. The appropriation for Treaty Four in 1885 was $58,473.49, in 1886 it was $55,686.45; in Treaty Six in 1885 the appropriation was $127,392.26, in 1886 it was $98,915.65; in Treaty Seven in 1885 the appropriation was $287,589.32, in 1886 it was $384,473.29, CHC, *Sessional Papers*, 1886, 1887. The people of Treaty Seven received all of the increased appropriations because they were not implicated in the rebellion.

107 CHC, *Sessional Papers*, vol. 5, no. 6, 1882, xxiv.

108 NA, RG 10, vol. 3751, file 30,249, Dewdney to MacPherson, acting SGIA, 18 June 1881.

109 Indian History Film Project (Saskatchewan Indian Federated College Library, Regina, Saskatchewan), IH 245, interview with Tom Yellowhorn, Peigan, 7 Mar. 1975; IH 234, 234a, interview with Useless Good Runner, Blood Elder; M.K. Lux, Peigan field notes, Alan Pard interview, Dec. 1999; IH233, 233a, interview with George First Rider, Blood Elder.

110 NA, MG 29, D65, vol. 8, Maclean Papers, 'Daily Journal Fort Macleod, 1880–1888,' entry for 25 June 1883, 52.

111 CHC, *Sessional Papers,*, vol. 4, no. 5, 1883, 176.

112 Noel Dyck, 'The Administration of Federal Indian Aid in the North-West Territories, 1879–1885' (MA thesis, University of Saskatchewan, 1970), 55; NA, RG 10, vol. 3696, file 150,040, Wadsworth to Dewdney, 14 Aug. 1884; vol. 9418, Annuity Paylists, 1884.

113 GAI, M8458, Lucien M. and Jane R. Hanks fonds, box 2, file 46, 'Many Guns Interview,' 1938.

114 Quoted in Gail Pat Parsons, 'Puerperal Fever, Anticontagionists, and Miasmatic Infection, 1840–1860: Toward a New History of Puerperal Fever in Antebellum America,' *Journal of the History of Medicine* 52, no. 4 (October 1997), 438.

115 NA, RG 10, vol. 9417, Annuity Paylists for Treaties 4, 6, and 7, Blackfoot Reserve, 1884; the sixty-one deaths were from all causes, CHC, *Sessional Papers*, Report of Acting Agent W. Pocklington, vol. 3, no. 3, 1884, 87.

116 GAI, M4421, R.N. Wilson fonds, vol. 2, 'Bad Head Winter Count.'

117 Kennedy, *Recollections of an Assiniboine Chief*, 72.

118 Treaty Seven Elders and Tribal Council, *The True Spirit and Original Intent of Treaty Seven*, 140–1.

119 NA, RG 10, vol. 3653, file 8675, Pocklington to commissioner, 8 Aug. 1883; CHC, *Sessional Papers*, vol. 3, no. 3, 1885, 88.

120 Robert Kim-Farley, 'Measles,' in Kiple, ed., *Cambridge World History of Human Disease*, 873.

121 NA, RG 10, vol. 9419, Annuity Paylists, Stoney, 1887. There were sixty-four deaths from all causes in a population of 614; vols. 9420, 9421, 9422; CHC, *Sessional Papers*, vol. 13, no. 15, 1888, 103, 193.

122 The appropriation for the Blackfoot in 1886 was $142,034.77, and in 1887 it was $87,729.29, CHC *Sessional Papers*, vol. 5, no. 6, 1887, 170, and vol. 13, no. 15, 1888, 174; NA, RG 10, vol. 3712, file 25,550-5, Inspector's Reports, Blackfoot Reserves, 1885–87.

123 NA, RG 10, vol. 3770, file 3395-2, Blackfoot Reports, 8 Feb. 1887.

124 David Breen, *The Canadian Prairie West and the Ranching Frontier, 1874–1924* (Toronto: University of Toronto Press, 1983), 8.

125 CHC, *Sessional Papers*, vol. 3, no. 3, 1885, 159–61. The expenditures were for 'Supplies for the Destitute' and did not include annuities or wages and expenses for department employees; CHC, *Sessional Papers*, 1885–1892. For example, in 1886 in Treaty Seven the total expenditure reported under the 'Supplies for the Destitute' was $384,473.29 for a population of 6,294. Flour cost between $2.84 and $4.00 per sack, and beef cost $0.11 per pound. In Treaty Six the expenditure was $98,915.65 for a population of 6,329, with flour at $6.75 per sack and bacon at $0.15 per pound. In Treaty Four the population was 4,643 and the expenditure was $55,686.45, while flour cost $2.71 per sack and bacon $0.12 per pound.

126 Noel Dyck, 'An Opportunity Lost: The Initiative of the Reserve Agricultural Programme in the Prairie West,' in F. Laurie Barron and James B. Waldram,

eds., *1885 and After: Native Society in Transition* (Regina: Canadian Plains Research Center, 1986), 127.

127 For example, the per capita expenditure for Treaty Seven in 1887 was $42.95. The per diem was $0.11 per person, which was spent not just on rations but on freighting, medicines, blankets, tea, etc. The same year, the per diem for Treaty Six was $0.08, and for Treaty Four $0.03.

128 CHC, *Sessional Papers*, vol. 3, no. 3, 1885, 88.

129 In 1881 the total Blackfoot population was 2,761. In 1882 the population receiving annuities was lowered to 2,255. In 1883 it was lowered again to 2,158 – a loss of 603 people or 21.8 per cent of the population.

130 NA, RG 10, vols. 9414–16, Annuity Paylists Blackfoot, 1881–1883. The average death rate, 1883–1888, was 22.4 per thousand, and the average birth rate was 15.4 per thousand; vols. 9416–21, Annuity Paylists Blackfoot, 1883–1888.

131 Ibid., vol. 3644, file 7785-1, Dewdney to SGIA, 17 July 1883; vol. 3698, file 16,106, Pocklington to Dewdney, 30 Sept. 1884; vol. 3357, file 31,398-1, Reed to SGIA, 24 Jan. 1887.

132 Indian History Film Project, IH 226, Jim Black, Blackfoot elder, 18 June 1974; IH 245, Tom Yellowhorn, Peigan elder, 7 March 1975.

133 Jefferson, *Fifty Years on the Saskatchewan*, 36.

134 NA, RG 10, vol. 3949, file 126,345, Lindsay to Forget, 31 May 1895.

135 Blackfoot elder Jim Black related the story and suggested that the English translation of Ajawana was 'Scrapings,' not 'Scraping Hide or High' as the newspapers reported (IH 226, Indian History Film Project). Hugh Dempsey states that his name was Atsa'oan or Scraping High, *Amazing Death of Calf Shirt* (Saskatoon: Fifth House, 1994), 186.

136 NA, RG 10, vol. 3912, file 111,762, MacDonnell to Alex McGibbon, 29 May 1895; John McCrea to McGibbon, 31 May 1895; Baker to McGibbon, 1 June 1895; MacDonell to McGibbon, 29 May 1895; Baker to McGibbon, 1 June 1895; Reed to Forget, 6 Apr. 1895.

137 Arthur J. Ray, *The Canadian Fur Trade in the Industrial Age* (Toronto: University of Toronto Press, 1990), 30.

138 In this period the total expenditure for relief supplies ranged from a low in 1885 of $478,038 to a high in 1886 of $541,825.26, CHC, *Sessional Papers*, 'Supplies for the Destitute,' 1883 to 1887; Ray, *The Canadian Fur Trade in the Industrial Age*, 40.

139 CHC *Debates*, 27 Apr. 1882, 1186.

140 Morris, *Treaties of Canada*, 211.

141 Dion, *My Tribe the Crees*, 114.

2: 'Help Me Manitou': Medicine and Healing in Plains Cultures

1 Quoted in Katherine Pettipas, 'Severing the Ties That Bind: The Canadian Indian Act and the Repression of Indigenous Religious Systems in the Prairie Region, 1896–1951' (PhD dissertation, University of Manitoba, 1988), 137.

2 Charles Rosenberg, 'The Therapeutic Revolution,' in Charles Rosenberg, ed., *Explaining Epidemics* (Cambridge: Cambridge University Press, 1992), 10–11.

3 David Young et al., *Cry of the Eagle: Encounters with a Cree Healer* (Toronto: University of Toronto Press, 1989), 25.

4 M.K. Lux, Peigan field notes, Alan Pard interview, Dec. 1999.

5 Saskatchewan Archives Board (hereafter SAB), Mandelbaum field notes, Notebooks vol. I, 1934, Qu'Appelle Agency, Informant Sam Seer, 142.

6 See Glenbow-Alberta Institute (GAI), M8458, Lucien M. and Jane R. Hanks fonds, box 2, file 61, informant Mary White Eagle, 'Some others have vowed just saying it [vowing to take a bundle] ie no sickness. This is the original old way,' 10.

7 Quoted in Beverly Hungry Wolf, *The Ways of My Grandmothers* (New York: Quill, 1980), 34.

8 GAI, M37, Fran Fraser Collection, Mrs Rose Ayoungman, 8–9.

9 Claude E. Shaeffer, *Blackfoot Shaking Tent*, Occasional Paper No. 5 (Calgary: Glenbow Museum, 1969); Michael S. Kennedy, ed., *The Assiniboines: From the Accounts of the Old Ones Told to First Boy (James Larpenteur Long)* (Norman: University of Oklahoma Press, 1961), 163; David G. Mandelbaum, *The Plains Cree: An Ethnographic, Historical, and Comparative Study* (Regina: Canadian Plains Research Center, 1979), 176. The Plains Cree have a number of vowed ceremonies: the Thirst Dance, the Smoking Tipi (*pihtwowikamik*), the Masked or Wihtiko Dance (*wihtikokancimuwin*), the Give Away Dance, the Prairie Chicken Dance, the Horse, Elk, Bee, and Bear dances, the Pipestem Bundle Dance, and the Round Dance.

10 Hugh Dempsey, *Blackfoot Ghost Dance*, Occasional Paper No. 3 (Calgary: Glenbow-Alberta Institute, 1968), 3.

11 Mandelbaum, *The Plains Cree*, 162, 232; GAI, M8458, Hanks fonds, box 2, file 48; Mike Mountain Horse, *My People the Bloods* (Calgary: Glenbow Museum and Blood Tribal Council, 1989), 67.

12 John C. Hellson, *Ethnobotany of the Blackfoot Indians* (Ottawa: Mercury Series, 1977), 62, 63.

13 M.K. Lux, Blood field notes, Dec. 1999.

14 Kennedy, ed., *The Assiniboines*, 158.

15 M.K. Lux, Blood field notes, Dec. 1999.

16 William E. Farr, 'Introduction' to Walter McClintock, *The Old North Trail: Life Legends and Religion of the Blackfeet Indians* (Lincoln: University of Nebraska Press, 1999), xiv.
17 McClintock, *The Old North Trail*, 244–50.
18 M.K. Lux, Peigan field notes, Alan Pard interview, Dec. 1999.
19 M.K. Lux, Assiniboine field notes, Kaye Thompson interview, Dec. 2000.
20 Mandelbaum, *The Plains Cree*, 162, 163, 168.
21 GAI, M37, Fran Fraser Collection, Rose Ayoungman, 9.
22 GAI, M243 Esther Schiff Goldfrank fonds, Mrs Jessie Creighton, 265.
23 Mandelbaum, *The Plains Cree*, 150–3.
24 SAB, Mandelbaum field notes, Notebook V, Fine Day, Aug. 1934, 117.
25 Mandelbaum, *The Plains Cree*, 183.
26 SAB, Mandelbaum field Notes, Notebook II, 1935, 10.
27 Pettipas, *Severing the Ties That Bind*, 58–9.
28 Clark Wissler, *A Blackfoot Source Book* (New York: Garland Publishing, 1986), 432.
29 Mike Mountain Horse, *My People the Bloods*, 57.
30 M.K. Lux, Peigan field notes, Alan Pard interview, Dec. 1999.
31 John Hellson, *Ethnobotany of the Blackfoot Indians*, 70–3.
32 M.K. Lux, Assiniboine field notes, Kaye Thompson interview, Jan. 1998.
33 Freda Ahenakew and H.C. Wolfart, eds., *Our Grandmother's Lives as Told in Their Own Words* (Saskatoon: Fifth House, 1992), 157.
34 Dianne Meili, *Those Who Know: Profiles of Alberta's Native Elders* (Edmonton: NeWest Press, 1991), 135–6.
35 Hellson, *Ethnobotany of the Blackfoot Indians*, 65.
36 M.K. Lux, Assiniboine field notes, Violet Ashdohonk interview, Jan. 2000.
37 See Young et al., *Cry of the Eagle*.
38 NA, MG 29, D65, vol. 8, MacLean Papers, 'Daily Journal Fort Macleod 1880–1888,' entry for Sunday 2 Sept. 1883, 54.
39 Raymond J.A. Huel, *Proclaiming the Gospel to the Indians and the Metis* (Edmonton: University of Alberta Press, 1996), 76.
40 CHC, *Sessional Papers*, vol. 3, no. 3, 1885, 158.
41 GAI, M2816, vol. 8, Dewdney Papers, Lacombe to Dewdney, 7 Apr. 1889, 2187.
42 GAI, M1234, Tims Papers, file 7, Reed to Tims, 21 April 1891.
43 Quoted in Jacqueline Gresko, 'White "Rites" and Indian "Rites": Indian Education and Native Responses in the West, 1879–1910,' in Anthony Rasporich, ed., *Western Canada: Past and Present* (Calgary: McClelland & Stewart West, 1975), 176.
44 GAI, M2476, McNeill to Commissioner, 5 Feb. 1904.

45 Pettipas, *Severing the Ties That Bind*, 109.
46 CHC, *Sessional Papers*, vol. 3, no. 3, 1885, 74; vol. 13, no. 15, 1888, 97; vol. 4, no. 4, 1886, 76; vol. 5, no. 6, 1887, 122.
47 See John Duffy, 'Medicine and Medical Practices among the Aboriginal American Indians,' *International Record of Medicine* 171 (1958), 347.
48 NA, RG 10, vol. 3855, file 79,963, Orton to SGIA, 16 June 1891. George Orton was born in 1837 in Guelph, Ontario, and was appointed to the Indian Department in Feb. 1888; SGIA to Orton, 9 July 1891.
49 NA, RG 10, vol. 3765, file 32,784, Battleford Agency Monthly Reports, 31 July 1890; CHC, *Sessional Papers*, vol. 10, no. 12, 1890, 78.
50 NA, RG 10, vol. 3770, file 3395-2, Blackfoot Reports, 3 Mar. 1888; Blackfoot Reports, 1 May 1889, 3 June 1889.
51 NA, RG 10, vol. 3765, file 32,784, Williams to commissioner, 30 June 1888; 31 Jan.1889, 28 Feb. 1889, 31 Mar. 1889.
52 CHC, *Sessional Papers*, vol. 13, no. 16, 1889, 95.
53 NA, MG 29, E–106, Reed Papers, vol. 16, Dewdney to Reed, 26 May 1890.
54 CHC, *Sessional Papers*, vol. 15, no. 18, 1891, 39, 44, 71.
55 NA, RG 10, vol. 3765, file 32,784, Williams to commissioner, 31 Jan., 28 Feb. and 31 Mar. 1890; NA, RG 10, vol. 9423, Annuity Paylists Thunderchild and Sweet Grass, 1890. At Red Pheasant the death rate was 31 per thousand, at Poundmaker's it was 48 per thousand, and at Mosquito's it was 65.5 per thousand.
56 CHC, *Sessional Papers*, vol. 15, no. 18, 1891, 151, 200; vols. 15, 25, nos. 18, 10, 1891, 1892.
57 CHC, *Sessional Papers*, NWMP Annual Report, vol. 11, no. 15, 1897, 65, 138; quoted in Pettipas, *Severing the Ties That Bind*, 116; CHC, *Sessional Papers*, vol. 10, no. 14, 1896, 67.
58 CHC, *Sessional Papers*, vol. 11, no. 14, 1897, Report of the DSGIA, xxxii.
59 Pettipas, *Severing the Ties That Bind*, 137; John Tobias, 'Payipwat,' *Dictionary of Canadian Biography* 13 (Toronto: University of Toronto Press, 1994), 818; CHC, *Sessional Papers*, vol. 11, no. 27, 1904, 207.
60 SAB, Mandelbaum field notes, vol. 1, Crooked Lakes, June 1934, 'General Remarks in Moose Mountain Agency,' 9.
61 CHC, *Sessional Papers*, vol. 10, no. 14, 1896, 199; vol. 11, no. 14, 1897, 166.
62 Robert Jefferson, *Fifty Years on the Saskatchewan* (Battleford, SK: Canadian North-West Historical Society Publications, 1929), 82.
63 M.K. Lux, Assiniboine field notes, Kaye Thompson interview, Jan. 1998.
64 William M. Graham, *Treaty Days: Reflections of an Indian Commissioner* (Calgary: Glenbow Museum, 1991), 44.
65 M.K. Lux, Assiniboine field notes, Jan. 2000.

66 CHC, *Sessional Papers*, vol. 11, no. 27, 1907, 'Report of the Deputy Superintendent General,' xxii.

67 SAB, Mandelbaum field notes, vol. I, 'General Remarks about the Sun Dance,' Crooked Lakes, 23 June 1934, 17.

68 See especially Martin, *Keepers of the Game*; John W. Grant, *Moon of Wintertime* (Toronto: University of Toronto Press, 1984).

69 SAB, Mandelbaum Field notes, notebook VII, 1934, 12.

70 Pettipas, *Severing the Ties That Bind*, 220–1; for similar notions of resistance and accommodation, see also Eugene Genovese, *Roll, Jordan, Roll: The World the Slaves Made* (New York: Vantage Books, 1976), 161–232.

71 NA, MG 29, D65, vol. 8, Maclean Papers, 'Daily Journal Fort Macleod, 1880–1888,' 9 Aug. 1885.

72 SAB, Mandelbaum field notes, Notebook vol. I, Crooked Lakes, 23 June 1934, 38; Mandelbaum, *The Plains Cree*, 183.

73 CHC, *Sessional Papers* vol. 11, no. 14, 1897, Reed Report, xxiv.

74 Mandelbaum, *The Plains Cree*, 139; Alex Johnston, *Plants and the Blackfoot*, Occasional Paper No. 4 (Edmonton: Provincial Museum of Alberta Natural History, 1982), 7; Anna Leighton, *Wild Plant Use by the Woods Cree of East-Central Saskatchewan*, Canadian Ethnology Service, Paper No. 101 (Ottawa: National Museum, 1985), 77.

75 Meili, *Those Who Know*, 54.

76 SAB, Mandelbaum field notes, Notebook IV, 1934, Fine Day interview, Battleford Agency, 6 Aug. 1934.

77 Patricia Jasen, 'Race, Culture, and the Colonization of Childbirth in Northern Canada,' *Social History of Medicine* 10, no. 3 (1997), 388; Daniel Williams Harmon, *A Journal of Voyages and Travels in the Interior of North America*, introduction W.L. Grant (Toronto: Courier Press, 1911), 93.

78 Margaret A. Macleod, ed., *The Letters of Letitia Hargrave* (Toronto: The Champlain Society, 1947), 97.

79 Regina Flannery, *Ellen Smallboy: Glimpses of a Cree Woman's Life* (Montreal: McGill-Queen's University Press, 1995), 31; Flannery's interviews were conducted in the 1930s, when Ellen Smallboy was eighty years old.

80 SAB, X.2, Pioneer Questionnaire, file 8, Health.

81 Sarah Preston, 'Competent Social Behaviour within the Context of Childbirth: A Cree Example,' in William Cowan, ed., *Papers of the Thirteenth Algonquian Conference* (Ottawa: Carleton University Press, 1982), 212.

82 Freda Ahenakew and H.C. Wolfart, eds., *Our Grandmother's Lives as Told in Their Own Words* (Saskatoon: Fifth House, 1992), 75.

83 David Smits, '"The Squaw Drudge": A Prime Index of Savagism,' *Ethnohistory* 29, no. 4 (1982), 281–306.

84 Harmon, *A Journal of Voyages*, 97–8; According to Jennifer H. Brown, Harmon's wife was Elizabeth Duval. *Strangers in Blood: Fur Trade Company Families in Indian Country* (Vancouver: University of British Columbia Press, 1980), 107.

85 Harmon, *A Journal of Voyages*, 298.

86 Alice B. Kehoe, 'The Shackles of Tradition,' and Alan Klein, 'The Political-Economy of Gender: A Nineteenth-Century Plains Indian Case Study,' in Patricia Albers and Beatrice Medicine eds., *The Hidden Half: Studies of Plains Indian Women* (Lanham: University Press of America, 1983).

87 Jasen, 'Race, Culture, and the Colonization of Childbirth,' 391.

88 M.K. Lux, Assiniboine field notes, Kay Thompson interview, Jan. 1998.

89 CHC, *Sessional Papers*, vol. 14, no. 27, 1908, 267.

90 NA, RG 10, vol. 1542, Hyde to McLean, 25 Feb. 1913.

91 NA, RG 10, vol. 1541, Agent Dilworth to D.C. Scott, 3 May 1916.

92 Wendy Mitchinson, *The Nature of Their Bodies* (Toronto: University of Toronto Press, 1991), 164.

93 M.K. Lux, Assiniboine field notes, Kaye Thompson interview, Jan. 1998.

94 SAB, X.2, Pioneer Questionnaire, file 8, Health, Mrs Maggie Whyte, 1883, Indian Head, Saskatchewan; Mrs Ellen W. Hubbard, 1894, Grenfell, Saskatchewan.

95 NA, MG 29, C20, Mrs David McDougall.

96 SAB, X.2, Pioneer Questionnaire, file 8, Health, Robert Webster Widdess, 1883, Rocanville, Saskatchewan; Mrs Jane Victoria Carmichael, born 1887, Rocanville, Saskatchewan.

97 M.K. Lux, Assiniboine field notes, Jan. 2000.

98 SAB, X.2 Pioneer Questionnaire, file 8, Health, Charles Cantlon Bray, 1883, Wolseley, Saskatchewan; John Hellson, *Ethnobotany of the Blackfoot Indians*, 65; Anna Leighton, *Wild Plant Use by the Woods Cree of East-Central Saskatchewan*, 23.

99 SAB, X.2, Pioneer Questionnaire, file 8, Health, Peter Fraser, 1891, Kamsack, Saskatchewan; Mrs Elizabeth Webster, 1884, Balcarres, Saskatchewan; M.K. Lux, Assiniboine field notes, Jan. 2000.

100 SAB, X.2, Pioneer Questionnaire, file 8, Health, Mrs Ellen Mott, 1887, South Qu'Appelle; Andrew Cass Hunt, 1883, Earlswood, Saskatchewan; Mrs Jane Victoria Carmichael, 1887, Rocanville, Saskatchewan; Mr H.M. Harrison, 1903, Baljennie, Saskatchewan; Mrs Mary Edith Moore, 1899, Kajewski, Saskatchewan.

101 Leighton, *Wild Plant Use by the Woods Cree*, 51; M.K. Lux, Assiniboine field notes, Kaye Thompson interview, Jan. 1998.

102 NA, MG 27 I F12, James Clinskill reminiscences, 80–1.

103 CHC, *Sessional Papers*, vol. 9, no. 14, 1895, 65; vol. 10, no. 14, 1896, 137; M.K. Lux, Assiniboine field notes, Kaye Thompson interview, Jan. 1998; Ahenakew and Wolfart, *Our Grandmother's Lives*, 219, 263.

104 For fur trade era, see Brown, *Strangers in Blood*; Sylvia Van Kirk, *Many Tender Ties: Women in Fur Trade Society, 1670–1870* (Winnipeg: Watson and Dwyer, n.d.).

105 CHC, *Sessional Papers* vol. 25, no. 10, 1892, 163; vol. 11, no. 14, 1897, xxiv; vol. 11, no. 14, 1900, Report, Touchwood Hills Agent S. Swinford, 183.

106 For examples of women's work, see CHC, *Sessional Papers*, vol. 10, no. 14, 1896, 62; vol.12, no. 14, 1899, 150–1, 154; vol. 11, no. 14, 1900, 129, 139, 181.

107 CHC, *Sessional Papers*, vol. 11, no. 14, 1897, 140; Sarah Carter, *Capturing Women: The Manipulation of Cultural Imagery in Canada's Prairie West* (Montreal: McGill-Queen's University Press, 1997), 160.

108 M.K. Lux, Assiniboine field notes, Kaye Thompson interview, Jan. 1998.

109 M.K. Lux, Blood field notes, Dec. 1999.

3: 'I Was in Darkness' Schools and Missions

1 J.R. Miller, *Shingwauk's Vision* (Toronto: University of Toronto Press, 1996), 102–3.

2 Peter Erasmus, *Buffalo Days and Nights* (Calgary: Fifth House, 1999), 153.

3 M.K. Lux, Blood field notes, Dec. 1999.

4 NA, MG 29, D 65, vol. 7, Rev. John Maclean Papers, Medical Record, Blood Reserve, 1885.

5 Ann Carmichael, 'Erysipelas,' in Kiple, ed., *The Cambridge World History of Human Disease*, 720; NA, MG 29, D 65, vol. 7, Maclean Papers, Medical Record, 24 May 1885.

6 Miller, *Shingwauk's Vision*, 127; see especially 'Part Two: Experiencing Residential Schools,' 151–343.

7 M.K. Lux, Assiniboine field notes, Kaye Thompson interview, Jan. 1998.

8 Quoted in Beverly Hungry Wolf, *Daughters of the Buffalo Women* (Skookumchuck, BC: Canadian Caboose Press, 1996), 25.

9 M.K. Lux, Assiniboine field notes, Kaye Thompsons interview, Jan. 1998; Peigan field notes, Alan Pard interview, December 1999.

10 NA, RG 10, vol. 3765, file 31,161, Dewdney to SGIA, 17 Oct. 1885.

11 CHC, *Sessional Papers*, vol. 10, no. 14, 1894, 91–7.

12 Pettipas, *Severing the Ties That Bind*, 138; NA, RG 10, vol. 3965, file 149,874, Benson to Maclean, 24 Mar. 1902.

13 CHC, *Sessional Papers*, vol. 13, no. 16, 1889, 94; vol. 5, no. 6, 1887, 139–42; vol. 10, no. 12, 1890, 296.

14 Dan Kennedy (Ochankugahe), *Recollections of an Assiniboine Chief* (Toronto: McClelland & Stewart, 1972), 54.

15 Provincial Archives of Alberta (PAA), 71.220/3412, box 81, Oblate Collection, St Joseph's [Dunbow] Industrial School, Sick Book, 1888–1915.

16 GAI, M1380, McDougall Orphanage, Letter Book II, p. 45, Niddrie to Rev. Sutherland, 24 July 1901; file 3, Commissioner Laird to Principal 11 Apr. 1900.

17 NA, RG 10, vol. 3917, file 116,575-5, Seymour to commissioner, 9 Sept. 1895; vol. 3957, file 140,754-1, Lindsay to commissioner, 6 June 1896.

18 NA, RG 10, vol. 1543, file 14,839, Tom Many Feathers to agent, 2 June 1907; Riou to agent, 19 June 1907; Agent Wilson to commissioner, 15 July 1907, 8 Apr. 1908.

19 Miller, *Shingwauk's Vision*, 129.

20 NA, RG 10, vol. 3957, file 140,754-1, Dr Macadam to commissioner, 5 June 1896; Dr Hicks, Red Deer school, to commissioner, 6 June 1896; surgeon Spencer, Brandon Industrial school, to commissioner, 11 June 1896; Allingham to commissioner, 4 June 1896.

21 NA, RG 10, vol. 3957, file 140,754-1, DSGIA to Forget, 10 July 1896.

22 GAI, M1234, file 27, Tims Papers, 'Hospital at Blackfoot Reserve, First Report.'

23 CHC, *Sessional Papers*, vol. 9, no. 14, 1895, 131; vol. 10, no. 14, 1896, 274; vol. 11, no. 14, 1897, 213.

24 Quoted in Hugh A. Dempsey, *Crowfoot: Chief of the Blackfeet* (Halifax: Goodread Biographies, 1988), 147.

25 H.W. Gibbon Stocken, *Among the Blackfoot and Sarcee*, introduction by G. Barrass (Calgary: Glenbow Museum, 1976), 38, 36. The medicine chest is on display at the Glenbow Museum in the Missionaries exhibit.

26 NA, RG 10, vol. 3909, file 107,557, Begg to commissioner, 25 Ap. 1894.

27 GAI, M1234, file 27, Tims Papers, 24 Feb. 1898; 'Hospital at Blackfoot Reserve, First Report.'

28 Gibbon Stocken, *Among the Blackfoot and Sarcee*, 55.

29 Anglican Church of Canada, General Synod Archives, *Letter Leaflet of the Women's Auxiliary to the Board of Domestic and Foreign Missions*, Miss Alice Turner, Blackfoot Home to Diocesan President, Mar. 1895, 581.

30 GAI, M2463, Alice Turner Papers, 'My Dear Girls,' Alice Turner to Women's Auxiliary Branches, 21 Aug. 1899.

31 NA, RG 10, vol. 1627, McLean to McNeill, 24 Jan. 1899.

32 University of Alberta Archives, Heber C. Jamieson papers, 25/1 Box 1, file 8, 'J.D. Lafferty.'

33 NA, RG 10, vol. 3909, file 107,557, Lafferty to Minister of the Interior, Dec. 1899.

34 Ibid., Sifton to Smart, 29 Dec. 1899.

35 GAI, M1234, file 27, Tims Papers, 'Hospital at the Blackfoot Reserve, First Report..'

36 NA, RG 10, vol. 3909, file 107,557, Lafferty to Sifton, Dec. 1899.

37 NA, RG 10, vol. 9432, Annuity Paylists Blackfoot, 1899; the *Sessional Papers* report twenty-nine births and fifty-one deaths, vol. 11, no. 12, 1901, 136.

38 NA, RG 10, vol. 3675, file 11,422-2, 17458, Macdonald to Privy Council, 30 Dec. 1884.

39 GAI, M4096, Jane Megarry, 'Blackfoot Hospital, Queen Victoria Jubilee Hospital,' n.d.

40 CHC *Sessional Papers*, vol. 17, no. 27, 1910, 'Report of the Chief Medical Officer,' 272–3.

41 GAI, M4096, Jane Megarry, 'Blackfoot Hospital, Queen Victoria Jubilee Hospital,' n.d.

42 NA, RG 10, vol. 3993, file 186,790, Lafferty to Sifton, 23 June 1899; Markle to secretary DIA, 17 Oct. 1905.

43 GAI, M1234, file 27, Gibbon Stocken Report, 24 Feb. 1898.

44 GAI, M1234, file 27, Gibbon Stocken to the Women's Auxiliary, 5 Feb. 1904.

45 NA, RG 10, vol. 9433, Annuity Paylists Blackfoot, 1900. The *Sessional Papers*, vol. 11, no. 27, 1902, 128, erroneously reported twenty-six births and thirty-seven deaths.

46 CHC, *Sessional Papers*, vol. 11, no. 27, 1904, 146. Statistics reported in the Sessional Papers in the post-1900 period must be viewed with extreme caution since there is no other source of verification.

47 NA, RG 10, vol. 3909, file 107,557, Gibbon Stocken to R.B. Bennett, 27 Feb. 1912; Rose to Secretary DIA, 27 Apr. 1912.

48 Ibid., Gibbon Stocken to Gooderham, 20 Nov. 1912; Gibbon Stocken to Gooderham, 8 Dec. 1913; Gooderham to Pedley, 9 Dec. 1913.

49 GAI, M4738, box 1, file 3, G.H. Gooderham, 'The Hospital'; GAI, M3974, Gooderham Family papers, G.H. Gooderham, 'Twenty-five Years as an Indian Agent to the Blackfoot Band,' Jan. 1972, 7.

50 David Hall, 'Clifford Sifton and Canadian Indian Administration, 1896–1905,' in Ian Getty and Antoine Lussier, eds., *As Long as the Sun Shines and Water Flows* (Vancouver: University of British Columbia Press, 1983), 121–2.

51 CHC, *Sessional Papers*, vol. 12, no. 14, 1899, DSGIA Report, xix–xx; vol. 11, no. 14, 1898, xxvii.

52 NA, RG 10, vol. 3965, file 150,000-4, A. Naessens, Dunbow school, to commissioner, 23 Mar. 1901; E. Matheson, Battleford school, to commissioner, 15 Mar. 1901; Ferrier to commissioner, 22 Mar. 1901; Dagg to commissioner, 12 Mar. 1901; Hugonnard to commissioner, 21 Mar. 1901; Laird to secretary DIA, 25 Sept. 1901.

53 Ibid., Lafferty to Laird, 18 July 1905; Laird to Pedley, 3 May 1906.

54 CHC, *Debates*, 1904, 6946–56, 18 July 1904.

55 Henry James Morgan, *The Canadian Men and Women of the Time* (Toronto: Briggs, 1912), 164; Heather MacDougall, '"Enlightening the Public": The Views and Values of the Association of Executive Health Officers of Ontario, 1886–1903,' in Charles Roland, ed., *Health, Disease, and Medicine* (McMaster University: Hannah Conference on the History of Medicine, 1982), 459.

56 NA, RG 10, vol. 4037, file 317,021, P.H. Bryce, *Report on the Indian Schools of Manitoba and the North-West Territories* (Ottawa: Government Printing Bureau, 1907), 18, 17; Benson to SGIA, 6 Nov. 1907.

57 Miller, *Shingwauk's Vision*, 139. For the political machinations between Blake, Bryce, and the government, see 137–40.

58 Anglican Church of Canada, General Synod Archives, MM 29.7.T38, T.W. Tims, 'The Call of the Red Man for Truth, Honesty and Fair Play'; PAA, 85.136, box ed530/31, Missionary Society of the Church of England in Canada (MSCC), Minutes of the Board of Management, Toronto 30 Apr. 1908.

59 NA, RG 10, vol. 4037, file 317,021, Bryce Recommendations, 4 June 1907. Years later, Bryce made his recommendations public in his pamphlet *The Story of a National Crime: Being an Appeal for Justice to the Indians of Canada* (Ottawa: James Hope and Sons, 1922), 4. The pamphlet is a scathing attack on the department and especially on D.C. Scott and the failure to act on Bryce's recommendations. Bryce especially took offence at not being appointed to head the newly created Department of Health in 1918.

60 NA, RG 10, vol. 4037, file 317,021, Bryce Recommendations, 4 June 1907.

61 Ibid., agent at Duck Lake to SGIA, 21 Nov. 1907; Inspector Chisholm, North Saskatchewan inspectorate, to SGIA, 27 Nov. 1907; Laird to SGIA, 7 Dec. 1907; Jackson to SGIA, 15 Dec. 1907.

62 Ibid., Hogbin to SGIA, 22 Nov.1907; Haynes to SGIA, 23 Nov. 1907; Matheson to SGIA, 10 Dec. 1907.

63 Ibid., Dodds to SGIA, 13 Dec. 1907; Swinford to SGIA, 4 Dec. 1907; Principal, Birtle school to SGIA, 8 Dec. 1907.

64 Ibid., Balter to SGIA, 4 Dec. 1907; Hallam to SGIA, 27 Dec. 1907; Hugonnard to SGIA, 17 Dec. 1907.

65 NA, RG 10, vol. 3957, file 140,754-1, Lafferty to McLean, Dec. 1908.

66 Ibid., Pedley to Oliver, 19 Apr. 1909.

67 CHC, *Sessional Papers*, vol. 15, no. 27, 1909, 164; vol. 17, no. 27, 1910, 131; NA RG 10, vol. 3957, file 140,754-1, Pedley to Oliver, 19 Apr. 1909; Supplementary Estimates, 1907–8.

68 NA RG 10, vol. 3957, file 140,754-1, Bryce to Pedley, 5 Nov. 1909. The Mantoux and Pirquet's (or von Pirquet's) tests are the current methods for diagnosing tuberculosis sensitivity.

69 Ibid., Lafferty to Bryce, Calgary, 22 Jan. 1910; D.C. Scott, memo, 'Notes on Dr. Bryce's Report with Suggestions for Further Action,' 7 March 1910.

70 See E. Brian Titley, *A Narrow Vision: Duncan Campbell Scott and the Administration of Indian Affairs in Canada* (Vancouver: UBC Press, 1986).

71 Ibid., Bryce to Pedley, 5 Nov. 1909, 24.

72 Quoted in Linda Bryder, *Below the Magic Mountain: A Social History of Tuberculosis in Twentieth-Century Britain* (Oxford: Clarendon Press, 1988), 57.

73 NA, RG 10, vol. 3957, file 140,754-1, Bryce to Pedley, 5 Nov. 1909, 25; Bryder, 65.

74 Ibid., D.C. Scott, 'Notes on Dr. Bryce's Report with Suggestions for Further Action,' 7 Mar. 1910.

75 Ibid., Lafferty to Pedley, 22 June 1910.

76 Ibid., Scott to DSGIA, 28 Mar. 1911.

77 Ibid.

78 Bryce, *The Story of a National Crime*, 5–6.

79 CHC, *Sessional Papers*, vol. 19, no. 27, 1911, 'Report of the Deputy Superintendent,' xxii.

80 NA, RG 10, vol. 3957, file 140,754-1, Lafferty to McLean, Dec. 1908.

81 M.K. Lux, Assiniboine field notes, Kaye Thompson interview, Jan. 1998.

82 NA, RG 10, vol. 1543, Agent Wilson to McLean, 23 Dec. 1910.

83 Eleanor Brass, *I Walk in Two Worlds* (Calgary: Glenbow Museum, 1987), 21, 22.

84 Quoted in Jean Goodwill and Norma Sluman, *John Tootoosis* (Winnipeg: Pemmican, 1984), 98.

85 J. R. Miller, 'Owen Glendower, Hotspur, and Canadian Indian Policy,' *Ethnohistory* 37, no. 4 (Fall 1990), 404.

86 GAI, M1356, Calgary Indian Mission papers, Box 1, file 2, Agent to Tims, 14 Aug. 1909; Tims to Agent, 24 Aug. 1909; file 6, McLean to Tims, 17 Feb. 1917; Memo, n.d. (1917); file 3, Tims to Secretary DIA, 28 Apr. 1917.

87 Georgina Feldberg, *Disease and Class: Tuberculosis and the Shaping of Modern North American Society* (New Brunswick, NJ: Rutgers University Press, 1995), 61–2.

88 NA, RG 10, vol. 4092, file 546,898, Dr F.A. Corbett to Graham, 7 Dec. 1920; vol. 3957, file 140,754-1, Lafferty to McLean, Dec. 1908; S. Gould to Scott, 17 Jan. 1921.

89 Diamond Jenness, *The Sarcee Indians of Alberta*, Bulletin no. 90 (Canada: Department of Mines and Resources, Mines and Geology Branch, National Museum of Canada, 1938); *Indians of Canada*, 6th ed. (National Museum of Canada, 1963), 261.

90 NA, RG 10, vol. 3957, file 140,754-1, Scott to Lougheed, 11 Dec. 1920; Graham to Scott, 24 June 1922; GAI, M1356, Calgary Indian Missions, Box 1, file 6, Gooderham Recollections, 9 Nov. 1962; M742, McGill papers, Box 4, file 36, 'Correspondence, 1928–41.'

91 See especially Miller, *Shingwauk's Vision*.

4: 'Indifferent to Human Life and Suffering': Medical Care for Native People to 1920

1 Brooke Claxton, Minister of Health and Welfare, CHC, *Sessional Papers*, 'Joint Committee of the Senate and House of Commons Appointed to Consider the Indian Act,' Minutes of Proceedings and Evidence, no. 1, 28–30 May 1946, 65.

2 CHC, *Sessional Papers*, vol. 8, no. 10, 1878, xxx, 147; NA, RG 10, vol. 3678, file 11,683, Hagarty to Vankoughnet, 27 Sept. 1879. See also Chapter 1 for Hagarty's vaccination trip.

3 Noel Dyck, 'The Administration of Federal Indian Aid in the North-West Territories, 1879–1885' (MA thesis, University of Saskatchewan, 1970), 43.

4 NA, RG 10, vol. 3704, file 17,858, Dewdney Report, 1879.

5 NA, RG 10, vol. 3768, file 33,642, Qu'Appelle Chiefs' Address.

6 CHC, *Sessional Papers*, vol. 5, no. 6, 1887, 110; vol. 13, no. 15, 1888, 82.

7 CHC, *Commons Debates*, 4th Session, 5th Parliament, 15 Apr. 1886, 718–30, 719; NA, RG10, vol. 3743, file 29,488, part 2, Dewdney to SGIA, 1 May 1886.

8 A.N. Lalonde, 'Colonization Companies in the 1880s,' in D.H. Bocking, ed, *Pages from the Past: Essays in Saskatchewan History* (Saskatoon: Western Producer Prairie Books, 1979), 19, 18, 17; Donald McLean, '1885: Métis Rebellion or Government Conspiracy?' in Laurie Barron and James Waldram, eds., *1885 and After* (Regina: Canadian Plains Research Center, 1986), 85, 86.

9 CHC *Debates*, 15 Apr. 1886, 739–40; James Whorton, 'Dyspepsia,' in Kiple, ed., *The Cambridge World History of Human Disease*, 696–8.

10 NA, RG 18, B1, vol. 1025, file 3533, Crozier to Dewdney, 2 Nov. 1885; Joseph

Dion, *My Tribe the Crees* (Calgary: Glenbow, 1979), 114; NA, RG 18, B1, vol. 1038, file 68, Supt Perry to NWMP commissioner Irvine, 19 Feb. 1886.

11 NA, RG 10, vol. 3599, file 1500, 'Petition to J.A. Macdonald from the inhabitants of Prince Albert and a large number on the Mistawasis reserve,' 1 May 1882.

12 NA, RG 10, vol. 3632, file 6326, DSGIA to Girard, 19 May 1883; David H. Breen, *The Canadian Prairie West and the Ranching Frontier, 1874–1924* (Toronto: University of Toronto Press, 1983), 9, 14.

13 NA, RG 10, vol. 3632, file 6326, DSGIA to SGIA, 30 Sept. 1885; Vankoughnet to SGIA, 2 Sept. 1887; Thomas White to Langevin, 11 Apr.1888.

14 Quoted in Breen, *The Canadian Prairie West and the Ranching Frontier,* 48; NA, RG 10, vol. 3632, file 6326, Langevin to Vankoughnet, 12 May 1888; Wadsworth to Secretary DIA, 20 July 1900.

15 NA, RG 10, vol. 3632, file 6326, Agent James Wilson to Commissioner, 3 Feb. 1897.

16 NA, MG 29, E 106, vol. 17, Reed Papers, Kennedy to Dewdney, 2 Nov. 1889 (marked 'Private'); CHC, *Sessional Papers,* vol. 6, no. 6f, 1891, Table IV, Annual Report of the Department of Agriculture, Mortality Statistics; Herbert Brown Ames, *The City below the Hill* (1897; reprint, Toronto: University of Toronto Press, 1972), 81.

17 NA, MG 29, E 106, vol. 17, Kennedy to Dewdney, 2 Nov. 1889; NA, RG 10, vol. 3632, file 6326, Wilson to commissioner, 3 Feb. 1897.

18 Ibid., Henderson to Dewdney, 1 Dec. 1885; vol. 3811, file 54,550, Report of Inspector McGibbon, 15 Jan. 1889.

19 CHC, *Sessional Papers,* vol. 3, no. 3, 1885, 159; vol. 4, no. 4, 1886; vol. 5, no. 6, 1887; vol. 13, no. 15, 1888; vol. 13, no. 16, 1889; vol. 10, no. 12, 1890; vol. 15, no. 18, 1891. For example, in 1884 the total cost for medicine and medical attendance was $4,641.53, or a per capita expenditure of $0.26, based on a total population of Treaties Four, Six, and Seven of 17,839. The per capita expenditure by 1891 had risen to $0.91 based on a total population of 15,259.

20 NA, MG 29, E106, vol. 17, Reed Papers, Mitchell to Reed, 20 Sept.1891; Hilda Neatby, 'The Medical Profession in the North-West Territories,' in S.E.D. Shortt, ed., *Medicine in Canadian Society: Historical Perspectives* (Montreal: McGill-Queen's University Press, 1981), 166; see also NA, RG 10, vol. 3632, file 6326, DSGIA to Girard, 19 May 1883, on Girard's desire to establish a private practice; GAI, M7283, Box 1, file 4, Edwards to Mrs Edwards, 30 Nov. 1897, on Edwards's attempts to establish a private practice.

21 NA, MG 29, E106, vol. 17, Reed Papers, Macdowell to Reed, 12 May 1890; CHC, *Sessional Papers,* vol. 9, no. 14, 1895.

22 NA, RG 10, vol. 3765, file 32,784, Battleford reports, A.M. McNeill, acting agent, 31 May 1890.

23 NA, MG 29, E106, vol. 17, Reed Papers, McGirr to Reed, 16 Apr. 1891.

24 NA, RG 10, vol. 9423, Annuity Paylists, 1890; GAI, M2816, Dewdney Papers, vol. 8, Birth and Death Rates, Treaties Four, Six, and Seven, 1890, 2198.

25 NA, RG 10, vol. 3790, file 44,666, McColl to DSGIA, 21 Apr. 1890; Reed to Dewdney, 5 Apr. 1890.

26 Carter, *Lost Harvests*, 161–2; J.R. Miller, *Skyscrapers Hide the Heavens* (Toronto: University of Toronto Press, 1989), 201.

27 *Statutes of Canada*, 39 Vic., chap. 18, 1880.

28 Frantz Fanon, 'Medicine and Colonialism,' in John Ehrenreich, ed., *The Cultural Crisis of Modern Medicine* (New York: Monthly Review Press, 1978).

29 Pettipas, *Severing the Ties That Bind*, 98.

30 Quoted in Carter, *Lost Harvests*, 213; and 209–29 for Reed's 'peasant farming' policy.

31 CHC, *Sessional Papers*, vol. 11, no. 14, 1897, Reed Report, xxiv; John Maclean, *The Indians of Canada: Their Manners and Customs* (1898; reprint, Toronto: Coles Publishing, 1970), 322.

32 CHC, *Sessional Papers*, vol. 10, no. 12, 1890, 161; NA, RG10, vol. 3853, file 78,004, Sinclair to Reed, 2 Jan. 1891.

33 CHC, *Sessional Papers*, vol. 25, no. 10, 1892, 163.

34 NA, MG 29, E 106, vol. 16, Petition from the Headmen of Pasquah and Muscowpetung to the House of Commons, 24 Feb. 1893.

35 Ibid., Reed to SGIA Daly, 13 March 1893; NA, RG 10, vol. 3900, file 99,275, Department Circular, 1893.

36 NA, RG 10, vol. 9426, Annuity Paylist, Muscowpetung Agency, 1893; vol. 9427, Annuity Paylist, Muscowpetung Agency, 1894.

37 NA, RG 10, vol. 3949, file 126,345, Seymour to commissioner, 28 May 1895.

38 NA, RG 10, vol. 9427, Annuity Paylist, Stoney Reserve, 1894; vol. 3917, file 116,493, Petition from Morley and Stoney Plain reserves, July 1894; Reed to McDougall, 30 July 1894.

39 Ibid., vol. 3912, file 111,777-1, memo, McGibbon meeting with minor chiefs, 3 June 1895.

40 Ibid., vol. 3949, file 126,345, Reed to Forget, 14 Feb. 1895.

41 Ibid., Stewart to Commissioner, 12 Mar. 1895; vol. 3855, file 79,963, Orton to DSGIA, 16 June 1891; vol. 3949, file 126,345, Girard to Commissioner, 1 Apr. 1895.

42 NA, RG 10, vol. 3949, file 126,345, Lindsay to Reed, 31 May 1895; CHC, *Sessional Papers*, vol. 11, no. 14, 1897, 201; GAI, M1837, file 23, Sarcee Indian

Agency Files, Ration Tickets, 1895; an average of 192 people were on the ration list.

43 NA, RG 10, vol. 3949, file 126,345, Patrick to Commissioner, 17 June 1895; vol. 3984, file 168,921, 'List of Employees No Longer in Service since June 1896.'

44 D.J. Hall, 'Clifford Sifton and the Canadian Indian Administration, 1896–1905,' *Prairie Forum* 2, no. 2 (1977), 129.

45 CHC, *Debates*, 9 July 1903, 6329–30; NA, RG10, vol. 3957, file 140,745-1, Macrae to McLean, 6 Feb. 1903.

46 Henry James Morgan, 'Bryce, Peter Henderson,' in H.J. Morgan, ed., *The Canadian Men and Women of the Time* (Toronto: Briggs, 1912), 164; Valverde, *Age of Light, Soap, and Water*, 49; Neil Sutherland, 'To Create a Strong and Healthy Race: School Children in the Public Health Movement, 1880–1914,' in S.E.D. Shortt, ed., *Medicine in Canadian Society: Historical Perspectives* (Montreal: McGill-Queen's University Press, 1981), 361–2.

47 CHC, *Sessional Papers*, Report of the Medical Officer, vol. 12, no. 27, 1905, 271; CHC, *Debates*, 18 July 1904, 6960.

48 NA, RG 10, vol. 1627, Secretary to the Commissioner to Lash, 10 July 1899; vol. 3632, file 6326, Wilson to SGIA, 3 Feb. 1901.

49 NA, RG 10, vol. 3756, file 31,161, Ashdown to Secretary, 30 Aug. 1904; Carthew to DSGIA, 13 Nov. 1904; Graham to Pedley, 25 Nov. 1904.

50 CHC, *Sessional Papers*, vol. 11, no. 27, 1904, 238; vol. 11, no. 27, 1905, xix.

51 Carter, *Lost Harvests*, 237.

52 Allotment in severalty and forced enfranchisement, as set out in the 1857 Gradual Civilization Act, had been consistently opposed by Native people east of Lake Superior. The people of the west were exempt from the act until the superintendent general considered them sufficiently civilized; John Tobias, 'Protection, Civilization, Assimilation: An Outline of Canada's Indian Policy,' *Western Canadian Journal of Anthropology* 6, no. 2 (1976), 23.

53 CHC, *Sessional Papers*, vol. 12, no. 27, 1906, 189; Stewart Raby, 'Indian Land Surrenders in Southern Saskatchewan,' *Canadian Geographer* 17, no. 1 (1973), 39.

54 NA, RG 10, vol. 1547, Blood Agent Reports, Pedley to Hyde, 9 Aug. 1911; R.N. Wilson, 'Our Betrayed Wards' (Ottawa, 1921), 42.

55 Lucien Hanks and Jane Richardson Hanks, *Tribe under Trust: A Study of the Blackfoot Reserve of Alberta* (Toronto: University of Toronto Press, 1950), 50.

56 Hugh Dempsey, 'One Hundred Years of Treaty Seven,' in Ian A.L. Getty and Donald B. Smith, eds., *One Century Later: Western Canadian Reserve Indians Since Treaty Seven* (Vancouver: University of British Columbia Press, 1978), 27.

57 M.K. Lux, Assiniboine field notes, Jan. 1998; Jan. 2000.

58 GAI, M4421, R.N. Wilson fonds, V.I 'Religion, Feb. 4, 1891' pp. 57–8.

59 An Act to Amend the Indian Act, 4–5 George V, chap. 35, June 1914.

60 CHC, *Sessional Papers*, vol. 14, no. 27, 1908, 267.

61 NA, RG 10, vol. 1540, Blood Reserve, Monthly Hospital Returns, 4 Feb. 1908; CHC, *Sessional Papers*, vol. 12, no. 27, 1907, 281.

62 Patricia Anne Roome, 'Henrietta Muir Edwards: The Journey of a Canadian Feminist' (PhD dissertation, Simon Fraser University, 1996), 76.

63 Roome, 113, 133.

64 GAI, M7283, Edwards and Gardiner Family fonds, box 1, file 4, Edwards to Henrietta Edwards, 30 Nov. 1897; 5 Nov. 1897; box 1, file 14, Edwards to daughter Alice, 13 Oct. 1901.

65 NA, RG 10, vol. 1541, Dr Steele, medical officer, Blood reserve, to agent Ostrander, 14 Apr. 1920.

66 Roome, 'Henrietta Muir Edwards,' 192, 186.

67 NA, RG 10, vols. 1540–2, Blood Reserve, Medical Officer's Monthly Reports; the monthly reports are extant from 1905 to 1910, become sporadic in 1911 and 1912, more complete in 1914, and then none until 1923; GAI, M1781, Box 1, 2, files 4, 6, Battleford Agency, Monthly Reports, 1908–1919.

68 A. Finkel, M. Conrad, and V. Strong-Boag, *History of the Canadian Peoples*, vol. 2 (Toronto: Copp Clark Pitman, 1993), 226; in 1943 in Saskatchewan the infant mortality rate was 52 per thousand births, by 1990 the Canadian rate was 7.9 per thousand births, 513; Edward Stockwell, 'Infant Mortality,' in Kiple, ed., *The Cambridge World History of Human Disease*, 225.

69 NA, RG 10, vol. 1540, Blood Medical Reports, Edwards, 5 June 1906; CHC, *Sessional Papers*, 1906–1910, Annual Reports, Chief Medical Officer.

70 Mary Karasch, 'Ophthalmia,' in Kiple, ed., *The Cambridge World History of Human Disease*, 898–9; CHC, *Sessional Papers*, Annual Reports, Chief Medical Officer, 1906–1909.

71 John Kemink et al., 'Mastoiditis,' in Kiple, ed., *The Cambridge World History of Human Disease*, 866.

72 CHC, *Sessional Papers*, Annual Reports, Chief Medical Officer, 1906–1909.

73 GAI, M1781, Box 1, file 4, Battleford Agency, Medical Reports, 1909–1914, Moosomin Reserve, Reports of dispenser A.E Rotsey, Jan. 1913–Mar. 1914.

74 CHC, *Sessional Papers*, Annual Reports, Chief Medical Officer, 1906–1910, 268. Given that Bryce reported 65 deaths in a population of 1, 168, the death rate should have been 55.6 per thousand, but Bryce reported the births and deaths for a nine-month period and then extrapolated the death rate for a twelve-month period, thereby arriving at the death rate of 74.1 per thousand; vol. 14, no. 27, 1907, 276.

75 GAI, M1781, Box 2, file 6, Battleford Agency, Agent's Monthly Reports, 1908–1919.

76 NA, RG 10, vol. 1540, Blood Reserve, Monthly Medical Reports, 1906, 1907; vol. 1542, Agent Hyde to McLean, 15 Nov. 1912; 3 July 1907.

77 GAI, M7289, Box 1, George Everett Learmonth, Case Book 1904–6. George Everett Learmonth (1876–1957) graduated from McGill in medicine in 1901. After a brief stint as a ship's doctor on various Liverpool-based lines, he studied tropical diseases in West Africa. He established his private practice in High River in 1903, and remained there until 1916, when he joined the Canadian Army Medical Corps. After discharge in 1919 he resumed private practice in Calgary until his retirement in 1951.

78 Jacalyn Duffin, *Langstaff: A Nineteenth-Century Life* (Toronto: University of Toronto Press, 1993), 114.

79 GAI, M7289, Box 1, George Everett Learmonth, Case Book 1904–6, 5 Oct. 1905; 25 May 1905; 7 Sept. 1912; 28 June 1905; 19 July 1905.

80 Alex Johnston, *Plants and the Blackfoot* (Occassional Paper no. 4. Edmonton: Provincial Museum, 1982); John Hellson, *Ethnobotany of the Blackfoot Indians,* Canadian Ethnology Service Paper No. 19 (Ottawa: National Museum, 1979); Anna Leighton, *Wild Plant Use by the Woods Cree of East-Central Saskatchewan,* Canadian Ethnology Service, Paper No. 101 (Ottawa: National Museum, 1985).

81 NA, RG 10, vol. 1540, Blood Reserve, Monthly Medical Reports, 3 July 1907; Wilson to McLean, 3 Apr. 1911.

82 NA, RG 10, vol. 1540, Blood Reserve Medical Reports, Hyde to McLean, 18 July 1911; CHC *Sessional Papers,* vol. 21, no. 27, 1913, 'Agency Reports, Dr Wheeler, Birtle Hospital and Boarding School,' 81.

83 NA, RG 10, vol. 1540, Blood Reserve Medical Reports, Wilson to McLean, 3 Apr. 1911.

84 Ibid., vol. 1542, Hyde to McLean, 25 Feb. 1913; vol. 1540, Legal to McLean, 9 Jan. 1913.

85 Ibid., vol. 1541, Dilworth to Tupper, 1 Mar. 1917; GAI, Box 1, file 4, Battleford Agency, Medical Reports, Agent Day to J.D. McLean, 18 Oct. 1910; Rotsey to Agent, 31 Mar. 1913; NA, RG 10, vol. 1541, Faunt to Graham, 20 Oct. 1920.

86 NA, RG 10, vol. 1541, Dilworth to Tupper, Sept. 1916; Tupper, 'Message to the Blood People,' 1916.

87 NA, RG 10, vol. 1541, 'Things Every Blood Indian Should Know,' [1916]; Dilworth to D. C. Scott, 3 May 1916.

88 Ibid., Blood Reserve Monthly Medical Reports, Apr., June 1919; vol. 1542, Blood Reserve, Monthly Hospital Reports; Kennedy to Graham, 7 Apr. 1923.

89 M.K. Lux, Peigan field notes, Dec. 1999.

90 NA, RG 10, vol. 1544, Blood Reserve, Monthly Hospital Reports, 1923; vol. 1541, Blood Reserve, Monthly Medical Reports, 5 Apr. 1920; vol. 1542, Kennedy to Graham, 7 Apr. 1923.

91 Ibid., vol. 1540, Blood Reserve, Monthly Medical Reports, 5 Apr. 1920; vol. 10,243, file 1/1–16–3, agent Rowland to Scott, 15 Dec. 1915; vol. 1547, Blood Reserve Reports, Dilworth to McLean, 2 July 1914.

92 NA RG 10, vol. 1542, Blood Reserve, Annual Medical Report, Kennedy, 7 Apr. 1923.

93 Ibid., Blood Reserve, Annual Medical Report, Dr Kennedy to commissioner, 7 Apr. 1923; Sister Mary Superior to agent Faunt, 15 May 1923; Graham to Scott, 6 June 1923.

94 Ibid., E. Smith to Faunt, May 1924; Faunt to secretary, 23 May 1924; Kennedy to Faunt, 21 June 1924.

95 GAI, M742, Harold W. McGill Papers, Box 4, file 36, Memo to Superintendent, 13 July 1935; Correspondence files, 1928–41.

96 M.K. Lux, Peigan field notes, Dec. 1999; Blood field notes, Dec. 1999; Assiniboine field notes, Feb. 1998; Jan. 2000.

97 CHC, *Sessional Papers*, vol. 23, no. 17, 1914, 296.

98 CHC *Sessional Papers*, vol. 19, no. 27, 1911, 'Report of the Deputy Superintendent General,' xxii.

99 NA, RG 10, vol. 1547, J.D. McLean, 'Circular to Medical Officers,' 27 May 1912; McLean, 'Circular to Medical Officers,' 2 Dec. 1912.

100 NA, RG 10, vol. 1595, Laird to Agent Jones, 5 Mar. 1902; GAI, M1781, Box 2, file 6, Battleford Agency Monthly Reports; NA, RG 10, vol. 1595, Chisholm to Agent Sibbald, 15 Jan. 1913; vol. 1393, Petition Piapot reserve to Nichol, 9 Mar. 1914; RG 18, B1, vol. 1, file 80, part 2, Birks to Commanding Officer, 25 Nov. 1918.

101 CHC, *Sessional Papers*, vol. 23, no. 27, 1915, xxiv.

102 NA, RG 10, vol. 1595, Smallpox at John Smith reserve, 1913.

103 'No Smallpox on Reserve,' *Moon* (Melfort, Saskatchewan), 16 Apr. 1913.

104 NA, RG 18, vol. 1749, file 1914, 73, Inspector Proby to Commanding Officer, 12 Feb. 1914; RG 10, vol. 1393, Petition, Piapot reserve to Nichol, 9 Mar. 1914; CHC, *Sessional Papers*, vol. 23, no. 27, 1915, xviii; NA, RG 10, vol. 1393, McLean to Nichol, 11 Jan. 1915.

105 NA, RG 10, vol. 1393, Oswald to Nichol, 31 Mar. 1915; Rock Thunder to Nichol, 20 Feb. 1916; Mountain Horse, *My People the Bloods*, 5; CHC, *Sessional Papers*, vol. 12, no. 27, 1907, 284.

106 M.K. Lux, 'The Impact of the 1918 Influenza Epidemic in Saskatchewan'

(MA thesis, University of Saskatchewan, 1989), 100–5; *Saskatoon Daily Star,* 5 Nov. 1918, 3.

107 M.K. Lux, 'Prairie Indians and the 1918 Influenza Epidemic,' *Native Studies Review* 8, no. 1 (1992), 23–34.

108 E.A. Robertson, MD, Cpt. CAMC, 'Clinical Notes on the Influenza Epidemic Occurring in the Quebec Garrison,' *Canadian Medical Association Journal* 9 (Feb. 1919), 156.

109 CHC, *Debates,* vol. 138, 4062 (25 June 1919); Saskatchewan Bureau of Public Health (SBPH), *Annual Reports 1918–1919,* 126.

110 D. Ann Herring, '"There Were Young People and Old People and Babies Dying Every Week": The 1918–1919 Influenza Pandemic at Norway House,' *Ethnohistory* 41, no. 1 (1994), 87, 96.

111 NA, RG 18, vol. 568, file 12-1919, F. Fish, University of Alberta, 1 Dec. 1918.

112 Quoted in Beverly Hungry Wolf, *Daughters of the Buffalo Women* (Skookumchuck, BC: Canadian Caboose Press, 1996), 124.

113 NA, RG 10, vol. 1541, Steele to Dilworth, 8 Oct. 1918; Dilworth to McLean, 3, 26 Dec. 1918; GAI, Battleford Agency, Agent's Monthly Report, 14 Jan. 1919; NA, RG10, vol. 4069, file 427,063, Indians in the Prairie Provinces, 1918; SBPH, *Annual Reports, 1919–1920,* 102.

114 NA, RG 10, vol. 3921, file 116,818-1B, Woodsworth to Secretary, Department of Indian Affairs, 25 Nov. 1918; GAI, M1356, file 3, Tims papers, 'Memo, Secretary DIA' 10 Jan. 1919.

115 NA, RG 18 RCMP, vol. 568, file 15-1919, Influenza – Indians Saskatchewan and Alberta, 1919 Comptroller to N.W. Rowell, MP, President of the Privy Council, 14 Jan. 1919; J.H. Birks to Officer Commanding RNWMP, Edmonton, 20 Nov. 1918.

116 Dion, *My Tribe the Crees,* 149–50.

117 NA, RG 10, vol. 3826, file 60,511-4a, Onion Lake Petition to Scott, 6 Mar. 1919; Sibbald to Secretary, 27 June 1919; RG 18, vol. 568, file 15-1919, Loggin, Staff Sergeant, F Division, RNWMP, Prince Albert, 12 June 1919.

5: 'A Menace to the Community': Tuberculosis

1 NA, RG 10, vol. 3958, file 140,754-3, Wodehouse to Dr D.A. Carmichael, Department of Soldier's Civil Re-Establishment, 4 Sept. 1924.

2 Ibid., vol. 3957, file 140,745-1, 'Tuberculosis Congress at Berlin, 24–6 May 1899,' Report on the proceedings by Edward Farrell, MD.

3 Georgina Feldberg, *Disease and Class: Tuberculosis and the Shaping of Modern North American Society* (New Brunswick, NJ: Rutgers University Press, 1995).

4 The declining rates of tuberculosis in Britain are treated in Linda Bryder,

Below the Magic Mountain: A Social History of Tuberculosis in Twentieth-Century Britain (Oxford: Clarendon Press, 1988), 2, and F.B. Smith, *The Retreat of Tuberculosis, 1850–1950* (London: Croom Helm, 1988), 1; Thomas Mc-Keown, *The Modern Rise of Population* (London: Edward Arnold, 1976), 92, links the declining rates of tuberculosis with general declines in all infectious diseases. In the United States the rates of tuberculosis infection and death had been falling steadily before any measures were taken against it, see Rene and Jean Dubos, *The White Plague: Tuberculosis, Man and Society* (Boston: Little, Brown, 1952), 185.

5 George Jasper Wherrett, *The Miracle of the Empty Beds: A History of Tuberculosis in Canada* (Toronto: University of Toronto Press, 1977), xvi, 41, 249–50.

6 NA, RG 10, file 407-3-6, part 2, Submission of the Alberta Indian Association to the Special Joint Committee of the Senate and House of Commons appointed to examine and consider the Indian Act, 1945, appendix B, xx, (hereafter Joint Committee).

7 NA, RG 10, vol. 3957, vol. 140,754-1, Secretary Treasurer Saskatchewan Medical Association, 28 March 1906; Battleford Board of Trade to Department of Indian Affairs, 5 June 1906; Fisher to Frank Oliver, 29 June 1906; CHC, *Sessional Papers*, vol. 12, no. 27, 1907, 'Report of the Chief Medical Officer,' 275.

8 NA, RG 10, vol. 3993, file 186,790, Markle to secretary, 17 Oct. 1905; CHC *Sessional Papers*, vol. 12, no. 27, 1906, 'Report of the Chief Medical Officer,' 277.

9 NA, RG 10, vol. 3993, file 186,790, Lafferty to Pedley, 19 Apr. 1906.

10 NA, RG 10, vol. 3957, file 140,745-1, 'Tuberculosis Congress at Berlin, 24–6 May 1899,' report on the proceedings by Edward Farrell, MD.

11 NA, RG 10, vol. 3957, file 140,754-1, Pedley to Oliver, 19 Apr. 1909; Bryce to Jacobs, 24 Apr. 1908; PAA 85.136, box ed 530/31, 'Memorandum for the Board of Management of Missionary Society of the [Anglican] Church in Canada' (MSCC), 1908, 11.

12 NA, RG 10, vol. 1540, Circular to all agents, March 1902; McLean to Lawrence, 22 March 1901.

13 Sarah Carter, 'Demonstrating Success: The File Hills Farm Colony,' *Prairie Forum* 16, no. 3 (1991), 157; NA, RG 10, vol. 1394, File Hills, Qu'Appelle Agency, Monthly Reports, Medical Employees, 1911–1922, Nurse Emily Mac-Mullen to J.D. McLean, 26 Apr. 1915; and Graham to Secretary, 21 June 1914, 13; Eleanor Brass, *I Walk in Two Worlds* (Calgary: Glenbow Museum, 1987).

14 NA, RG 10, vol. 1394, Dryer to Graham, 26 Sept. 1919; Deacon to Graham, 31 Dec. 1920; McLean to Deacon, 28 June 1921; Paget to Deacon, 29 Nov. 1921; Knoke to Graham, 15 Apr. 1915; Graham to McLean, 26 Apr. 1915;

GAI, M742, McGill papers, Box 5, file 58, Memo McGill to Hon. Superintendent General, 5 Sept.1933.

15 CHC, *Sessional Papers*, vol. 12, no. 27, 1907, Annual Report of the Chief Medical Officer, 274, 276; I. Burney Yeo, MD, *A Manual of Medical Treatment or Clinical Therapeutics*, vol. 1 (Chicago: W.T. Keener, 1905) 12th ed., 678.

16 NA, RG 10, vol. 4077, file 454,016, McLean to Grain, 5 Jan. 1914; Grain to Scott, 18 Jan.1914; Grain to Scott, memo, 24 Mar. 1914; vol. 4084, file 495,800, Grain to Scott, 5 Aug. 1916; vol. 1394, McLean to Graham, 7 May 1917.

17 NA, RG 10, vol. 4076, file 451,868, Grain personnel file, 12 Feb. 1919; McLean to SGIA, 16 May 1922.

18 Department of Health Act (S.C. 1919, chap. 24).

19 CHC, *Sessional Papers*, vol. 23, no. 27, 1916, 'Report of the DSGIA,' xxiii–xxv.

20 NA, RG 10, vol. 4084, file 495,800, Graham to Scott, 2 Nov. 1918.

21 C. Stuart Houston, *R.G. Ferguson: Crusader against Tuberculosis* (Toronto: Hannah Institute and Dundurn Press, 1991), 54.

22 NA, RG 10, vol. 4084, file 495,800, Graham to Scott, 22 June 1923.

23 Carter, *Lost Harvests*, 249–51.

24 NA, RG 10, vol. 4084, file 495,800, Graham to Scott, 11 July 1923; Graham to Scott, 28 Sept. 1923; Scott to Graham, 12 Oct. 1923.

25 M.K. Lux, Assiniboine field notes, Alice Ironstar interviews, Jan. 2000.

26 NA, RG 10, vol. 4092, file 546,898, Scott to Graham, 27 Aug.1924; Graham to Scott, 9 Dec. 1925.

27 Saskatchewan Anti-Tuberculosis Commission, *Report*, 1922, 19, 60.

28 NA, RG 10, v. 3958, file 140,754-3, Wodehouse to Dr D.A. Carmichael, Department of Soldier's Civil Re-Establishment, 4 Sept. 1924; Minutes, Canadian Tuberculosis Association meeting, 8 Dec. 1925; NA, RG 29, vol. 1225, file 311-T7-16, Scott to Amyot, 18 Feb. 1926.

29 NA, RG 29, vol. 1228, file 311-T7-24, Associate Committee on Tuberculosis Research, 21 Oct. 1925; Dominion of Canada, *National Research Council Report of the President and Financial Statement, 1926–27* (Ottawa: King's Printer, 1928), 44.

30 Bryder, *Below the Magic Mountain*, 138; Smith, *The Retreat of Tuberculosis*, 196; Feldberg, *Disease and Class: Tuberculosis and the Shaping of Modern North American Society*, 135.

31 Feldberg, 152.

32 Armand Frappier, 'Fifty Years of Study and Use of BCG Vaccine in Canada, 1924–1974' (paper distributed by the Institut Armand-Frappier), Oct. 1979, 10.

33 Dominion of Canada, *National Research Council Report of the President and*

Financial Statement, 1928–29 (Ottawa: King's Printer, 1930), 29; 1932 Report, 95.

34 Houston, *R.G. Ferguson*, 99.

35 Dominion of Canada, *National Research Council Report of the President and Financial Statement, 1928–29* (Ottawa: King's Printer, 1930), 44; R.G. Ferguson, *Tuberculosis Among the Indians of the Great Canadian Plains* (London: Adlard and Son, 1928), 9.

36 Quoted in Houston, *R.G. Ferguson*, 51.

37 SAB, A638, Saskatchewan Lung Association (SLA), VII.48 'Correspondence,' Cook to Parkinson, deputy minister, Department of Soldier's Civil Re-Establishment, 20 June 1922.

38 SAB, A638, SLA, VII.45, Ferguson Papers, 'Notes Taken by Dr. Ferguson at File Hills Indian School February 12, 1927.'

39 Michael Worboys, 'Tuberculosis and Race in Britain and Its Empire, 1900–50,' in Waltraud Ernst and Bernard Harris, eds., *Race, Science and Medicine, 1700–1960* (London: Routledge, 1999), 146.

40 Ferguson, *Tuberculosis among the Indians of the Great Canadian Plains*, was reprinted from the Transactions of the NAPT 1928 conference; SAB A638, SLA, IX.29, Lyle Cummins, 'Tuberculosis among the Indians of the Great Canadian Plains' where 'South African Natives' is written over 'Great Canadian Plains.' The misprinted title was repeated in Michael Worboys, 'Tuberculosis and Race in Britain and Its Empire, 1900–50,' 165, n43.

41 Lyle Cummins, 'Tuberculosis among the "Indians of the Great Canadian Plains" [*sic*]' (reprint), *Annual Report of the NAPT* (London: NAPT, 1928), 7.

42 Ferguson, *Tuberculosis among the Indians of the Great Canadian Plains*, 18, 24, 47.

43 Worboys, 'Tuberculosis and Race in Britain and Its Empire, 1900–50,' 146.

44 SAB, A638, SLA, IX.50, Ferguson Papers, Indian Research.

45 Ferguson, *Tuberculosis among the Indians of the Great Canadian Plains*, 2, 33, 36, 42, 24.

46 Houston, *R.G. Ferguson*, 60; SAB, A638, SLA, VIII.157, Barnett to Stark, 20 May 1966.

47 SAB, A638, SLA, VII.47, Ferguson Papers, Ferguson to Tory, 2 Sept. 1930.

48 M.K. Lux, Assiniboine field notes, Feb. 1998, Jan. 2000.

49 SAB, A638, SLA, VII.5, Ferguson Papers, 'A Memorandum Dictated in 1922 after the Completion of the Anti-Tuberculosis Commission Report'; VII.47, Memorandum from E.L. Stone, Director of Medical Services, Department of Indian Affairs, to D.C. Scott, DSGIA, 20 Apr. 1929.

50 NA, RG 10, vol. 1015, Battleford Agency, Monthly Medical Reports, secretary to Dr Cameron, 20 Aug. 1934.

51 In 1930 the general death rate was 23.54 per thousand; by 1932 it was 22.5 per thousand; while the infant mortality in 1930 was 216 per thousand, by 1932 it jumped to 302.3 due to epidemics of whooping cough and influenza. By 1933 it was down to 137.9 per thousand. The birth rate was 34.9 per thousand in 1930, and 45.08 in 1932. SAB, A638, SLA, VII.5, Ferguson Papers, 'Tuberculosis Research among the Indians of the Qu'Appelle Indian Health Unit,' Progress Reports, 1930, 1933; SLA, VII.50c, Ferguson Papers, Ferguson to Saskatchewan Minister of Public Health J.M. Uhrich, 26 Mar. 1935.

52 SAB, A638, SLA, IX.53, Ferguson Papers, Ferguson to H.M. Tory, 3 Jan.1931.

53 SAB, A638, SLA, VII.50b, Ferguson Papers, 'Resolution Passed at the Annual Meeting of Persons Directing Research under the Auspices of the Associate Committee on Tuberculosis, Mar. 21, 1933.'

54 See C. Stuart Houston, 'Ferguson's BCG Research – Canada's First Randomized Clinical Trial?' *Clinical Investigation of Medicine* 16, no. 1 (1993), 90; the schoolchildren were in groups 'B' and 'Bx.' SAB, A638, SLA, IX.60, Ferguson Papers, 'Year End Reports to the National Research Council – Qu'Appelle Indian Research, 31 Dec. 1946.'

55 R.G. Ferguson and A.B. Simes, 'BCG Vaccination of Indian Infants in Saskatchewan,' *Tubercle* 30, no. 1 (Jan. 1949), 2, 7, 5.

56 J.W. Hopkins, 'BCG Vaccination in Montreal,' *American Review of Tuberculosis* 43, no. 5 (May 1941), 591. The Montreal trials were conducted by Dr Baudouin from 1926 to 1938. For the first seven years of the Qu'Appelle trial, the non-tuberculosis death rate was 184.7 per thousand for the vaccinated group, and 240.7 per thousand for the control group. The Montreal trials showed a seven-year non-tuberculosis death rate of 86 per thousand for the vaccinated group and 73 per thousand for the controls. The method of accumulating the death rates is Hopkins's. 'BCG Vaccination in Montreal,' Table 4b, 592.

57 Feldberg, *Disease and Class*, 168–75.

58 Institut Pasteur's *Notice sur le BCG*, SAB, A638, SLA, VII.25, Ferguson Papers, 'The Indian Tuberculosis Problem and Some Preventive Measures,' June 1933.

59 Marion M. Torchia, 'Tuberculosis among American Negroes: Medical Research on a Racial Disease, 1830–1950,' *Journal of the History of Medicine* 32, no. 3 (July 1977); 'The Tuberculosis Movement and the Race Question,' *Bulletin of the History of Medicine* 49 (1975).

60 Todd Benson, 'Race, Health, and Power: The Federal Government and American Indian Health, 1909–1955' (PhD dissertation, Stanford University, 1994).

61 NA, RG 29, vol. 1225, file 311-T7-16, D.A. Volume, 'The Indian and Tuberculosis,' 4.

62 SAB, A638, SLA, VII.5, Ferguson Papers, 'Report of Indian Boarding School Children in Saskatchewan,' 1933–37.

63 NA, RG 29, vol. 1225, file 311-T7-16, Stewart to Bracken, 14 Nov. 1934.

64 PAA, 73.315/37, Box 2, Baker Memorial Sanatorium, 1917–1937, Baker to Secretary, 15 Sept. 1930; McGill to Baker, 1 Feb. 1934.

65 PAA, 73.351/35, Riou to Baker, 29 Nov. 1937; GAI, M742, box 4, file 36, J. Guy to McGill, 19 Mar. 1935.

66 Personal interview, Dr G. Monks, hospital physician, 1949–51, 18 Mar. 1998.

67 GAI, M742, McGill Papers, box 4, file 36, Marcotte to McGill, 21 Mar. 1935; E.L. Stone, memo to McGill, 6 Dec. 1935.

68 M.K. Lux, Assiniboine field notes, Jan. 2000.

69 M.K. Lux, Assiniboine field notes, Jan. 1998.

70 Personal interview, Dr G. Monks, 18 Mar. 1998.

71 NA, RG 10, vol. 1225, file 311-T7-16, McGill to Agents, 14 Jan.1937; SAB, A638, SLA, VII.27, Ferguson Papers, Ferguson to Gardner, 8 Feb. 1937.

72 SAB, A638, IX.52 SLA Ferguson Papers, 'Meeting of the Indian Advisory Committee, Mar. 10, 1938,' 1, 4.

73 NA, RG 10, vol. 1225, file 311-T7-16, McGill to Agents, 1 Dec. 1937.

74 Ibid., 'Report of the Advisory Committee for the Control and Prevention of Tuberculosis Among the Indians,' May 1945.

75 CHC, *Sessional Papers*, 'Joint Committee,' Minutes of Proceedings and Evidence, no. 1, 28–30 May 1946, 65.

76 NA, RG 29, vol 1225, file 311-T7-16, J. Allison Glen to His Worship John W. Fry, 24 Oct. 1945.

77 Katherine McCuaig, *The Weariness, the Fever, and the Fret: The Campaign against Tuberculosis in Canada, 1900–1950* (Montreal: McGill-Queen's University Press, 1999) 72; Houston, *R.G. Ferguson*, 87.

78 M.K. Lux, Blood field notes, Dec. 1999.

79 NA, RG 29, vol. 1225, file 311-T7-16, Report of the Advisory Committee, 3; Wherrett, *Miracle of the Empty Beds*, Table 7, 116.

80 M.K. Lux, Assiniboine field notes, Jan. 1998.

81 T. Kue Young, *Health Care and Cultural Change: The Indian Experience in the Central Subarctic* (Toronto: University of Toronto Press, 1988), 45.

82 Pat Sandiford Grygier, *A Long Way from Home: The Tuberculosis Epidemic among the Inuit* (Montreal: McGill-Queen's University Press, 1994); Young, *Health Care and Cultural Change*, 95, 129.

Conclusion

1 Hilda Neatby, 'The Medical Profession in the North-West Territories,' in

S.E.D. Shortt, ed., *Medicine in Canadian Society: Historical Perspectives* (Montreal: McGill-Queen's University Press, 1981), 172.

2   Mariana Valverde, *The Age of Light, Soap, and Water: Moral Reform in English Canada, 1885–1925* (Toronto: McClelland & Stewart, 1991), 107; see also Howard Palmer, *Patterns of Prejudice: A History of Nativism in Alberta* (Toronto: McClelland & Stewart, 1982); Angus McLaren, *Our Own Master Race: Eugenics in Canada 1885–1945* (Toronto: McClelland & Stewart, 1990).

3   Friesen, *The Canadian Prairies*, 273.

4   Diamond Jenness, *The Indians of Canada*, 6th ed. (Ottawa: National Museum of Canada Bulletin 65, 1963), 260–4.

5   Eleanor Brass, *I Walk in Two Worlds* (Calgary: Glenbow Museum, 1987), 31, 45.

Bibliography

Note on Sources

The oral history method relies on the knowledge of elders. While some of the oral history cited herein has been published, printed, or recorded, much of it was collected through personal interviews with elders. As such, it is a personal and, in some ways, a private exchange. Consent, therefore, from elders is necessary before their names and their stories may be used. As a function of their humility, not all elders were comfortable with having their names disclosed. That wish must be respected. Reference notes identify the place and the time of interviews. Elders are identified in the text where consent has been received.

PRIMARY SOURCES

Archival Collections

Anglican Church of Canada
   General Synod Archives
Glenbow-Alberta Institute Archives
   Battleford Agency, Monthly Reports, 1908–19
   Calgary Indian Missions Reports
   Dewdney Papers
   D.C. Duvall Papers
   Edwards and Gardiner Family fonds
   Fran Fraser Collection
   Esther Schiff Goldfrank fonds
   Gooderham Family Papers
   Lucien M. and Jane R. Hanks fonds

Robert Jefferson Papers
Dr G.R. Johnson Papers
Dr G.E. Learmonth Papers
Dr N.J. Lindsay Papers
McDougall Orphanage
Dr H.W. McGill Papers
Jane Megarry Papers
Sarcee Indian Agency Files
Tims Papers
Alice Turner Papers
R.N. Wilson fonds

National Archives of Canada
    Robert Bell Papers
    Canadian Lung Association
    Dominion Council of Health, Record Group 17
    James Clinskill Papers
    Department of Indian Affairs. Record Group 10
        Black Series Central Registry Files
        Deputy Superintendent Letterbooks
    Department of External Affairs, Record Group 25
    Augustus Jukes Papers
    Jean L'Heureux Papers
    John MacLean Papers
    Minto Papers
    National Health and Welfare, Record Group 29
    Department of Agriculture Health Records
    Records of the Royal Canadian Mounted Police. Record Group 18
    Hayter Reed Papers

Public Archives of Alberta
    Anglican Church, Dioceses of Calgary
        Missionary Society of the Church of England in Canada
    Blood Reserve Hospital Register
    Baker Memorial Sanatorium
    Oblate Collection – Ecole Dunbow

Saskatchewan Archives Board
    Ferguson Papers
    Mandelbaum Field Notes

Saskatchewan Anti-Tuberculosis Commission, *Report.* 1922
Saskatchewan Lung Association Records
Saskatchewan Department of Public Health
Pioneer Questionnaire
    Charles Cantlon Bray, 1883, Wolseley, Saskatchewan
    Mrs Jane Victoria Carmichael, 1887, Rocanville, Saskatchewan
    Peter Fraser, 1891, Kamsack, Saskatchewan
    Mr H.M. Harrison, 1903, Baljennie, Saskatchewan
    Mrs Ellen W. Hubbard, 1894, Grenfell, Saskatchewan
    Andrew Cass Hunt, 1883, Earlswood, Saskatchewan
    Mrs Mary Edith Moore, 1899, Kajewski, Saskatchewan
    Mrs Ellen Mott, 1887, South Qu'Appelle
    Mrs Elizabeth Webster, 1884, Balcarres, Saskatchewan
    Mrs Maggie Whyte, 1883, Indian Head, Saskatchewan
    Robert Webster Widdess, 1883, Rocanville, Saskatchewan

University of Alberta Archives
    Heber C. Jamieson Papers

Oral History

Personal interviews
    Elder Alan Pard, Peigan First Nation, Brocket, Alberta
    Elders, Blood First Nation, Stand Off, Alberta
    Elders Kaye Thompson, Alice Ironstar, Violet Ashdohonk, Carry the Kettle
        First Nation, Sintaluta, Saskatchewan
    Rosabelle Gordon Pasqua First Nation, Fort Qu'Appelle, Saskatchewan
    Dr G. Monks, Fort Qu'Appelle Indian Hospital, physician, 1949–51

Indian History Film Project, Saskatchewan Indian Federated College Library,
    Regina, Saskatchewan
    IH 226, Jim Black, Blackfoot Elder, 18 June 1974
    IH 233, 233a, George First Rider, Blood Elder, n.d
    IH 234, 234a, Useless Good Runner, Blood Elder, n.d
    IH 245, Tom Yellowhorn, Peigan, 7 March 1975

Published Sources

Ames, Herbert Brown. *The City below the Hill: A Sociological Study of a Portion of the*

City of Montreal, Canada. 1897. Reprint, Toronto: University of Toronto Press, 1972.

Bryce, P.H. *Report on the Indian Schools of Manitoba and the North-West Territories.* Ottawa: Government Printing Bureau, 1907.

– *Report on Tuberculosis in Ontario.* Toronto: Warwick Brothers and Rutter, 1894.

– *The Story of a National Crime: Being an Appeal for Justice to the Indians of Canada.* Ottawa: James Hope and Sons, 1922.

Butler, William. *The Great Lone Land: A Narrative of Travel and Adventure in the North-West of America.* London: Sampson Low, Marston, Low and Searle, 1872.

Canada. *National Research Council Report of the President and Financial Statement, 1926–27.* Ottawa: King's Printer, 1928.

– *National Research Council Report of the President and Financial Statement, 1928–29.* Ottawa: King's Printer, 1930.

– Parliament. House of Commons. *Debates.*

– Parliament. House of Commons. *Sessional Papers.*

Cochin, Louis. *The Reminiscences of Louis Cochin, OMI.* Battleford, SK: Canadian North-West Historical Society Publications, 1927.

Cowie, Isaac. *The Company of Adventurers.* Winnipeg: William Briggs, 1913.

Cox, R. *Adventures on the Columbia River.* New York: J. and J. Harper, 1832.

Cummins, Lyle. 'Tuberculosis among the "Indians of the Great Canadian Plains" [*sic*].' (reprint). *Annual Report* of the National Association for the Prevention of Tuberculosis. London, 1928.

Denny, Cecil. *The Law Marches West.* Toronto: J.M. Dent, 1939.

Erasmus, Peter. *Buffalo Days and Nights.* Calgary: Fifth House, 1999.

The Facts Respecting Indian Administration in the North-West. Ottawa: Department of Indian Affairs, 1886.

Ferguson, R.G. *Studies in Tuberculosis.* Toronto: University of Toronto Press, 1955.

– *Tuberculosis among the Indians of the Great Canadian Plains.* London: Adlard and Son, 1928.

Ferguson, R.G., and A.B. Simes. 'BCG Vaccination of Indian Infants in Saskatchewan.' *Tubercle* 30, no. 1 (Jan. 1949): 5–11.

Fine Day. 'Incidents of the Rebellion as Related by Fine Day.' In *The Cree Rebellion of 1884.* Ed. Campbell Innis, Canadian North-West Historical Society. Battleford: Saskatchewan Herald, 1926.

Gates, Reginald Ruggles. *Heredity and Eugenics.* London: Constable, 1923.

– *Heredity in Man.* New York: Macmillan, 1928, 1931.

– 'A Pedigree Study of Amerindian Crosses in Canada.' *Journal of the Royal Anthropological Institute of Great Britain and Ireland* 58 (1928): 511–32.

Gibbon Stocken, H.W. *Among the Blackfoot and Sarcee.* Introduction by G. Barrass. Calgary: Glenbow Museum, 1976.

Graham, William M. *Treaty Days: Reflections of an Indian Commissioner.* Calgary: Glenbow Museum, 1991.

Harmon, Daniel Williams. *A Journal of Voyages and Travels in the Interior of North America.* Toronto: Courier Press, 1911.

Hopkins, W. 'BCG Vaccination in Montreal.' *American Review of Tuberculosis* 43, no. 5 (May 1941).

Hrdlicka, Ales. *Tuberculosis among Certain Indian Tribes of the United States.* Washington: Bureau of American Ethnology, Bulletin 42, 1909.

Hutchinson, Woods. 'Varieties of Tuberculosis According to Race and Social Condition.' *New York Medical Journal* 86 (1907): 624–76.

Jefferson, Robert. *Fifty Years on the Saskatchewan.* Battleford, SK: Canadian North-West Historical Society Publications, 1929.

– 'Incidents of the Rebellion as Related by Robert Jefferson.' In *The Cree Rebellion of 1884*, edited by Campbell Innes, Canadian North-West Historical Society Publications. Battleford: Saskatchewan Herald, 1926.

Maclean, John. *Canadian Savage Folk: The Native Tribes of Canada.* Toronto: William Briggs, 1896.

– *The Indians of Canada: Their Manners and Customs.* Toronto: Coles Publishing, 1970.

Matthews, Percy W. *Notes on Diseases among the Indians Frequenting York Factory, Hudson's Bay.* Montreal: Gazette Publishing, 1885.

Meriam, Lewis, ed. *The Problem of Indian Administration.* 1928. Reprint, Washington: Brookings Institution, 1971.

Morgan, Henry James. *The Canadian Men and Women of the Time.* Toronto: W. Briggs, 1912.

Morris, Alexander. *Treaties of Canada with the Indians of Manitoba and the North-West Territories.* 1880. Reprint, Saskatoon: Fifth House, 1991.

Orton, S.J. 'Scrofula Amongst the Indians of Manitoba and Western Canada.' *Lancet* 5 (1893): 214–15.

Palliser, John. *The Journals, Detailed Reports, and Observations Relative to the Exploration, by Captain John Palliser.* London: G.E. Eyre and W. Spottiswoode, 1863.

Robertson, E.A., M.D., Cpt. CAMC. 'Clinical Notes on the Influenza Epidemic Occurring in the Quebec Garrison.' *Canadian Medical Association Journal* 9 (February 1919), 155–9.

Saskatchewan. Saskatchewan Bureau of Public Health. *Annual Reports.*

Stone, E.L. 'Tuberculosis at Norway House.' *Public Health Journal* 16 (1925): 76–81.

Université de Montréal, Institute of Microbiology and Hygiene. *Notes on BCG.* 1951.

Wilson, R.N. *Our Betrayed Wards.* Ottawa: Privately Published, 1921.

Yeo, I. Burney, MD. *A Manual of Medical Treatment or Clinical Therapeutics* 1, 12th
ed. Chicago: W.T. Keener, 1905.

SECONDARY SOURCES

Acherknecht, Erwin A. *Medicine and Ethnology: Selected Essays.* Switzerland: Verlag
Huber, 1971.
Adair, John, and Kurt Deuschle. *The People's Health: Medicine and Anthropology in a
Navajo Community.* New York: Appleton-Century-Crofts, 1970.
Ahenakew, Edward. *Voices of the Plain Cree.* Ed. Ruth M. Buck. Regina: Canadian
Plains Research Center, 1995.
Ahenakew, Freda, and H.C. Wolfart, eds. and trans. *Our Grandmother's Lives as
Told in Their Own Words.* Saskatoon: Fifth House, 1992.
Alchon, Suzanne Austin. *Native Society and Disease in Colonial Ecuador.* Cambridge
Latin American Studies 71. Cambridge: Cambridge University Press, 1991.
Andrews, Isabel. 'The Crooked Lakes Reserves: A Study of Indian Policy in Prac-
tice from the Qu'Appelle Treaty to 1900.' MA Thesis, University of
Saskatchewan, 1972.
Badgley, Robin F. 'Social Policy and Indian Health Services.' *Anthropological
Quarterly* 46, no. 3 (1971): 150–9.
Barkan, Elazar. *The Retreat of Scientific Racism: Changing Concepts of Race in Britain
and the United States between the World Wars.* Cambridge: Cambridge University
Press 1992.
Barron, F. Laurie. 'Indian Agents and the North-West Rebellion.' In *1885 and
After: Native Society in Transition,* edited by F. Laurie Barron and James B.
Waldram, 139–54. Regina: Canadian Plains Research Center, 1986.
Barron, F. Laurie, and James B. Waldram, eds. *1885 and After: Native Society in
Transition.* Regina: Canadian Plains Research Center, 1986.
Beal, Bob, and Rod Macleod. *Prairie Fire: The 1885 North-West Rebellion.* Edmon-
ton: Hurtig, 1984.
Benson, Todd. 'Race, Health, and Power: The Federal Government and Ameri-
can Indian Health, 1909–1955.' PhD dissertation, Stanford University, 1994.
Berger, Carl. *Science, God, and Nature in Victorian Canada.* Toronto: University of
Toronto Press, 1983.
Bolt, Christine. *Victorian Attitudes to Race.* London: Routledge and Kegan Paul,
1971.
Bonnichsen, Robson, and Stuart Baldwin. *Cypress Hills Ethnohistory and Ecology.*
Archaeological Survey of Alberta, Occasional Paper No. 10. Alberta Culture
Historical Resources Division, 1978.
Boyd, Robert. 'Demographic History, 1774–1874.' In *Handbook of North American*

Indians: The Northwest Coast, edited by Wayne Suttles, 133–48. Washington: Smithsonian Institute, 1990.
– 'The Introduction of Infectious Diseases among the Indians of the Pacific Northwest, 1774–1874.' PhD dissertation, University of Washington, 1985.
Brass, Eleanor. *I Walk in Two Worlds.* Calgary: Glenbow Museum, 1987.
Breen, David. *The Canadian Prairie West and the Ranching Frontier, 1874–1924.* Toronto: University of Toronto Press, 1983.
Brown, S.H. Jennifer. *Strangers in Blood: Fur Trade Company Families in Indian Country.* Vancouver: University of British Columbia Press, 1980.
Brown, S.H. Jennifer, and Robert Brightman. *The Orders of the Dreamed: George Nelson on Cree and Northern Ojibwa Religion and Myth, 1823.* Manitoba Studies in Native History 3. Winnipeg: University of Manitoba Press, 1988.
Bryan, Liz. *The Buffalo People: Prehistoric Archaelogy on the Canadian Plains.* Edmonton: University of Alberta Press, 1991.
Bryder, Linda. *Below the Magic Mountain: A Social History of Tuberculosis in Twentieth-Century Britain.* Oxford: Clarendon Press, 1988.
Campbell, Gregory. 'Changing Patterns of Health and Effective Fertility among the Northern Cheyenne of Montana, 1886–1903.' *American Indian Quarterly* 15, no. 3 (1991): 339–58.
– 'Plains Indian Historical Demography and Health: An Introductory Overview.' *Plains Anthropologist* 34, no. 2 (1989): v–xiii.
Carmichael, Ann G. 'Erysipelas.' In *The Cambridge World History of Human Disease,* edited by Kenneth Kiple, 720–1. Cambridge: Cambridge University Press, 1993.
– 'Infection, Hidden Hunger, and History.' In *Hunger and History: The Impact of Changing Food Production and Consumption Patterns on Society,* edited by Robert I. Rotberg and Theodore K. Rabb, 51–66. Cambridge: Cambridge University Press, 1985.
Carter, Sarah. *Capturing Women: The Manipulation of Cultural Imagery in Canada's Prairie West.* Montreal: McGill-Queen's University Press, 1997.
– 'Demonstrating Success: The File Hills Farm Colony.' *Prairie Forum* 16, no. 3 (1991): 157–83.
– *Lost Harvests: Prairie Indian Reserve Farmers and Government Policy.* Montreal: McGill-Queen's University Press, 1990.
Coates, Ken S. *Best Left as Indians: Native-White Relations in the Yukon Territory, 1840–1973.* Montreal: McGill-Queen's University Press, 1991.
Cole, Douglas, and Ira Chaikin. *An Iron Hand upon the People: The Law against the Potlatch on the Northwest Coast.* Vancouver: Douglas and McIntyre, 1990.
Crosby, Alfred. *Ecological Imperialism: The Biological Expansion of Europe, 900–1900.* Cambridge: Cambridge University Press, 1986.

– 'Virgin Soil Epidemics as a Factor in the Aboriginal Depopulation in America.' *William and Mary Quarterly*, 3rd series, 33, no. 2 (1976): 289–99.

Cuthand, Stan. 'The Native Peoples in the 1920s and 1930s.' In *One Century Later: Western Canadian Reserve Indians Since Treaty Seven*, edited by Ian I.A. Getty and Donald B. Smith, 31–42. Vancouver: University of British Columbia Press, 1978.

Decker, Jody. 'Tracing Historical Diffusion Patterns: The Case of the 1780–82 Smallpox Epidemic among the Indians of Western Canada.' *Native Studies Review* 4, nos. 1, 2 (1988): 1–24.

– '"We Shall Never Be Again the Same People": The Diffusion and Cumulative Impact of Acute Infectious Diseases Affecting the Natives on the Northern Plains of the Western Interior of Canada, 1774–1839.' PhD dissertation, York University, 1989.

Dempsey, Hugh. *Amazing Death of Calf Shirt and Other Stories*. Saskatoon: Fifth House, 1994.

– *Big Bear: The End of Freedom*. Vancouver: Douglas and McIntyre, 1984.

– *Blackfoot Ghost Dance*. Occasional Paper No. 3. Calgary: Glenbow-Alberta Institute, 1968.

– *A Blackfoot Winter Count*. Occasional Papers No. 1, Calgary: Glenbow-Alberta Institute, 1965.

– *Crowfoot: Chief of the Blackfeet*. Halifax: Goodread Biographies, 1988.

– 'One Hundred Years of Treaty Seven.' In *One Century Later: Western Canadian Reserve Indians Since Treaty Seven*, edited by Ian A.L. Getty and Donald B. Smith, 20–30. Vancouver: University of British Columbia Press, 1978.

– *Red Crow, Warrior Chief*. Saskatoon: Western Producer Prairie Books, 1980.

Densmore, Francis. *Indian Use of Wild Plants for Crafts, Food, Medicine, and Charms*. Washington: Smithsonian Institution, 1923.

Dion, Joseph F. *My Tribe the Crees*. Calgary: Glenbow-Alberta Institute, 1993.

Dirks, Robert. 'Famine and Disease.' In *Cambridge World History of Human Disease*, edited by Kenneth Kiple, 157–63. Cambridge: Cambridge University Press, 1993.

Dobyns, Henry. *Their Number Become Thinned*. Knoxville: University of Tennessee Press, 1983.

Dubos, Rene, and Jean Dubos. *The White Plague: Tuberculosis, Man and Society*. Boston: Little, Brown and Co., 1952.

Duffin, Jacalyn. *Langstaff: A Nineteenth-Century Life*. Toronto: University of Toronto Press, 1993.

Duffy, John. 'Medicine and Medical Practices among the Aboriginal American Indians.' In *International Record of Medicine* 171 (1958): 331–49.

Dyck, Noel. 'The Administration of Federal Indian Aid in the North-West Territories, 1879–1885.' MA thesis, University of Saskatchewan, 1970.

– 'An Opportunity Lost: The Initiative of the Reserve Agricultural Programme in the Prairie West.' In *1885 and After: Native Society in Transition*, edited by F. Laurie Barron and James B. Waldram, 121–37. Regina: Canadian Plains Research Center, 1986.

Ernst, Walfraud, and Bernard Harris, eds. *Race, Science and Medicine*. London: Routledge, 1999.

Ewers, John C. *The Blackfeet: Raiders on the Northwestern Plains*. Norman: University of Oklahoma Press, 1958.

Fanon, Frantz. 'Medicine and Colonialism.' In *The Cultural Crisis of Modern Medicine*, edited by John Ehrenreich. New York: Monthly Review Press, 1978.

Feldberg, Georgina D. *Disease and Class: Tuberculosis and the Shaping of Modern North American Society*. New Brunswick, NJ: Rutgers University Press, 1995.

Finkel, Alvin, Margaret Conrad, and Veronica Strong-Boag. *History of the Canadian Peoples*. Vol. 2. Toronto: Copp Clark Pitman, 1993.

Fischer, David. *Historians' Fallacies*. New York: Harper and Row, 1970.

Fisher, A.D. 'Introducing "Our Betrayed Wards" by R.N. Wilson.' *Western Canadian Journal of Anthropology* 4, no.1 (1974): 21–59.

Fisher, Robin. *Contact and Conflict: Indian-European Relations in British Columbia, 1774–1890*. Vancouver: University of British Columbia Press, 1977.

Fisher, Robin, and Kenneth Coates, eds. *Out of the Background: Readings on Canadian Native History*. Toronto: Copp Clark Pitman, 1988.

Flannery, Regina. *Ellen Smallboy: Glimpses of a Cree Woman's Life*. Montreal: McGill-Queen's University Press, 1995.

Foster, J. E. 'The Saulteaux and the Numbered Treaties: An Aboriginal Rights Position?' In *The Spirit of the Alberta Indian Treaties*, edited by Richard T. Price. 161–80. 3rd ed. Edmonton: University of Alberta Press, 1999.

Frappier, Amand. *Fifty Years of Study and Use of BCG Vaccine in Canada, 1924–1974*. Montreal: Institut Armand-Frappier, 1979.

Friesen, Gerald. *The Canadian Prairies: A History*. Toronto: University of Toronto Press, 1984.

Genovese, Eugene. *Roll, Jordan, Roll: The World the Slaves Made*. New York: Vantage Books, 1976.

Getty, Ian A.L., and Antoine S. Lussier, eds. *As Long as the Sun Shines and Water Flows: A Reader in Canadian Native Studies*. Vancouver: University of British Columbia Press, 1983.

Getty, Ian A.L., and Donald B. Smith, eds. *One Century Later: Western Canadian Reserve Indians Since Treaty Seven*. Vancouver: University of British Columbia Press, 1978.

Gidney, R.D., and W.P.J. Millar. 'The Reorientation of Medical Education in Late Nineteenth-Century Ontario: The Proprietary Medical Schools and the

Founding of the Faculty of Medicine at the University of Toronto.' *Journal of the History of Medicine and Allied Sciences* 49, no. 1 (1994): 52–78.

Goodwill, Jean, and Norma Sluman. *John Tootoosis*. Winnipeg: Pemmican Press, 1984.

Gough, Anna F. 'Public Health in Canada: 1867 to 1967.' *Medical Services Journal* 23 (1967): 32–41.

Graham-Cumming, G. 'Health of the Original Canadians, 1867–1967.' *Medical Services Journal* 23 (February 1967): 115–66.

Grant, John. *Moon of Wintertime*. Toronto: University of Toronto Press, 1984.

Gresko, Jacqueline. 'White "Rites" and Indian "Rites": Indian Education and Native Responses in the West, 1879–1910.' In *Western Canada: Past and Present*, edited by Anthony Rasporich, 163–82. Calgary: McClelland & Stewart West, 1975.

Grygier, Pat Sandiford. *A Long Way from Home: The Tuberculosis Epidemic among the Inuit*. Montreal: McGill-Queen's University Press, 1994.

Hall, D.J. 'Clifford Sifton and the Canadian Indian Administration, 1896–1905.' *Prairie Forum* 2, no. 2 (1977): 127–51.

Hanks, Lucien, and Jane Richardson Hanks. *Tribe Under Trust: A Study of the Blackfoot Reserve of Alberta*. Toronto: University of Toronto Press, 1950.

Heber, R. Wesley. 'Indian Medicine in Northern Saskatchewan.' *Western Canadian Anthropologist* 7 (1990): 95–108.

Hellson, John. *Ethnobotany of the Blackfoot Indians*. National Museum of Man, Canadian Ethnology Service Paper No. 19. Ottawa: National Museums of Canada, 1979.

Henige, David. *Numbers from Nowhere: The American Indian Contact Population Debate*. Norman: University of Oklahoma Press, 1998.

– 'Primary Source by Primary Source: On the Role of Epidemics in New World Depopulation.' *Ethnohistory* 33, no. 3 (1986): 293–312.

Herring, D. Ann. '"There Were Young People and Old People and Babies Dying Every Week": The 1918–1919 Influenza Pandemic at Norway House.' *Ethnohistory* 41, no. 1 (1994): 73–105.

– 'Toward a Reconsideration of Disease and Contact in the Americas.' *Prairie Forum* 17, no. 2 (1992): 153–65.

Hickey, Lynn, Richard Lightening, and Gordon Lee. 'T.A.R.R. Interview with Elders Program' and 'Interviews with Elders.' In *The Spirit of the Alberta Indian Treaties*, edited by Richard T. Price. 3rd ed., 103–12. Edmonton: University of Alberta Press, 1999.

Houston, C. Stuart. 'Ferguson's BCG Research – Canada's First Randomized Clinical Trial?' *Clinical Investigation of Medicine* 16, no. 1 (1993): 89–91.

– *R.G. Ferguson: Crusader against Tuberculosis.* Toronto: Hannah Institute and Dundurn Press, 1991.

Huel, Raymond J.A. *Proclaiming the Gospel to the Indians and the Metis.* Edmonton: University of Alberta Press, 1996.

Hungry Wolf, Beverly. *Daughters of the Buffalo Women.* Skookumchuck, BC: Canadian Caboose Press, 1996.

– *The Ways of My Grandmothers.* New York: Quill, 1980.

Irwin, Lee. 'Cherokee Healing: Myth, Dreams, and Medicine.' *American Indian Quarterly* 16 (1992): 237–57.

Jackson, Robert H. 'The Dynamic of Indian Demographic Collapse in the San Francisco Bay Missions, Alta California, 1776–1840.' *American Indian Quarterly* 16 (1992): 141–56.

Jasen, Patricia. 'Race, Culture, and the Colonization of Childbirth in Northern Canada.' *Social History of Medicine* 10, no. 3 (1997): 383–400.

Jenness, Diamond. *The Indians of Canada.* 6th ed. Ottawa: National Museum of Canada, Bulletin 65, 1963.

– *The Sarcee Indians of Alberta.* Ottawa: National Museum of Canada Bulletin, no. 90, 1938.

Johnston, Alex. *Plants and the Blackfoot.* Occasional Paper No. 4. Edmonton: Provincial Museum of Alberta Natural History, 1982.

Johnston, William D. 'Tuberculosis.' In *The Cambridge World History of Human Disease,* edited by Kenneth Kiple, 1059–68. Cambridge: Cambridge University Press, 1993.

Karasch, Mary. 'Opthalmia.' In *The Cambridge World History of Human Disease,* edited by Kenneth Kiple, 897–906. Cambridge: Cambridge University Press, 1993.

Kehoe, Alice B. 'The Shackles of Tradition.' In *The Hidden Half: Studies of Plains Indian Women,* edited by Patricia Albers and Beatrice Medicine. Lanham: University Press of America, 1983.

Kelm, Mary-Ellen. *Colonizing Bodies: Aboriginal Health and Healing in British Columbia, 1900–50.* Vancouver: UBC Press, 1998.

Kemink, John, et al. 'Mastoiditis.' In *The Cambridge World History of Human Disease,* edited by Kenneth Kiple, 865–71. Cambridge: Cambridge University Press, 1993.

Kennedy, Dan (Ochankugahe). *Recollections of an Assiniboine Chief,* edited by James Stevens. Toronto: McClelland & Stewart, 1972.

Kennedy, Jacqueline Judith. 'Qu'Appelle Industrial School: White "Rites" for the Indians of the Old North-West.' MA thesis, Carleton University, 1970.

Kennedy, Michael S. *The Assiniboines: From the Accounts of the Old Ones Told to First Boy (James Larpenteur Long).* Norman: University of Oklahoma Press, 1961.

Kim-Farley, Robert J. 'Measles.' In *The Cambridge World History of Human Disease*, edited by Kenneth Kiple, 871–5. Cambridge: Cambridge University Press, 1993.

Kiple, Kenneth F., ed. *The Cambridge World History of Human Disease*. Cambridge: Cambridge University Press, 1993.

Klein, Alan. 'The Political-Economy of Gender: A Nineteenth-Century Plains Indian Case Study.' In *The Hidden Half: Studies of Plains Indian Women*, edited by Patricia Albers and Beatrice Medicine, 143–75. Lanham: University Press of America, 1983.

Krech, Shepard. 'The Influence of Disease and the Fur Trade on Arctic Drainage Lowlands Dene, 1800–1850.' *Journal of Anthropological Research* 39 (1983): 123–46.

Kuhnlein, Harriet V., and Nancy J. Turner. *Traditional Plant Foods of Canadian Indigenous Peoples*. Philadelphia: Gordon and Beach, 1991.

Kunitz, Stephen J. *Disease and Social Diversity: The European Impact on the Health of Non-Europeans*. New York: Oxford University Press, 1994.

Lalonde, A.N. 'Colonization Companies in the 1880s.' In *Pages from the Past: Essays in Saskatchewan History*, edited by D.H. Bocking, 16–30. Saskatoon: Western Producer Prairie Books, 1979.

Lee, David. 'Piapot: Man and Myth.' *Prairie Forum* 17, no. 2 (1992): 251–62.

Leighton, Anna. *Wild Plant Use by the Woods Cree of East-Central Saskatchewan*. Canadian Ethnology Service, Paper No. 101. Ottawa: National Museum of Canada, 1985.

Leighton, J.D. 'A Victorian Civil Servant at Work: Lawrence Vankoughnet and the Canadian Indian Department, 1874–1893.' In *As Long as the Sun Shines and Water Flows*, edited by Ian A.L. Getty and Antoine S. Lussier, 104–19. Vancouver: University of British Columbia Press, 1983.

Levine, Lawrence. *Black Culture, Black Consciousness*. New York: Oxford University Press, 1977.

Lewis, Maurice H. 'The Anglican Church and Its Mission Schools Dispute.' *Alberta Historical Review* 14, no. 4 (1966): 7–13.

Lewis, Oscar. *The Effects of White Contact upon Blackfoot Culture, with Special Reference to the Role of the Fur Trade*. New York: J.J. Augustin, 1942.

Lux, M.K. 'The Impact of the 1918 Influenza Epidemic in Saskatchewan.' MA thesis, University of Saskatchewan, 1989.

– 'Prairie Indians and the 1918 Influenza Epidemic,' *Native Studies Review* 8, no. 1 (1992): 23–34.

MacDougall, Heather. '"Enlightening the Public": The Views and Values of the Association of Executive Health Officers of Ontario, 1886–1903.' In *Health, Disease, and Medicine*, edited by Charles Roland, 436–64. McMaster University: Hannah Conference on the History of Medicine, 1982.

Macfarlane, Alan. *Reconstructing Historical Communities.* Cambridge: Cambridge University Press, 1977.

Macleod, Margaret A., ed. *The Letters of Letitia Hargrave.* Toronto: The Champlain Society, 1947.

Mandelbaum, David. *The Plains Cree: An Ethnographic, Historical, and Comparative Study.* Regina: Canadian Plains Research Center, 1979.

Marcy, Peter T. 'Factors Affecting the Fecundity and Fertility of Historical Populations: A Review.' *Journal of Family History* 6, no. 3 (1981): 309–26.

Martin, Calvin. *Keepers of the Game.* Berkeley: University of California Press, 1978.

McArthur, Norma. *Island Populations of the Pacific.* Canberra: Australian National University Press, 1967.

McClintock, Walter. *The Old North Trail or Life: Legends and Religion of the Blackfeet Indians.* Lincoln: University of Nebraska Press, 1999.

McCuaig, Katherine. *The Weariness, the Fever, and the Fret: The Campaign against Tuberculosis in Canada, 1900–1950.* Montreal: McGill-Queen's University Press, 1999.

McGrath, J. 'Biological Impact of Social Disruption Resulting from Epidemic Disease.' *American Journal of Physical Anthropology* 84 (1991): 407–20.

McKeown, Thomas. 'Food, Infection, and Population.' In *Hunger and History: The Impact of Changing Food Production and Consumption Patterns on Society,* edited by Robert I. Rotberg and Theodore K. Rabb, 29–50. Cambridge: Cambridge University Press, 1985.

– *The Modern Rise of Population.* London: Edward Arnold, 1976.

McLaren, Angus. *Our Own Master Race: Eugenics in Canada 1885–1945.* Toronto: McClelland & Stewart, 1990.

McLean, Donald. '1885: Metis Rebellion or Government Conspiracy?' In *1885 and After: Native Society in Transition,* edited by Laurie Barron and James B. Waldram, 79–104. Regina: Canadian Plains Research Center, 1986.

McNeill, William. *Plagues and Peoples.* New York: Anchor Press, 1979.

Meili, Dianne. *Those Who Know: Profiles of Alberta's Native Elders.* Edmonton: NeWest Press, 1991.

Migliore, Sam. 'Etiology, Distress, and Classification: The Development of a Tri-Axial Model.' *Western Canadian Anthropologist* 7, no. 1 (fall 1990): 3–35.

Miller, J.R. 'Owen Glendower, Hotspur, and Canadian Indian Policy.' *Ethnohistory* 37, no. 4 (1990): 386–415.

– *Shingwauk's Vision.* Toronto: University of Toronto Press, 1996.

– *Skyscrapers Hide the Heavens: A History of Indian-White Relations in Canada.* Rev. ed. Toronto: University of Toronto Press, 1991.

Milloy, John. *The Plains Cree: Trade, Diplomacy and War, 1790–1870.* Winnipeg: University of Manitoba Press, 1988.

Mitchinson, Wendy. *The Nature of Their Bodies: Women and Their Doctors in Victorian Canada.* Toronto: University of Toronto Press, 1991.

Mountain Horse, Mike. *My People the Bloods.* Calgary: Glenbow Museum, 1989.

Neatby, Hilda. 'The Medical Profession in the North-West Territories.' In *Medicine in Canadian Society: Historical Perspectives,* edited by S.E.D. Shortt, 165–88. Montreal: McGill-Queen's University Press, 1981.

Newson, Linda. *Indian Survival in Colonial Nicaragua.* Norman: University of Oklahoma Press, 1987.

Owram, Douglas. *Promise of Eden: The Canadian Expansionist Movement and the Idea of the West, 1856–1900.* Toronto: University of Toronto Press, 1980.

Palmer, Howard. *Patterns of Prejudice: A History of Nativism in Alberta.* Toronto: McClelland & Stewart, 1982.

Parsons, Gail Pat. 'Puerperal Fever, Anticontagionists, and Miasmatic Infection, 1840–1860: Toward a New History of Puerperal Fever in Antebellum America.' *Journal of the History of Medicine* 52, 4 (October 1997): 424–52.

Patterson, David K. *Pandemic Influenza, 1700–1900: A Study in Historical Epidemiology.* New Jersey: Row and Littlefield, 1986.

Peterson, Hans J. 'Imasees and His Band: Canadian Refugees after the North-West Rebellion.' *Western Canadian Journal of Anthropology* 8, no. 1 (1978): 21–37.

Pettipas, Katherine. 'Severing the Ties That Bind: The Canadian Indian Act and the Repression of Indigenous Religious Systems in the Prairie Region, 1896–1951.' PhD dissertation, University of Manitoba, 1988.

– *Severing the Ties That Bind.* Winnipeg: University of Manitoba Press, 1994.

Preston, Samuel H. 'The Changing Relation between Mortality and Level of Economic Development.' *Population Studies* 29, no. 2 (1975): 231–48.

Preston, Samuel H., and Michael R. Haines. *Fatal Years: Child Mortality in Late Nineteenth-Century America.* Princeton: Princeton University Press, 1991.

Preston, Sarah. 'Competent Social Behaviour within the Context of Childbirth: A Cree Example.' *Papers of the Thirteenth Algonquian Conference,* edited by William Cowan, 211–17. Ottawa: Carleton University Press, 1982.

Raby, Stewart. 'Indian Land Surrenders in Southern Saskatchewan.' *Canadian Geographer* 17, no. 1 (1973): 36–52.

Ranger, Terrence. 'The Influenza Pandemic in Southern Rhodesia: A Crisis of Comprehension.' *Society for the Social History of Medicine Bulletin* 39 (1986): 38–43.

Ray, Arthur J. *The Canadian Fur Trade in the Industrial Age.* Toronto: University of Toronto Press, 1990.

– 'The Diffusion of Disease in the Western Interior.' In *Medicine in Canadian Society: Historical Perspectives*, edited by S.E.D. Shortt, 45–73. Montreal: McGill-Queen's University Press, 1981.

– *Indians in the Fur Trade: Their Role as Hunters, Trappers and Middlemen in the Lands Southwest of the Hudson's Bay, 1660–1870.* Toronto: University of Toronto Press, 1974.

Rice, Jon F. 'Health Conditions of Native Americans in the Twentieth Century.' *The Indian Historian* 10, no. 4 (1977): 14–18.

Roe, F.G. *The North American Buffalo: A Critical Study of the Species in its Wild State.* Toronto: University of Toronto Press, 1951.

Roome, Patricia Anne. 'Henrietta Muir Edwards: The Journey of a Canadian Feminist.' PhD dissertation, Simon Fraser University, 1996.

Rosenberg, Charles. *The Cholera Years: The United States in 1832, 1849, and 1866.* Chicago: University of Chicago Press, 1962.

– 'The Therapeutic Revolution: Medicine, Meaning, and Social Change in Nineteenth-Century America.' In *Explaining Epidemics and Other Studies in the History of Medicine*, edited by Charles Rosenberg, 9–31. Cambridge: Cambridge University Press.

Rotberg, Robert I., and Theodore K. Rabb. *Hunger and History: The Impact of Changing Food Production and Consumption Patterns on Society.* Cambridge: Cambridge University Press, 1985.

Shaeffer, Claude E. *Blackfoot Shaking Tent.* Occasional Paper No. 5. Calgary: Glenbow Museum, 1969.

Shortt, S.E.D., ed. *Medicine in Canadian Society: Historical Perspectives.* Montreal: McGill-Queen's University Press, 1981.

Sigerist, H.E. *A History of Medicine.* Vol. 1. New York: Oxford University Press, 1951.

Smith, F.B. *The Retreat of Tuberculosis, 1850–1950.* London: Croon, Helm, 1988.

Smits, David. '"The Squaw Drudge": A Prime Index of Savagism.' *Ethnohistory* 29, no. 4 (1982): 281–306.

Snow, Dean, and K. Lanphear. 'European Contact and Indian Depopulation in the Northeast: The Timing of the First Epidemics.' *Ethnohistory* 35, no. 1 (1987): 15–35.

Stanley, G.F.G. *The Birth of Western Canada: A History of the Riel Rebellions.* 1936. Reprint, Toronto: University of Toronto Press, 1960.

Stepan, Nancy. *The Idea of Race in Science: Great Britain, 1800–1960.* London: Macmillan, 1982.

Stockwell, Edward. 'Infant Mortality.' In *The Cambridge World History of Human Disease*, edited by Kenneth Kiple, 224–9. Cambridge: Cambridge University Press, 1993.

Stonechild, A. Blair. 'The Indian View of the 1885 Uprising.' In *1885 and After:*

Native Society in Transition, edited by F. Laurie Barron and James B. Waldram, 155–70. Regina: Canadian Plains Research Center, 1986.

Stonechild, Blair, and Bill Waiser. *Loyal Till Death: Indians and the North-West Rebellion*. Calgary: Fifth House, 1997.

Sundstrom, Linea. 'Smallpox Used Them Up: References to Epidemic Disease in Northern Plains Winter Counts, 1714–1920.' *Ethnohistory* 44, no. 2 (spring 1997): 305–43.

Sutherland, Neil. 'To Create a Strong and Healthy Race: School Children in the Public Health Movement, 1880–1914.' In *Medicine in Canadian Society: Historical Perspectives*, edited by S.E.D. Shortt, 361–94. Montreal: McGill-Queen's University Press, 1981.

Tarasoff, Koozma. *Persistent Ceremonialism: The Plains Cree and Saulteaux*. National Museum, Mercury Series, Canadian Ethnology Service paper no. 69. Ottawa: National Museum of Canada, 1980.

Taylor, Carl E. 'Synergy among Mass Infections, Famines and Poverty.' In *Hunger and History: The Impact of Changing Food Production and Consumption Patterns on Society*, edited by Robert I. Rotberg and Theodore K. Rabb, 285–304. Cambridge: Cambridge University Press, 1985.

Taylor, John F. Counting: The Utility of Historic Population Estimates in the Northwestern Plains, 1800–1880.' *Plains Anthropologist* 34, no. 2 (1989): 17–30.

– 'Sociocultural Effects of Epidemics on the Northern Plains, 1734–1850.' *Western Canadian Journal of Anthropology* 7, no. 4 (1977): 55–81.

Taylor, John Leonard. 'Two Views on the Meaning of Treaties Six and Seven.' In *The Spirit of the Alberta Indian Treaties*, edited by Richard Price. 3rd ed. 9–45. Edmonton: University of Alberta Press, 1999.

Thistle, Mel. *The Inner Ring: The Early History of the National Research Council of Canada*. Toronto: University of Toronto Press, 1966.

Thistle, Paul. *Indian-European Trade Relations in the Lower Saskatchewan River Region to 1840*. Winnipeg: University of Manitoba Press, 1986.

Thompson, E.P. 'The Moral Economy of the English Crowd in the Eighteenth Century.' *Past and Present* 50 (1971): 76–136.

Thornton, Russell. *American Indian Holocaust and Survival*. Norman: University of Oklahoma Press, 1987.

Thornton, Russell, Gary Sandefur, and C. Matthew Snipp. 'American Indian Fertility Patterns: 1910 and 1940 to 1980.' *American Indian Quarterly* 15, no. 3 (1991): 359–67.

Titley, Brian. 'The Fate of the Sharphead Stoneys.' *Alberta History* 39, no. 1 (1991): 1–8.

– *A Narrow Vision: Duncan Campbell Scott and the Administration of Indian Affairs in Canada*. Vancouver: UBC Press, 1986.

Tobias, John. 'Canada's Subjugation of the Plains Cree.' In *Out of the Background: Readings on Canadian Native History*, edited by Robin Fisher and Kenneth Coates, 190–218. Toronto: Copp Clark Pitman, 1988.

– 'Payipwat.' *Dictionary of Canadian Biography* 13: 818. Toronto: University of Toronto Press, 1994.

– 'Protection, Civilization, Assimilation: An Outline of Canada's Indian Policy.' *Western Canadian Journal of Anthropology* 6, no. 2 (1976): 13–30.

Torchia, Marion M. 'Tuberculosis among American Negroes: Medical Research on a Racial Disease, 1830–1950.' *Journal of the History of Medicine* 32, no. 3 (July 1977): 252–88.

– 'The Tuberculosis Movement and the Race Question.' *Bulletin of the History of Medicine* 49 (1975): 152–68.

Tough, Frank. 'Native People and the Regional Economy of Northern Manitoba: 1870–1930s.' PhD dissertation, York University, 1987.

Treaty Seven Elders and Tribal Council, with Walter Hildebrandt, Sarah Carter, and Dorothy First Rider. *The True Spirit and Original Intent of Treaty Seven.* Montreal: McGill-Queen's University Press, 1996.

Trigger, Bruce. 'The Historians' Indian: Native Americans in Canadian Historical Writing from Charlevoix to the Present.' In *Out of the Background: Readings on Canadian Native History*, edited by Robin Fisher and Ken Coates, 19–44. Toronto: Copp Clark Pitman, 1988.

– *Natives and Newcomers.* Montreal: McGill-Queen's University Press, 1985.

Van Kirk, Sylvia. *Many Tender Ties: Women in Fur Trade Society, 1670–1870.* Winnipeg: Watson and Dwyer, n.d.

Valverde, Mariana. *The Age of Light, Soap, and Water: Moral Reform in Canada, 1885–1925.* Toronto: McClelland & Stewart, 1991.

Waldrum, James B., et al. *Aboriginal Health in Canada: Historical Cultural and Epidemiological Perspectives.* Toronto: University of Toronto Press, 1995.

Watetch, Abel. *Payepot and His People.* Regina: Saskatchewan History and Folklore Society, 1959.

Weaver, Sally M. *Medicine and Politics among the Grand River Iroquois: A Study of the Non-Conservatives.* National Museum of Man, Publications in Ethnology, no. 4. Ottawa: National Museum of Canada, 1972.

Wherrett, George Jasper. *The Miracle of the Empty Beds: A History of Tuberculosis in Canada.* Toronto: University of Toronto Press, 1977.

Whorton, James. 'Dyspepsia.' In *The Cambridge World History of Human Disease*, edited by Kenneth F. Kiple, 696–8. Cambridge: Cambridge University Press, 1993.

Wissler, Clark. *A Blackfoot Source Book.* New York: Garland Publishing, 1986.

- 'Population Changes among the Northern Plains Indians.' *Yale University Publications in Anthropology* 1 (1936): 3–20. Reprint, New Haven, CT: Human Relations Area Files, 1970.

Wood, C.S. *Human Sickness and Health: A Biocultural View.* California: Mayfield, 1979.

Worboys, Michael. 'Tuberculosis and Race in Britain and Its Empire, 1900–50.' In *Race, Science and Medicine, 1700–1960,* edited by Waltraud Ernst and Bernard Harris, 144–66. London: Routledge, 1999.

Young, David, Grant Ingram, and Lise Swartz. *Cry of the Eagle: Encounters with a Cree Healer.* Toronto: University of Toronto Press, 1989.

Young, T. Kue. *Health Care and Cultural Change: The Indian Experience in the Central Subarctic.* Toronto: University of Toronto Press, 1988.

Illustration Credits

Glenbow Archives, Calgary, Alberta: Blackfoot grave, NA-249-80; Women waiting at ration house, NA-943-42 (RCMP Museum, Regina); Young boy, NA-943-39 (RCMP Museum, Regina); Blackfoot Old Woman, NA-4035-157; Ration issue at Upper Agency, NA-100-25; Dr O.C. Edwards, NA-4035-7; Dr O.C. Edwards's granddaughter, NA-4035-52; Boys on Sarcee reserve, NA-192-13; Blackfoot healers, ND-24-15; Patients in the new Blood hospital, ND-27-10

Saskatchewan Archives Board: Stoney people c. 1900, S-B2862; Dr R.G. Ferguson, R-A14776; Provincial sanitorium, R-B10315; Indian 'sanitorium,' R-A14847; Native family with public health nurse R-B6926(2)

Index

Striped Gopher, 28
Stuyimi, 76–7
subdivision, reserves, 160
Sun Dance. *See* dances
surrender, reserves lands, 160–4
sweat lodge, 72, 77, 101
Sweet Grass, Chief, 22, 25, 28–9
Sweet Grass reserve, 58, 87
Swinford, S., 126

Take the Coat, Chief, 40, 81
tent hospitals, 124, 193–4, 200
The Clothes, 52
therapeutics, 5, 71–3, 101, 166, 171–3
Thirst Dance. *See* dances
Thompson, Hazel, 219
Thompson, Kaye (Assiniboine elder), 133, 180, 218–19
thoracoplasty, 222
Thunderchild, Chief (Kapitikow), 21, 36
Thunderchild, reserve, 49; death rates at, 58, 87
Tims, John William, 68, 83, 111–12, 123, 134–5
tobacco, as sacrifice, 72, 99–100
Todd, William, 15
Toma, Joseph, 26
Toronto Women's Auxiliary (Anglican church), 112
Touchwood Hills agency, 34, 87, 88, 194
Treaties, 20; Aboriginal influence on, 23; Aboriginal understandings of, 20, 23–4, 31–2, 70; and education, 104, 105; government understanding of, 20, 22–4, 32, 70; Royal Proclamation, (1763), 22
Treaty One, 23
Treaty Two, 23
Treaty Three, 23, 25

Treaty Four, Qu'Appelle Treaty, 4, 23–5, 33; Aboriginal understanding of, 23–4
Treaty Four reserves, birth and death rates at, 46–7 Tables 1.1, 1.3; causes of death at, 41; population distribution, 46–7 Tables 1.2, 1.4; ration policy for, 65–6; vaccinations at, 33–4
Treaty Six, 4, 25–9, 33, 51; medicine chest clause of, 27
Treaty Six reserves, 51; agriculture at, 49; birth and death rates, 50 Table 1.5, 57 Table 1.7; chief's council (1884), 52–3; Edmonton chiefs, 56; population distribution, 50 Table 1.6, 57 Table 1.8; population loss at, 56, 58; ration policy for, 65–6; and Riel Rebellion, 53–5
Treaty Seven, 4, 29–32; Aboriginal understanding of, as peace treaty, 31–2; anniversary, 78; interpreters at, 31
Treaty Seven reserves, conditions at, 58–64; birth and death rates, 61, Table 1.9, 63 Table 1.11; paylists at, 66–7; population distribution, 61 Table 1.10, 63 Table 1.12; ration policy at, 65–6; repression of dances, 88
Tremont, Barney, 54
Trigger, Bruce, 13
Tsuu T'ina. *See* Sarcee
tuberculin, 129, 135
tuberculosis, 4, 5, 41–2, 45; Aboriginal death rates, 192, 201; Aboriginal treatment of, 80; at Battleford agency, 171; at Blood reserve, 84, 145, 170–1; department circular, 197–8; diagnosis of, 129–30; of lymph glands (scrofula), 44, 67, 68;